Handbook of
Voice Assessments

Handbook of
Voice Assessments

ESTELLA P.-M. MA, PhD
EDWIN M.-L. YIU, PhD

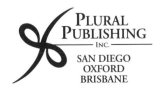

PLURAL
PUBLISHING
INC.
SAN DIEGO
OXFORD
BRISBANE

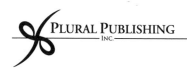

PLURAL PUBLISHING
INC.

5521 Ruffin Road
San Diego, CA 92123

e-mail: info@pluralpublishing.com
Web site: http://www.pluralpublishing.com

49 Bath Street
Abingdon, Oxfordshire OX14 1EA
United Kingdom

FSC
Mixed Sources
Product group from well-managed
forests and other controlled sources

Cert no. SW-COC-002283
www.fsc.org
© 1996 Forest Stewardship Council

ISBN-13: 978-1-59756-364-2
ISBN-10: 1-59756-364-1

Library of Congress Cataloging-in-Publication Data:

Handbook of voice assessments / [edited by] Estella Ma and Edwin Yiu.
    p. ; cm.
 Includes bibliographical references and index.
 ISBN-13: 978-1-59756-364-2 (alk. paper)
 ISBN-10: 1-59756-364-1 (alk. paper)
 1. Voice disorders—Handbooks, manuals, etc. I. Ma, Estella, 1975- II. Yiu, Edwin, 1958-
III. Title.
 [DNLM: 1. Voice Disorders—diagnosis—Handbooks. WV 39]
 RF510.H36 2010
 616.85'56—dc22

                   2011009652

Contents

Foreword

A handbook generally can be defined as a concise manual or reference book providing specific information or instruction about a subject. Handbooks can become landmark publications that define a field by consolidating expert knowledge that is made readily available to a wide audience. Ma and Yiu's *Handbook of Voice Assessments* is a handbook par excellence, certainly destined to be a landmark in the field of voice disorders. It is a concise volume that puts valuable information in the hands of readers. The contributions by experts from around the world provide a coverage of voice assessments that is extraordinary in its range and precise in its delivery. Critical information about various approaches to assessment is efficiently organized in seven major sections: aerodynamics, vocal fold movements, laryngeal muscle activities, acoustics, resonance, auditory-perceptual evaluation, and quality of life evaluation. All of these approaches have contributed to the contemporary understanding of voice disorders and surely will shape the field for years to come.

Furthermore, each of these has been demonstrated to be a useful tool for assessing voice disorders in the clinic. Even though an individual type of assessment can contribute importantly to clinical judgments of the type, etiology and severity of a voice disorder, professionals often rely on a synthesis of information gathered from different methods of assessment. Frequently, proficiency with any single method is not sufficient to ensure a competent assessment. In *Handbook*, clinical application is facilitated by specific advice and instruction, which form the substance of the book. As the editors note in their Preface, no other book that is currently available summarizes this "how to" information on voice assessments. This information not only is a guide to practitioners on how an assessment is to be performed, but also is a major step in standardization of assessment procedures, which is a boon to the clinical endeavor.

Recent advances in the clinical art and science of voice assessments have ushered in a new era for voice practitioners. The prospects for refined analysis and assessment are truly exciting, and, thanks to this new book, are eminently feasible as well. *Handbook for Voice Assessments* is structured for efficiency. The uniform format across chapters enables readers to find information quickly and follow detailed instructions on a particular method of assessment. The contributors are acknowledged experts who offer first-hand discussions of why and how an assessment is performed. By organic metaphor, this book is muscular—it directs actions that target assessment goals. Readers are not hindered by extraneous material or excess verbiage. Theoretical issues are presented in a tightly written, single paragraph. *Handbook* is the next best thing to having a cadre of experts who are available on site to consult on a particular approach to assessment.

Estella Ma and Edwin Yiu, together with their distinguished team of contributors, have given us a book of great value. Their vision for a handbook to guide voice assessments impressively is realized to the great benefit of professionals in the field of voice.

Ray D. Kent, PhD

Preface

The conceptualization of *Handbook of Voice Assessments* arose from the recognized fact that there is no availability of a single volume of book that describes the practical issues and the procedural aspects of voice assessments. Practical suggestions on "the types of testing stimuli to be used," "the verbal instructions to be presented that could best elicit the target responses from clients," "precautions to be taken before and during the procedures," and "how to analyze the data collected for the most representative results" can hardly be found in the literature. These practical and instructional issues are critical in any evaluative procedures. In many instances, speech-language pathology students/clinicians or resident laryngologists can only gain these skills and knowledge through direct contacts with their clients or through their clinical educators or mentors. A sourcebook with practical voice assessment suggestions is needed to teach and equip professionals with basic clinical skills in voice assessment. This handbook is developed to have a dual feature of being a textbook and a sourcebook. It aims to maximize students' and clinicians' competence, knowledge, and effectiveness in voice assessments.

In the process of compiling and editing this handbook, the editors undertook a few principles in editing the chapters:

1. The description of a specific instrument in this handbook by no means implies the authors or the editors endorsed a particular system.
2. This handbook is not intended to be a technical manual for troubleshooting a specific instrument. Readers should refer to the technical manuals provided by the vendors for details on technical and operation information.
3. The terms "clients" and "patients" are used interchangeably in this handbook.
4. This handbook does not describe all the possible procedures in a specific type of voice assessments. Only newly developed or current popular procedures are described. For example, in recording a voice range profile, the use of computerized system to automate the profile generation process is the contemporary approach (as described in Chapter 19). The voice range profile can, nevertheless, be plotted manually using a tone generator and a sound level meter. This "old-fashioned" way of recording method for voice range profile is not detailed in this handbook.

This handbook embraces the current best practice and the latest research reports in voice assessments by leading recognized voice researchers and clinicians in the profession. We are proud to have contributing authors representing an international profile from Australia, China, Czech Republic, Hong Kong, Sweden, the

United Kingdom, and the United States. We would like to thank our contributors here who have been so accommodating in meticulously following the prescriptive framework set out by the editors. Their considerable inputs and efforts have allowed this handbook to become a reality.

We would also like to acknowledge the great support extended to us from our late Dr. Sadanand Singh and Professor Thomas Murry who have provided us with invaluable advice and insightful suggestions in making this a readable volume. Last but not least, our sincere thanks to Professor Ray Kent, who kindly has written a wonderful foreword for this handbook despite his "busy" retirement.

Estella Ma, Ph.D.
Edwin Yiu, Ph.D.

Contributors

Richard D. Andreatta, PhD
Laboratory of Speech-Orofacial
   Sensorimotor Physiology
Department of Rehabilitation Sciences
Division of Communication Sciences &
   Disorders
The Rehabilitation Sciences Doctoral
   Program
College of Health Sciences
University of Kentucky
Lexington, Kentucky
Chapter 15

Susan Baker Brehm, PhD
Associate Professor
Department of Speech Pathology and
   Audiology
Miami University
Voice Scientist
Department of Speech Pathology
Cincinnati Children's Hospital Medical
   Center
Oxford, Ohio
Chapter 2

Karen M.-K. Chan, PhD
Research Assistant Professor
Division of Speech and Hearing
   Sciences
The University of Hong Kong
Chapter 23

**Petrea Cornwell, BSpPath (Hons),
PhD**
Research Fellow

School of Health and Rehabilitation
   Sciences
Division of Speech Pathology
The University of Queensland
Speech Pathology Department
Princess Alexandra Hospital
Brisbane, Australia
Chapter 5

Maria Dietrich, PhD
Division of Communication Sciences
   and Disorders
Department of Rehabilitation Sciences
University of Kentucky College of
   Health Sciences
Lexington, Kentucky
Chapter 15

Ruth Epstein, PhD
Head of Speech-Language Therapy
   Services
Royal National Throat Nose and Ear
   Hospital
Director—MSc Voice Pathology
University College
London, England
Chapters 9 and 13

Bruce R. Gerratt, PhD
Professor
Division of Head and Neck Surgery
David Geffen School of Medicine
University of California, Los Angeles
Los Angeles, California
Chapter 21

Demin Han, MD
Professor
Department of Otolaryngology
Beijing Tongren Hospital
Capital Medical University
Beijing, China
Chapters 10 and 16

Barbara Jacobson
Assistant Professor
Department of Otolaryngology
Vanderbilt Voice Center
Nashville, Tennessee
Chapter 24

Jiangping Kong, PhD
Professor of Phonetics
Department of Chinese Language and
    Literature
Peking University
Beijing, China
Chapter 12

Jody Kreiman, PhD
Professor of Head and Neck Surgery
UCLA School of Medicine
Los Angeles, California
Chapter 21

Alice Lee, PhD
Lecturer
Department of Speech and Hearing
    Sciences
University College, Cork
Cork, Ireland
Chapter 20

Per-Åke Lindestad, MD, PhD
Assistant Professor
Department of Otolaryngology
Karolinska University Hospital
Stockholm, Sweden
Chapter 7

Estella P.-M. Ma, PhD
Assistant Professor, Division of Speech
    and Hearing Sciences
Co-Director, Voice Research Laboratory
Faculty of Education
The University of Hong Kong
Chapters 1, 3, 14, and 19

**Catherine Madill, PhD, BAppSc
(Speech Pathology) Hons1M, BA
Hons**
Lecturer
Department of Speech Pathology
Faculty of Health Sciences
University of Sydney
Australia
Chapter 18

Patricia McCabe, PhD
Senior Lecturer
Speech Pathology
Faculty of Health Sciences
The University of Sydney
Australia
Chapter 18

Clark A. Rosen, MD, FACS
Director
University of Pittsburgh Voice Center
Professor of Otolaryngology
University of Pittsburgh School of
    Medicine
Associate Professor of Communication
    Science and Disorders
University of Pittsburgh School of
    Health and Rehabilitation Sciences
Pittsburgh, Pennsylvania
Chapter 8

John S. Rubin, MD, FACS, FRCS
Honorary Senior Lecturer
University College of London
Consultant ENT Surgeon
Lead Clinician, Voice Disorders

Royal National Throat, Nose, and Ear
  Hospital
London, England
Chapter 9

Rahul Shrivastav, PhD
Associate Professor
Department of Speech, Language and
  Hearing Sciences
University of Florida
Gainesville, Florida
Chapter 22

Nancy Pearl Solomon, PhD, CCC-SLP
Adjunct Professor
University of Maryland and
Research Speech-Language Pathologist
Walter Reed Army Medical Center
Washington, D.C.
Chapter 4

František Šram, MD, CSc
Associate Professor
Voice Center Prague
Medical Healthcom, Ltd.
Prague, the Czech Republic
Chapter 11

Joseph Stemple, PhD
Professor
Department of Rehabilitation Sciences
University of Kentucky
Lexington, Kentucky
Chapter 2

Jan G. Švec, PhD
Research Scientist
Department of Experimental Physics
Laboratory of Biophysics
Palacky University Olomouc
Olomouc, The Czech Republic
Chapter 11

Adam P. Vogel, PhD
Research Fellow

Department of Otolaryngology
The University of Melbourne
Australia
Chapter 17

Barbara Weinrich, PhD
Professor
Department of Speech Pathology and
  Audiology
Miami University
Oxford, Ohio
Chapter 2

Tara L. Whitehill, PhD, CCC-SLP
Professor
Division of Speech and Hearing Sciences
Faculty of Education
Centre for Communication Disorders
University of Hong Kong
Hong Kong
Chapter 20

Amy Y.-H. Wong
Bachelor of Speech and Hearing Sciences
Speech Therapist
Tuen Mun Hospital
Hong Kong
Chapter 14

Wen Xu, MD
Associate Professor
Department of Otolaryngology
Beijing Tongren Hospital
Capital Medical University
Beijing, China
Chapters 10 and 16

VyVy N. Young, MD
Assistant Professor
Department of Otorhinolaryngology-
  Head and Neck Surgery
University of Maryland
Baltimore, Maryland
Chapter 8

Edwin M.-L. Yiu, PhD
Associate Dean, Faculty of Education
Professor, Voice Research Laboratory
The University of Hong Kong
Faculty of Education
Honorary Professor, Discipline of
  Speech Pathology
Faculty of Health Sciences
The University of Sydney
Chapters 1, 6, and 12

Richard I. Zraick, PhD, CCC-SLP
Associate Professor
Department of Audiology and Speech
  Pathology
University of AR for Medical Sciences
Little Rock, Arkansas
Chapter 24

CHAPTER 1

Introduction

ESTELLA P.-M. MA AND EDWIN M.-L. YIU

Voice assessment is essential in the management of voice disorders. It has four primary purposes: (1) to arrive at a diagnosis with severity levels for the voice problems; (2) to determine the underlying causes of the voice problems; (3) to facilitate the planning of voice treatment; and (4) to evaluate the outcomes of the voice treatment. Historically, clinical voice assessment was limited to auditory-perceptual voice quality evaluation per se. Instrumental analyses become more popular when technologies advance and more development is available on different types of acoustic or aerodynamic measurements. Contemporary clinical voice assessments target not just the extent of impairments of phonatory structures and functions, but also on assessing the impact of the impairment on daily communicative activities and participation in these activities. This handbook covers procedures spanning from perceptual and instrumental assessments that are impairment based to the impact on activities/participation that are disability based.

The seven sections of this handbook are broadly arranged using a phonatory physiology framework that covers aerodynamic forces, vocal fold vibrations, laryngeal muscle activities, acoustics, resonance, auditory-perceptual evaluation, and quality of life evaluation. Consistent formats and terminologies are used throughout. Each chapter begins with a succinct list of the purposes of the assessment method, followed by a description of the assessment procedures in a systematic format. Readers can follow directly the detailed examples of verbal instructions provided in the chapters. Each assessment method is illustrated by a pertinent case example to show the clinical application of the assessment method. We believe readers who are speech-language pathology students and clinicians, resident laryngologists, or other professionals with a variety of backgrounds and levels of expertise will find this handbook useful as a self-learning sourcebook.

In this introductory chapter, we highlight four general principles for good practice in clinical voice assessments in addition to the specific guidelines described for each assessment method detailed in individual chapters.

1. **Clinicians should apply the evidence-based practice framework in voice assessments.**
   Evidence-based practice (EBP) is the integral use of current best evidence, clinical expertise, and client values to guide clinical decision making (American Speech-Language-Hearing Association, 2005). When carrying out voice assessments, clinicians should follow the recording procedures and parameters that are derived and supported by scientific findings, whenever such evidence is available in the literature.

2. **Clinicians should use instrumentations with a critical mind.**
   With advances in technology, the instrumentation for voice assessments becomes more popular, affordable, and user friendly. Computer-assisted voice analysis programs can complete the analysis and present the results in the form of numbers in a few seconds. Although this can be very appealing, particularly in a busy clinic, clinicians should not rely on the numerical values alone. They should know exactly what the voice parameters are assessing and interpret the assessment results in relation to the laryngeal anatomy and phonatory physiology. A good practice is to begin assessment with a hypothesis set out first for the client, and then use the assessment results to testify the hypothesis (Baken & Orlikoff, 1997; Behrman & Orlikoff, 1997).

3. **Clinicians should understand both the usefulness and limitations of voice measurement.**
   Although voice assessments are useful in clinical decision-making, they are not without limitations. Examples of limitations include acoustic perturbation analysis, which gives better calculation of frequency-related measures on periodic voices than on aperiodic voices (Titze, 1995). Another example relates to auditory-perceptual evaluation of vocal qualities, which has always been regarded as the gold standard in voice assessment (Kreiman, Gerratt, Kempster, Erma, & Berke, 1993). However, its subjective nature leads to concerns about the reliability of this procedure.

4. **Clinicians should consider modifying the assessment protocol for different client populations.**
   Special considerations need to be taken when assessing certain client populations, namely, professional singers, the pediatric population, the elderly population, and clients from different linguistic, cultural, and racial groups. Flexibility to deviate from the standard procedures may be necessary in these populations but caution also should be applied in the interpretation of the results obtained through nonstandard procedures. Some suggestions are given in the following sections:

   ■ **Professional singers.** Professional singers are different from the general population in various aspects, namely, they are more concerned about their voice quality (Benninger & Murry, 2006). A slight deviant in voice may lead to significant limitations in singing voice activities. Therefore, the voice assessment protocol should extend beyond speaking tasks and include singing tasks.

   ■ **The pediatric population.** There are substantial structural, histologic, and functional differences between the pediatric and adult larynx. Pediatric larynx locates at a higher position in the larynx (Rahbar & Healy, 2006) and their vocal folds are shorter in length (Kerschner & Merati, 2008). There also is a relatively higher percentage of the cartilaginous than the membranous portion of the vocal folds (Sasaki, Kim, & Hundal, 2006) in the pediatric larynx. Therefore, the normative data collected from the adult population cannot be generalized directly to children. Besides, clinicians should present instructions and testing stimuli that are age-appropriate to the receptive and expressive language levels of the children. Ways to motivate young children should also be considered when devising the assessment protocol.

■ **The elderly population.** In the elderly, there are age-related declines of laryngeal structures and vocal fold tissues. These declines include atrophy of laryngeal muscles, a degeneration of laryngeal mucosal glands, and an increase in vocal fold stiffness. Ossification and calcification of the laryngeal cartilages occurs with increasing age (Kahane, 1987; Kahane & Beckford, 1991). Similar to assessing young children, clinicians should apply the sets of normative data that are relevant to the elderly group.

■ **Different linguistic, cultural, and racial groups.** The literature has documented that voice measures can manifest differently in speakers of different language, cultural and racial groups (Andri-

anopoulos et al., 2001a; 2001b; Awan & Mueller, 1996; Chen, 2005; Xue, Hao, & Mayo, 2006; Yamazawa & Hollien, 1992). Different cultures also can influence the patient's perception of the functional impacts of voice-related disorders (Lam, Chan, Ho, Kwong, Yiu, & Wei, 2006; Yiu et al., in press). Clinicians should apply the sets of normative data that are relevant to the appropriate cultural and ethnic groups for meaningful normative comparisons.

REFERENCES

Andrianopoulos, M. V., Darrow, K. N., & Chen, J. (2001a). Multimodal standardization of voice among four multicultural populations: formant structures. *Journal of Voice, 15,* 61–77.

Andrianopoulos, M. V., Darrow, K. N., & Chen, J. (2001b). Multimodal standardization of voice among four multicultural populations: Fundamental frequency and spectral characteristics. *Journal of Voice, 15,* 194–219.

American Speech-Language-Hearing Association. (2005). *Evidence-based practice in communication disorders* [Position statement]. Retrieved from http://www.asha.org/members/ebp/

Awan, S. N., & Mueller, P. B. (1996). Speaking fundamental frequency characteristics of White, African American, and Hispanic kindergartens. *Journal of Speech and Hearing Research, 39*(3), 573–577.

Baken, R. J., & Orlikoff, R. F. (1997). Voice measurement: Is more better? *Logopedics, Phoniatrics, Vocology, 22,* 147–151.

Behrman, A., & Orlikoff, R. F. (1997). Instrumentation in voice assessment and treatment: What's the use? *American Journal of Speech-Language Pathology, 6*(4), 9–16.

Benninger, M. S., & Murry, T. (2006). Introduction. In M. S. Benninger & T. Murry (Eds.), *The performer's voice* (pp. 3–6). San Diego, CA: Plural Publishing.

Chen, S. H. (2005). The effects of tones on speaking frequency and intensity ranges in Mandarin and Min dialects. *Journal of the Acoustical Society of America, 117*, 3225–3230.

Kahane, J. C. (1987). Connective tissue changes in the larynx and their effects on voice. *Journal of Voice, 1*, 27–30.

Kahane, J. C., & Beckford, N. S. (1991). The aging larynx and voice. In D. N. Ripich (Ed.), *Handbook of geriatric communication disorders* (pp 165–186). Austin, TX: Pro-Ed.

Kerschner, J. E., & Merati, A. L. (2008). Science of voice production from infancy through adolescent. In C. J. Hartnick & M. E. Boseley (Eds.), *Pediatric voice disorders* (pp. 23–30). San Diego, CA: Plural Publishing.

Kreiman, J., Gerratt, B. R., Kempster, G. B., Erma, A., & Berke, G. S. (1993). Perceptual evaluation of voice quality: Review, tutorial, and a framework for future research. *Journal of Speech and Hearing Research, 36*, 21–40.

Lam, P. K. Y., Chan, K. M., Ho, W. K., Kwong, E., Yiu, E. M., & Wei, W. (2006). Cross-cultural adaptation and validation of the Chinese Voice Handicap Index-10. *Laryngoscope, 116*, 1192–1198.

Rahbar, R., & Healy, G. B. (2006). Voice disorders in the pediatric population. In J. S. Rubin, R. T. Sataloff, & G. S. Korovin (Eds.), *Diagnosis and treatment of voice disorders* (3rd ed., pp. 381–392). San Diego, CA: Plural Publishing.

Sasaki, C. T., Kim, Y.-H., & Hundal, J. (2006). Anatomy of the human larynx. In J. S. Rubin, R. T. Sataloff, & G. S. Korovin (Eds.), *Diagnosis and treatment of voice disorders* (3rd ed., pp. 31–46). San Diego, CA: Plural Publishing.

Titze, I. R. (1995). *Workshop on acoustic voice analysis: Summary statement.* Iowa City, IA: National Center for Voice and Speech.

Xue, S. A., Hao, G. J. P., & Mayo, R. (2006). Volumetric measurements of vocal tracts for male speakers from different races. *Clinical Linguistics and Phonetics, 20*, 691–702.

Yamazawa, H., & Hollien, H. (1992). Speaking fundamental frequency patterns of Japanese women. *Phonetica, 49*, 128–140.

Yiu, E. M.-L., Ho, E. M., Ma, E. P.-M., Verdolini, K., Branski, R., Richardson, K., & Li, N. Y.-K. (in press). Possible cross-cultural differences in the perception of impact of voice disorders. *Journal of Voice.*

SECTION I

Aerodynamics

CHAPTER 2

Aerodynamic Measurement of Vocal Function: Phonatory Aerodynamic System

JOSEPH STEMPLE, BARBARA WEINRICH, AND SUSAN BAKER BREHM

PURPOSES

- To assess the aerodynamic and respiratory components of vocal functions.
- To discriminate normal and disordered vocal function.
- To inform the glottal competence associated with specific voice disorders.
- To inform changes between pre- and postsurgical/therapy vocal function.
- To be used as a primary feedback tool in behavioral voice therapy.

THEORETICAL BACKGROUND

Multiple anatomic and physiologic systems are necessary to produce and perceive voice. The respiratory system provides the power necessary to drive the vibrating vocal folds, which are the voice source. The acoustic sound wave generated by the voice source is then filtered by the resonators (pharyngeal, oral, and nasal cavities) before it is released into the air and perceived by the auditory system of the listener. It is possible to make discrete and meaningful measures at each level of voice production/perception. These measures may inform both the voice clinician and researcher about various aspects of normal and disordered voice. When combined with the patient interview, these assessments often aid in the planning of successful voice treatment.

During normal phonation, vocal fold vibration is initiated and maintained by interactions between the respiratory and phonatory systems. Assessment of the aerodynamic aspects of voice production, therefore, has the potential to yield information related to laryngeal as well as respiratory function (Sapienza, 1996). Aerodynamic assessment is capable of producing a variety of measures related to airflow, air pressure, and lung volume. Some aerodynamic measures yield gross information regarding respiratory function during speech and airflow through the larynx during phonation. Other measures produce precise information related to the features of individual glottal cycles. Instrumentation for aerodynamic assessment varies widely as well, from rudimentary instruments, such as the stopwatch used for simple phonation time measures, to the sophisticated pneumotachograph used for finer measures of airflow and glottal cycles.

Two principle aerodynamic components, subglottic pressure and transglottic flow, reveal indirect information about the underlying valving activity of the larynx. The interaction of pressure and flow is an essential component of vocal fold vibration. Aerodynamic measures tend to relate more closely to the vocal fold valving capabilities than do acoustic analysis data (Bless, 1991; Hirano & Bless, 1993; Scherer, 1991). A number of airflow and pressure measures are available clinically. Additional derived (combination) measures that integrate pressure and flow in mathematic ratios (single measure) also have been examined, such as laryngeal resistance or glottal power (Hirano, 1981; Hoit & Hixon, 1992; Melcon, Hoit, & Hixon, 1989; Smitheran & Hixon, 1981). Other aerodynamic measures are specific to clinical tasks, such as phonation threshold pressure, which is the minimum subglottic pressure needed to initiate vocal fold vibration (Bless, Glaze, Biever-Lowery, Campos, & Peppard, 1993; Titze, 1991), or average transglottic flow, which is assessed under sustained vowel conditions (Fisher & Swank, 1997; Holmberg, Hillman, & Perkell, 1988).

In speech production, pressure and flow variations are both dynamic and transient because of rapid sequencing of speech and voice sounds. Momentary changes in oral pressure measured during production of specific individual plosive or fricative consonants are examples of transient or short-term aerodynamic measures (Iwata, 1988; Kitajima & Fujita, 1992; Netsell, 1969). Clinically, however, it often is useful to measure average airflow rate or flow volume during sustained productions of vowels or connected speech, reflecting long-term or average aerodynamic measures. Constraints that limit the clinical application of other instrumental measures also limit the utility of aerodynamic measures. These constraints include technologic error (such as calibration error) (Schutte, 1992), type of speech sample (variability in frequency and intensity) (Holmberg et al., 1988), and intrasubject variability (variations such as time of day and effort) (Higgins, Netsell, & Schulte, 1994).

Nonetheless, measures of intraoral pressure, transglottic flow, and derived measures, such as laryngeal resistance, have been used to discriminate normal and pathologic vocal function, to assess disorder severity, to aid management planning, and, in some cases, to suggest implications for the diagnostic source of the voice pathology. For example, an excessive average flow rate usually indicates an underlying glottal incompetence (such as those seen in presbylaryngeus and unilateral vocal fold paralysis). Increased subglottic pressure measures often are associated with hyperfunctional voice use patterns (such as muscle tension dysphonia and adductor spasmodic dysphonia) (Iwata, 1988). When aerodynamic measures provide a real-time visual display, clinicians can use these readings as primary treatment feedback tools to offer support for behavioral changes in vocal fold valving during voice production.

Aerodynamic results appear to correlate clearly with the theoretical understanding of vocal fold vibration. As a result, a movement toward increased clinical use of aerodynamic assessment seems appropriate. Such measures could provide clinicians with a sensitive indicator of pathology, feedback during therapy, and a measure of treatment effectiveness.

DESCRIPTION OF THE SYSTEM

The Phonatory Aerodynamic System (PAS), KayPENTAX Model 6600, Version 3.2.1, was designed and developed to obtain phonatory, acoustic/aerodynamic data (frequency, sound pressure, airflow, and air pressure) of speech and voice signals for use in the speech clinic or laboratory. The PAS is a sophisticated, yet user-friendly, instrument designed for both the ease of clinical assessment and the rigors of clinical research. The data obtained can be used to monitor airflow and laryngeal function during speech. The PAS is a sophisticated pnuemotach consisting of a tube with a series of mesh screens that detect the drop in pressure as air passes through the tube. The information obtained by the instrument is analyzed by software and stored on a computer hard drive. The data are easily retrieved and inserted into clinical reports as needed (Figure 2–1).

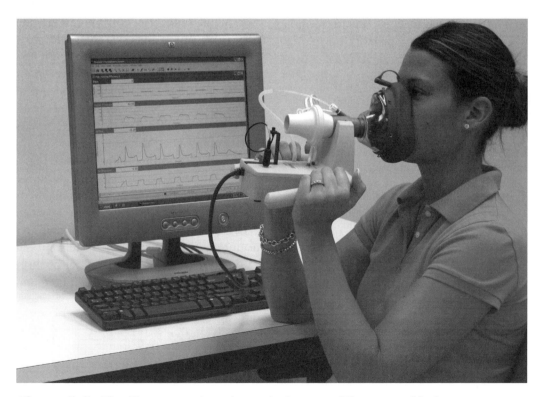

Figure 2-1. The Phonatory Aerodynamic System. (Photo provided as a courtesy of KayPENTAX)

EQUIPMENT AND MATERIALS

The components of the PAS external module are the PAS hand-held device, an integrated microphone, airflow head (pnuemotach), mask and airflow tubes, intraoral pressure kit with various tubes, and coupler. The mask and intraoral tube are the parts that have direct contact with the patient. When the mask is used to collect data, it must be held tightly against the patient's face to avoid air leakage. The intraoral tube is used to collect air pressure measures and should rest inside the patient's mouth without contact against the cheek or tongue.

The Microsoft Windows XP/Vista operating system is used to run the PAS program (Version 3.2), which is designed to have program functions executed by either pull-down menus, defined key commands, or selected icons on the toolbar. The KayPENTAX PAS instruction manual (2008) provides detailed information regarding *Using PAS, Menus, and Program Functions*.

TEST PROCEDURES

General Guidelines

The accuracy and efficiency of aerodynamic measures are dependent on the manner in which the tasks are performed and equipment is managed. Below are several general considerations for testing procedures.

Calibration

The clinician should turn on the hardware components of the PAS 15 minutes prior to calibration and data collection. When the PAS software program is opened, it provides a prompt window to calibrate the airflow head. Follow instructions provided at the prompt window on the computer screen. In addition, access **Options** and select **Calibrate Air Pressure Zerolevel**. It is recommended that this be performed every time the system is first turned on. The purpose of calibration is to adjust for changes in flow head "resistance" which may be affected by changes in humidity level and room temperature. If the system remains on for an entire workday, the system will prompt for recalibration at set time intervals. The default is 4 hours and this timing can be modified by accessing **Options**, then select **PAS Capture Display**, and then **Airflow Head Calibration Frequency**. Note that the calibration applies for the specific user who completes the calibration. If a new user signs onto the computer (via the Microsoft operating system), the new user should calibrate the PAS, even if less than 4 hours have passed. If an examiner removes a flow head for cleaning or to change to a previously cleaned flow head, calibration should be performed. There is variation between the flow heads, requiring the calibration to adjust. Also, when a flow head is cleaned between patients, there is a greater chance of damage or change to the flow head screen. So even if the "same" flow head is being re-mounted, the user should calibrate. In order to recalibrate without a prompt window, go to the **Options** menu and select **Calibrate Airflow Head**.

Mask Seal

The PAS hand-held device has two side handles, which the patient may hold during the examination to create a tight seal with the mask. It is essential that the patient understand the necessity to press the mask very tightly against his or her face for valid airflow measure. Patients with extremity weakness or coordination concerns may require assistance from the clinician to maintain a tight seal. This assistance also may be required for young children. To provide assistance, the clinician can hold one of the device handles, pressing the mask to the patient's face. The examiner can place his or her other hand against the back of the patient's head. This procedure will ensure a tight mask seal.

Explanation of Task Procedures

The PAS is designed to measure parameters during the expiratory phase. Due to health safety considerations with repeated use of the handheld device, patients should be instructed *not* to inspire through the device. Therefore, it is recommended that the clinician clearly explain and practice the appropriate breathing procedures prior to holding the mask against the patient's face. Specifically, the patient should be instructed to inspire prior to bringing the device to his or her face. The coordination of the inspiration and expiration with and without the device may be especially difficult for children. It is recommended that the clinician strictly follow the "expiratory phase only" into the device in all clinical activities with the PAS. If the clinician does not feel that the "expiratory phase only" can be followed in his or her setting, it is recommended that the procedures in Appendix 2-A be utilized for disinfecting the pneumotach between each patient. Additionally, if the clinician is using the nondisposable masks, these masks must be disinfected following guidelines in Appendix 2-A between

each patient. The disposable masks are intended to be for one-time use only. The intraoral tube should be replaced for each patient.

It is important to introduce the hand-held device to children or patients with cognitive impairments in a manner that does not alarm them. Some patients with complex medical histories may associate the device with surgical/anesthesia masks. These patients may need assurance that the mask will not put them to sleep and does not have a "funny smell." Using analogies, such as, "Today you can be an airplane pilot," may be helpful. More detailed explanation of all breathing and speaking tasks may be required for young children or patients with cognitive impairments. For example, during the *Vocal Efficiency* protocol these patients may require additional practice prior to the mask being held to the face. Often, these patients need reminders *not* to inspire between syllables, as well as additional coaching to perform the task at the appropriate rate. They may need to begin the task saying /a/ with the clinician tapping their arm when they should close their lips to produce a syllabic train of /papapa/ with an elongated /a/.

Multiple Measurements

Obtaining multiple measurements from an individual patient performing each protocol that is utilized for the assessment session is important. When patients do not fully understand the directions for a task, or feel slightly uncomfortable about their ability to perform a task, they may not perform to the best of their ability during the first trial. Learning effects should be considered and generally three trials of each task should be performed, with an average value recorded.

Standing Versus Sitting

The clinician's discretion is used to determine whether the patient should stand or sit for the testing protocol. This decision may be dictated by physical constraints of the patient. However, the clinician should be aware that values for parameters, such as vital capacity, vary slightly depending on body position. It is recommended that the clinician be consistent for repeated measurements with a given patient (e.g., pre/post-therapy measurements).

Troubleshooting

If values obtained from patients appear inaccurate or out of physiologic range, a first step would be to recalibrate. If recalibration does not produce a satisfactory change, the clinician should perform measurements of his or her airflow and pressure values. In order for self-measurements to be useful to clinicians in troubleshooting, they should obtain "normal" measures on themselves when becoming familiar with the PAS. (See Appendix C of the Kay-PENTAX (2008) PAS Instruction Manual for detailed troubleshooting information.)

PAS Protocols

The PAS program uses a variety of macros to configure graphics and execute protocols to capture data and display analysis of results. A macro is a single computer instruction that results in a series of instructions in machine language. The **PAS Protocols** menu provides the macros, which are the recommended method of performing program operations. The protocols provide the user with sufficient information to capture and analyze the data. The results are presented in a **PAS**

Analysis Results dialog box. There are seven predefined protocols (Vital Capacity, Air Pressure Screening, Maximum Sustained Phonation, Comfortable Sustained Phonation, Variation in Sound Pressure Level, Voicing Efficiency, and Running Speech) and four user profiles intended for user modification to meet specific analysis needs. The KayPENTAX (2008) PAS Instruction Manual provides information regarding *Clinical Significance, Equipment Setup, Assessment Task, Recommended Data Selection Strategy, Capture/Display Profile, Threshold,* and *Analysis Profile* for each of the protocols. The protocols can be used for pre- and post-treatment measures with a variety of patients presenting with voice disorders.

Vital Capacity

Vital capacity refers to the maximum amount of air available for respiration or phonation, whereas lung capacity is the total volume of air in the lungs. Residual air is the amount of air in the lungs after maximal exhalation. Vital capacity is a measure of clinical interest for patients experiencing difficulty with adequate respiratory volume needed to produce various speech tasks performed by lecturers, aerobic instructors, public speakers, and so forth, and/or singing tasks. Vital capacity, which is measured without phonation, is a measure that will help clinicians calculate expected adequate performance in a maximum phonation task, which is used with the therapeutic tasks of Vocal Function Exercises (Stemple, Lee, D'Amico, & Pickup, 1994).

Instructions: *"Inhale maximally, hold your breath briefly while placing the mask firmly against your face; then exhale maximally."*

Air Pressure Screening

A minimal amount of air pressure generated by the respiratory system is necessary to produce running speech. An approximate oral pressure at 5 cm H_2O held for 5 seconds is considered adequate for minimal demands to produce voice. Patients with motor speech disorders may have difficulty generating adequate air pressure for running speech. This is a performance screening task and there are no measurements obtained from this protocol.

> **Instructions:** *"Tightly seal your lips around both the intraoral tube and the leak tube which is inserted in the corner of your mouth. Then, while monitoring the computer screen, generate an oral pressure of at least 5 cm H_2O and hold that pressure for at least 5 seconds."*

Maximum Sustained Phonation

Assessing the patient's ability to efficiently manage an adequate air supply during phonation is referred to as a maximum performance task. This protocol provides frequency, sound pressure level, and airflow measurements that are taken during a sustained open vowel ("aaah"). The patient is instructed to take a deep breath and sustain the vowel at a comfortable pitch and loudness for as long as possible. This protocol provides information related to vocal fold function, as well as respiratory support, and is useful for pre/post-therapeutic measures, such as Vocal Function Exercises.

> **Instructions:** *"Take a deep breath; place the mask firmly against your face and produce the sustained tone 'aaah' with a comfortable pitch and loudness until you feel the need to take a breath."*

Comfortable Sustained Phonation

Clinical assessments of voice include measurements of mean airflow rate (the rate at which air passes between the vocal folds during phonation) used in sustained phonation to confirm laryngeal dysfunction noted in acoustic analysis and laryngeal imaging observations. Patients who demonstrate inadequate glottic closure will have higher than normal mean airflow rate, whereas those producing voice with too much laryngeal tension will have lower than normal mean airflow rate during sustained phonation (Iwata, 1988). This protocol provides measurements of frequency, sound pressure level, and airflow rate during a sustained vowel /a/ of 7 seconds. It is recommended that measures be taken during the middle 3 seconds of the sustained tone.

> **Instructions:** *"Take a breath; place the mask firmly against your face and produce the sustained tone 'aaah' with a comfortable pitch and loudness for 7 seconds."*

Variation in Sound Pressure Level

The ability to vary frequency, intensity, and airflow enables a speaker to provide suprasegmental and prosodic components to speech that enhance communication. Patients with monotonicity do not vary frequency and intensity measures of their voice. This protocol provides measurement of frequency, sound pressure level, and airflow during a syllable task (/pa-pa-pa/) repeated at different loudness levels.

Instructions: *"Take a breath; place the mask firmly against your face. Produce the syllable string 'pa-pa-pa' at your usual loudness level; then half your usual loudness level; then twice your usual loudness level."*

Voicing Efficiency

Subglottic pressure and ratio measures of glottal resistance and glottal efficiency are laryngeal function measures commonly described in the assessment of aerodynamic function. These measures are of clinical interest for patients who are using hypofunctional or hyperfunctional voices. The voicing efficiency protocol calculates the relationship of air pressure measurements from peak air pressure events (release of plosive consonant /p/, which is an estimate of glottal pressure) to average airflow and sound pressure level measurements from voiced segments (vowel /a/) of the syllable /pa/. The syllable train of "pa-pa-pa" should include five to seven repetitions, with approximately 1.5 seconds per syllable, and continuous airflow for "ah" throughout the production. These calculations yield voice efficiency measures that are useful when comparing pre- and post-treatment results. *Caveat:* As vocal frequency and amplitude affect subglottic pressure measures, the clinician should note the fundamental frequency and sound pressure level measurements of pretreatment and strive to capture those measures within a ±5% range during post-treatment measures. Young children, individuals with significant cognitive impairments, or patients with respiratory-compromise may have difficulty performing this task.

Instructions: *"Take a breath; place the mask firmly against your face*

with the pressure tube placed inside your mouth; then repeat the syllable 'pa' five to seven times on a single breath at a rate of 1.5 to 2 syllables per second."

Running Speech

Articulatory precision, coordination, timing, and laryngeal function are important behaviors for successful communication during running speech. Inspiratory volume and flow may diminish during running speech, which is characteristic of the fatigue experienced by patients with neurological or degenerative disorders. This protocol measures frequency, sound pressure level, and airflow during running speech.

Instructions: *"Place the mask firmly against your face. Read this passage in your normal speech."*

NORMATIVE AERODYNAMIC MEASURES

As with many instrumental measures of voice, a wide range of measures exist for the major aerodynamic categories including:

- airflow (measured in L/s or mL/s)
- air pressure (measured in cm H_2O)
- laryngeal airway resistance (measured in cm $H_2O/(L/s)$)

Airflow refers to the rate at which air passes between the vocal folds during phonation. Subglottic pressure (Ps) is the air pressure necessary to set the approximated folds into vibration and to maintain vibration. Laryngeal airway resistance (R_{law}) is the ratio of air pressure over airflow, which is a measure of glottal resistance. Below are normative data for these aerodynamic measures as reported in the following references (Hirano, 1981; Holmberg et al., 1988; Netsell, Lotz, DuChane, & Barlow, 1991; Smitheran & Hixon, 1981):

- Airflow (mL/s): 80–200 mL/s
- Air Pressure (cm H_2O): 5–8 cm H_2O
- Laryngeal Airway Resistance: 32–45 cm H_2O/(L/s)

CASE STUDY: UNILATERAL (RIGHT) TRUE VOCAL FOLD PARALYSIS (MALE)

Unilateral vocal fold paralysis most often is caused by injury or disruption of the recurrent laryngeal nerve. Less frequently, paralysis may be due to involvement of the external branch of the superior laryngeal nerve. Injury of the recurrent laryngeal nerve may be due to surgical or accidental trauma, heart disease, or neurogenic disease. In some cases, the cause is idiopathic. The paralyzed fold may remain at the midline position, causing minimal voice disturbance but minor obstruction of the airway during physical exertion. It is more common for the paralyzed fold to remain in an abducted or paramedian position. This positioning of the paralyzed fold results in a glottal gap, causing breathiness and soft intensity, due to difficulty building sufficient subglottic pressure. Treatment for unilateral vocal fold paralysis greatly depends on the position of the paralyzed fold. Intervention may be surgical, behavioral, or a combination of both.

Aerodynamic measures may be useful in documenting vocal function prior to and following intervention. When one observes the vocal folds under stroboscopic conditions, glottic closure is incomplete. Consequently, as voice is produced, excessive airflow occurs. Vocal fold paralysis often results in overall hyperfunctioning of the larynx with supraglottic activity to produce voice, which necessitates increased subglottic pressure. If airflow remains constant, laryngeal airway resistance increases. Along with perceptual assessment, stroboscopic observations, and acoustic analysis, aerodynamic assessment can add to the diagnostic process.

The following measures were taken with the PAS pre- and post-treatment on a 60-year-old male, who presented with unilateral vocal fold paralysis and subsequent medialization procedure. Perceptually, his voice was described as moderately dysphonic, characterized by a breathy hoarseness, with decreased intensity and pitch range. The PAS software protocols chosen to measure the aerodynamics of his vocal function included *Maximum Sustained Phonation*, *Comfortable Sustained Phonation*, and *Voicing Efficiency*. These protocols allow for measures that are sensitive to glottal gap and voice effort, and provide for ratio measures of voice efficiency. The protocols also provide important acoustic information studied simultaneously with aerodynamic measures. Pitch and loudness measures aid in the description of this patient's phonatory function. The specific measures of interest for this patient are highlighted in Table 2–1.

Examining these measures for the pre- and post-treatment data informs the clinician and the patient of the following information:

- There was a change in fundamental frequency.
- Vocal fold closure improved (increased maximum sustained phonation).
- Ability to develop subglottic air pressure improved.

Table 2-1. Pretreatment and Posttreatment Aerodynamic Measures of the Case Example

Parameters	Pretreatment	Post-treatment
Maximum Sustained Phonation		
Maximum SPL	82.05 dB	81.78 dB
Minimum SPL	60.88 dB	64.01 dB
Mean SPL	78.23 dB	75.95 dB
SPL Range	21.17 dB	17.17 dB
Mean SPL During Voicing	78.28 dB	75.95 dB
Mean Pitch	143.99 Hz	135.70 Hz
Phonation Time	4.98 sec	24.67 sec
Peak Expiratory Airflow	0.71 L/sec	0.26 L/sec
Mean Expiratory Airflow	0.64 L/sec	0.16 L/sec
Expiratory Volume	3.39 L	3.94 L
Comfortable Sustained Phonation		
Maximum SPL	79.51 dB	81.14 dB
Minimum SPL	64.79 dB	78.15 dB
Mean SPL	74.73 dB	79.72 dB
SPL Range	14.71 dB	2.99 dB
Mean Pitch	154.15 Hz	139.72 Hz
Phonation Time	4.08 sec	4.38 sec
Peak Expiratory Airflow	0.63 L/sec	0.29 L/sec
Mean Expiratory Airflow	0.55 L/sec	0.23 L/sec
Expiratory Volume	2.30 L	1.02 L
Voicing Efficiency		
Maximum SPL	81.42 dB	81.35 dB
Mean SPL	74.97 dB	80.02 dB
Mean SPL During Voicing	75.11 dB	80.02 dB
Mean Pitch	157.40 Hz	128.81 Hz
Pitch Range	160.22 Hz	345.0 Hz
Expiratory Airflow Duration	0.35 sec	0.51 sec
Peak Air Pressure	4.25 cm H_2O	5.53 cm H_2O
Mean Peak Air Pressure	3.54 cm H_2O	5.15 cm H_2O
Peak Expiratory Airflow	0.72 L/sec	0.25 L/sec
Target Airflow	0.62 L/sec	0.20 L/sec
Expiratory Volume	0.22 L	0.10 L
Mean Airflow During Voicing	0.57 L/sec	0.20 L/sec
Aerodynamic Power	0.214 watts	0.103 watts
Aerodynamic Resistance	5.61 cm H_2O/(L/s)	24.78 cm H_2O/(L/s)
Aerodynamic Efficiency	20.72 ppm	137.97 ppm
Acoustic Ohms	5.72 ds/cm^5	25.27 ds/cm^5

■ Glottal resistance improved

■ Mean expiratory airflow rate was decreased due to the reduced glottal gap

Because of the size of this patient's glottal gap pretreatment, he was not able to adequately build subglottic air pressure. He obviously did not compensate with a vocal hyperfunction as his mean peak air pressure remained below normal limits. His post-treatment measures were improved and close to normal limits.

REFERENCES

Bless, D. M. (1991). Assessment of laryngeal function. In C. N. Ford & D. M. Bless (Eds.), *Phonosurgery* (pp. 91–122). New York, NY: Raven Press.

Bless, D. M., Glaze, L. E., Biever-Lowery, D., Campos, G., & Peppard, R. C. (1993). Stroboscopic, acoustic, aerodynamic, and perceptual attributes of voice production in normal speaking adults. In I. R. Titze (Ed.), *Progress report 4* (pp. 121–134). Iowa City, IA: National Center for Voice and Speech.

Fisher, K. V., & Swank, P. R. (1997). Estimating phonation threshold pressure. *Journal of Speech, Language, and Hearing Research, 40*(5), 1122–1129.

Higgins, M. B., Netsell, R., & Schulte, L. (1994). Aerodynamic and electroglottographic measures of normal voice production: Intrasubject variability within and across sessions. *Journal of Speech and Hearing Research, 37*(1), 38–45.

Hirano, M. (1981). *Clinical examination of voice.* New York, NY: Springer-Verlag.

Hirano, M., & Bless, D. (1993). *Videostroboscopic examination of the larynx.* San Diego, CA: Singular Publishing Group.

Hoit, J. D., & Hixon, T. J. (1992). Age and laryngeal airway resistance during vowel production in women. *Journal of Speech and Hearing Research, 35*(2), 309–313.

Holmberg, E. B., Hillman, R. E., & Perkell, J. S. (1988). Glottal airflow and transglottal air pressure measurements for male and female speakers in soft, normal and loud voice. *Journal of the Acoustical Society of America, 84,* 511–529.

Iwata, S. (1988). Aerodynamic aspects for phonation in normal and pathologic larynges. In O. Fujimura (Ed.), *Vocal physiology* (pp. 423–431). New York, NY: Raven Press.

Kay Pentax. (2008) *Phonatory aerodynamic system instruction manual,* Lincoln Park, NJ: Kay Pentax, Inc.

Kitajima, K., & Fujita, F. (1992). Clinical report on preliminary data on intraoral pressure in the evaluation of laryngeal pathology. *Journal of Voice, 6*(1), 79–85.

Melcon, M. C., Hoit, J. D., & Hixon, T. J. (1989). Age and laryngeal airway resistance during vowel production. *Journal of Speech and Hearing Disorders, 54*(2), 282–286.

Netsell, R. (1969). Subglottal and intraoral air pressures during intervocalic contrast of /t/ and /d/. *Phonetica, 20*(1), 68–73.

Netsell, R., Lotz, W. K., DuChane, A. S., & Barlow, S. M. (1991). Vocal tract aerodynamics during syllable productions: Normative data and theoretical implications. *Journal of Voice, 5,* 1–9.

Sapienza, C. M. (1996). Glottal airflow: Instrumentation and interpretation. *Florida Journal of Communication Disorders, 16,* 3–7.

Scherer, R. C. (1991). Aerodynamic assessment in voice production. In *Assessment of speech and voice production: Research and clinical applications* (pp. 42–49). Bethesda, MD: National Institute on Deafness and Other Communicative Disorders.

Schutte, H. K. (1992). Integrated aerodynamic measurements. *Journal of Voice, 6*(2), 127–134.

Smitheran, J. R., & Hixon, T. J. (1981). A clinical method for estimating laryngeal airway resistance during vowel production. *Journal of Speech and Hearing Disorders, 46,* 138–146.

Stemple, J. C., Lee, L., D'Amico, B., & Pickup, B. (1994). Efficacy of vocal function exercises as a method of improving voice production. *Journal of Voice, 8*(3), 271–278.

Titze, I. R. (1991). Phonation threshold pressure: A missing link for glottal aerodynamics. In I. R. Titze (Ed.), *Progress report 1* (pp. 1–14). Iowa City, IA: National Center for Voice and Speech.

APPENDIX 2-A

PAS Disinfecting Instructions

INSTRUCTIONS (AS PROVIDED BY KAYPENTAX)

There are several components that may require cleaning and/or disinfecting. Only use cleaning/disinfecting solutions and processes that are compatible with the PAS component materials. Below is a list of the PAS parts and the material makeup.

PAS Parts	Material Makeup
Mask Adaptor:	Polypropylene
Ambu Re-Usable Mask:	Mask Dome: Polysulphone
Mask Cuff:	Silicone Rubber
Airflow Head-to-Mask Coupler:	Polypropylene
Male Luer Plug:	High-Density Polyethylene, PVC
Male Luer Connector:	Nylon
Luer Connector O-Ring:	Silicone
Airflow Head (Pneumotach):	Encasement: ABS Plastic (Acrylonitrile-Butadiene-Styrene)
	Resistive Material: Stainless Steel Mesh

DISINFECTING SOLUTION

The hospital disinfectant Dakins is recommended. Dakins is a proprietary product (Century Pharmaceuticals) of buffered 0.25% or 0.5% sodium hypochlorite (NaClO) solution. Because this solution is buffered, it is more tolerable to the skin. The 0.5% solution is recommended.

If Dakins is not available, use standard household bleach (which is a 5.25% sodium hypochlorite solution (NaClO)). Dilute the bleach to a 20:1 ratio for a 0.25% solution or 10:1 for a 0.5% solution. Wear gloves when handling bleach. Use distilled water instead of tap water to eliminate mineral buildup.

Either of these agents (Dakins or bleach) is an effective bactericide, fungicide, tuberculocide, sporicide, and virucide. When properly diluted, the solution should have no harmful effects on the mask components.

DISINFECTING PROCESS

Use the following procedure to disinfect the PAS parts listed above:

Remove the airflow tubes from the airflow head and set them aside. Wash the PAS components (mask, airflow head, and airflow head-to-mask coupler) in distilled water/liquid detergent to remove spit/sputum, coughed up material, and so forth, that could be on the mask or pneumotach mesh.

Immerse the PAS components in the disinfectant solution as described above for 5 to 10 minutes. Rinse well with distilled water and air dry on a rack. Low pressure forced air can be used to remove residual water and accelerate drying. You can also use a blow dryer to dry the airflow head more quickly, but do this sparingly as it can damage the pneumotach mesh. The airflow head must be completely dry to function properly.

CHAPTER 3

Monitoring Oral Airflow and Air Pressure During Speech Production: Aerophone II

ESTELLA P.-M. MA

PURPOSES

- To assess the glottal functions by determining the amount of oral airflow during phonation.
- To assess the adductory force of vocal folds by determining the intraoral pressure during phonation.

THEORETICAL BACKGROUND

Phonation initiates with a series of respiratory and laryngeal events that involve airflow from the lungs, subglottal pressure, vocal fold vibration, and elasticity of the vocal folds. Airflow rate and subglottal pressure are the two principal and commonly used measures to assess laryngeal aerodynamics (Schutte, 1992). Airflow rate is the amount of air that flows through the glottis over a certain duration of phonation and it can be measured by a pneumotachograph. Subglottal air pressure is the driving force beneath the adducted vocal folds during phonation (Colton, Casper & Leonard, 2006). It can be measured directly by tracheal puncture, or by a miniaturized pressure transducer that is placed through the nostrils to below the glottis, or indirectly by an esophageal balloon that is placed inside the esophagus at the midthoracic level. Both the direct and indirect methods to measure subglottal pressure are considered invasive. Later in 1981, Smitheran and Hixon developed a noninvasive method to provide an estimate of the subglottal pressure. With this method, subglottal pressure is estimated from the peak intraoral pressure obtained at the release of a bilabial plosive, usually the voiceless /p/ (although voiced /b/ has also been used) preceded and followed by vowels (e.g., /a/ or /i/). The basic principle is that at the time just before the bilabial plosive releases, the lips are closed and the vocal folds are abducted. Therefore, the pressure throughout the upper airway reaches a state of equilibrium, and the intraoral pressure presumably is equal to the subglottal pressure (Smitheran & Hixon, 1981). Studies have demonstrated that either the peak intraoral pressure taken at the point of the plosive release (e.g., Löfqvist, Carlborg, & Kitzing, 1982) or the intraoral pressure taken at the mid-vowel point between the two plosives (e.g., Hertegard, Gauffin, & Lindestad, 1995) can be a reliable estimate of subglottal pressure. However, Kitajima and Fujita (1990) caution that the peak intra-oral pressure would be a valid estimate of subglottal pressure only if it is below 25 cm H_2O. The ratio of subglottal pressure to the airflow rate gives rise to glottal resistance.

Aerodynamic measurements have been used to: (1) differentiate dysphonic from healthy voices (e.g., Giovanni et al., 2000; Ng, Gilbert, & Lerman, 1997; Tanaka & Gould, 1985); (2) differentiate among laryngeal pathologies (e.g., Hillman, Holmberg, Perkell, Walsh, & Vaughan, 1989, 1990; Iwata, von Leden, & Williams, 1972; Rosen, Lombard, & Murry, 2000; Tanaka & Gould, 1985); and (3) document changes following voice treatment (e.g., Hirano, 1989).

DESCRIPTION

Several commercial systems are available for performing aerodynamic measurements. These systems include the Aero-phone II from KayPENTAX (http://www.kaypentax.com) and the Glottal Enterprises MS-110 system (http://www.glottal.com/Products/ms110.htm). The newer generation of the Aerophone II is called the Phonatory Aerodynamic System (PAS), which is described in Chapter 2 by Stemple, Weinrich, and Brehm.

EQUIPMENT AND MATERIALS

■ The software of the Aerophone II is the Voice Function Analyzer. It can be installed in a personal computer to capture and analyze voice samples. The Voice Function Analyzer digitizes the voice signals and simultaneously displays the intensity, the pressure, and the airflow traces on the computer screen upon the client's phonation (Figures 3–1 and 3–2). The system can be connected to an external analogue pitch extractor and an AD conversion board in the computer to capture and display the pitch level. [**Note**: The figures shown in this chapter were taken from the older version of the software that runs using DOS operating system. The software has a newer version that runs using a Windows operating system.]

■ The hardware of the Aerophone II (Model 6800, KayPENTAX) is made up of four main components: (1) A face mask that covers the client's nose and mouth for channeling the client's airstream; (2) A flow head (pneumotach) for detecting any change in airflow through the face mask; (3) A pressure transducer for detecting any change of oral pressure during phonation; (4) A microphone placed at 15 centimeters from the face mask for detecting any change of sound pressure level dur-

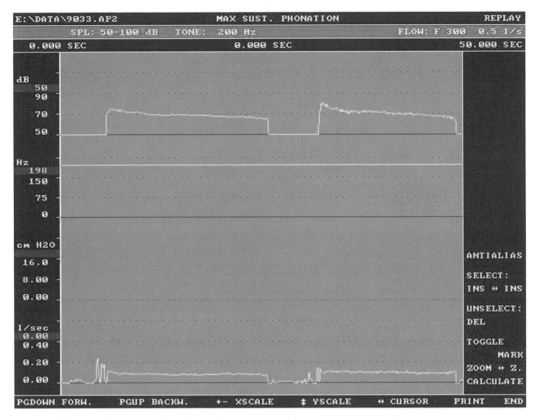

Figure 3-1. Main display screen of the Aerophone II under maximum sustained phonation task. (*Note:* Frequency trace was not displayed in this figure. User can connect the system to an external analogue pitch extractor and an AD conversion board in the computer for displaying the frequency trace).

ing phonation. The face mask, the flow head, and the pressure transducer are attached to a hand-held stand held by the client (Figure 3-3). The Aerophone II package provides two flow heads for various types of airflow measurement (F300LS for phonation tasks, namely, maximum and comfortable sustained phonation tasks; F1000LS for respiratory tasks, namely, maximum peakflow and vital capacity). The package also comes with a nose clamp for respiratory task, a 1-liter calibration syringe for calibration, and silicon rubber tubes for air pressure measurements.

■ Accessories for calibration: thermometer.
■ Other accessories: sterilizing solution (for cleaning the face mask and silicon tube).

TEST PROCEDURES

General Guidelines

■ **Phonational frequency and intensity levels.** It is recommended that the tasks be carried out using the client's most comfortable pitch and loudness levels to reveal the true phonatory

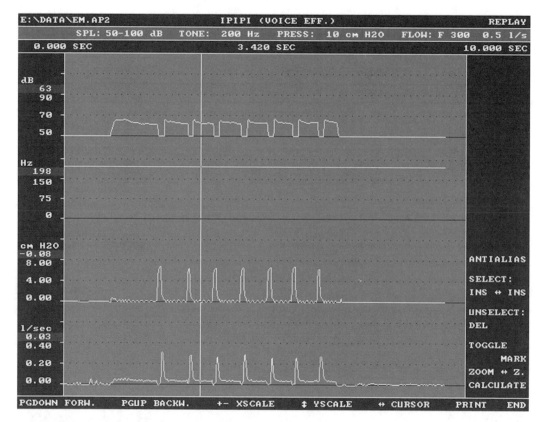

E:\DATA\EM.AP2   IPIPI (VOICE EFF.)   REPLAY
            SPL: 50-100 dB   TONE: 200 Hz   PRESS: 10 cm H2O   FLOW: F 300   0.5 l/s
        0.000 SEC   3.420 SEC   10.000 SEC

Figure 3–2. Main display screen of the Aerophone II under Voicing Efficiency (IPIPI) task. (*Note:* Frequency trace was not displayed in this figure. User can connect the system to an external analogue pitch extractor and an AD conversion board in the computer for displaying the frequency trace).

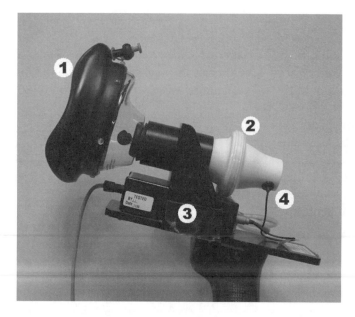

Figure 3–3. Hardware setup of Aerophone II (Model 6800, KayPENTAX): (1) A face mask that covers the client's nose and mouth for channeling the client's airstream; (2) A flow head for detecting any change in airflow through the face mask; (3) A pressure transducer for detecting any change of pressure of the phonation; and (4) A microphone for detecting any change of sound pressure level of the phonation.

behaviors of the client (Higgins, Netsell & Schulte, 1994; Hillman et al., 1990). However, the clinician should be aware that airflow rate and subglottal pressure levels vary with phonational frequency and intensity levels (Plant & Younger, 2000). Therefore, it is a good practice that the clinician also marks down the phonational frequency and intensity levels when recording voice samples for comparison purposes (e.g., pre- versus posttreatment recording).

- **Number of trials.** Higgins et al. (1994) contended that the more trials repeated, the more representative the measure would be and therefore the lower the intrasubject variability. Yiu, Yuen, Whitehill, and Winkworth (2004) demonstrated that aerodynamic measures based on at least five measurement trials were required to achieve a correct classification rate of over 90% in classifying between dysphonic and healthy voices. The author recommends at least five trials should be taken for aerodynamic measurement.

Calibration

The Aerophone II system needs to be calibrated every time before using. This is because air viscosity varies with relative humidity level and room temperature which may affect the aerodynamic measurements. The section below describes the calibration procedures:

1. Connect the calibration syringe with the airflow transducer using a disposable cardboard mouth tube. (Figure 3–4)
2. Select **Flow calibration** from the menu.
3. Enter the current room temperature in degree Celsius as read from the thermometer.
4. Press **Enter** to start the calibration process.
5. Push in the calibration syringe knob completely at a constant speed of within one second for the F1000LS flow head and four seconds for the F300LS flow head.

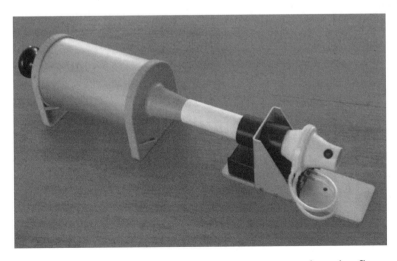

Figure 3–4. The calibration syringe connected to the flow head using a disposable cardboard mouth tube. (Photo provided as a courtesy of F-J Electronics)

6. Repeat Step 5 nine more times.
7. Press **END** to finish the calibration process.

Instructional Steps for Recording

Note: (1) The Aerophone II system offers a range of clinically relevant respiratory measurements, namely, peakflow and vital capacity. This chapter focuses on the procedures for phonatory measurements for airflow rate and air pressure; and (2) If peaking of either the airflow or pressure trace occurs during the recording, adjust the pressure setting (by pressing the **P** key) and the flow setting (by pressing the **F** key), accordingly.

Mean Airflow Rate

Maximum Sustained Phonation Task.

1. Select **Max. Sust. Phonation** from the menu.

   Instructions: *"Take a deep breath, then bring the face mask over your nose and mouth like this.* (The clinician then illustrates where to put the face mask.) *Please make sure that the mask covers your face firmly and that there is no air leakage. Say 'ah'* (or other vowels such as 'ee' or 'oo') *using your most comfortable pitch and loudness for as long as you possibly can until you run out of breath completely. Try to keep your pitch and loudness levels steady during the task. Now I will demonstrate the task to you."* (The clinician then gives a complete and full model of the MPT with the most comfortable pitch and loudness of his or her own.)

2. Press **ENTER** to start the recording.
3. Press **END** to finish the recording.
4. Give positive reinforcement to the client and repeat the task four more times.

   Instructions: *"Well done. Now please do this a second time, try to prolong the 'ah' longer this time. Remember to keep your pitch and loudness similar to those at the first trial."*

   [**Note:** (1) The Aerophone II package has a smaller face mask that can be used for young children or adult clients of small body size; and (2) Due to hygiene reasons, clients should not inspire through the face mask and flow head. Bring the mask to the client's face only when he or she is ready to expire or phonate.]

Most Comfortable Phonation Task.

1. Select **Most Comf. Phonation** from the menu.

   Instructions: *"Hold the face mask firmly over your nose and mouth. Say the sound 'ah'* (or other vowels such as 'ee' or 'oo') *for 5 seconds using your most comfortable pitch and loudness. Let's start."*

2. Press **ENTER** to start the recording.
3. Press **END** to finish the recording.
4. Repeat the task four more times.

Air Pressure Measurement

IPIPI (Voice Eff.) Task.

1. Attach a silicon rubber tube to the 3-way stopcock and then insert the tube through the sleeve hole in the face mask.

2. Select **IPIPI (Voice Eff.)** from the menu.

   Instructions: *"Place this tube centrally on top of your tongue, but do not bite it. Hold the face mask firmly over your nose and mouth. Say '/i/' followed with seven '/pi/' at a rate of 1.5 syllables per second using the most comfortable pitch and loudness level. Let's start."*

3. Press **ENTER** to start the recording.
4. Press **END** to finish the recording.
5. Repeat the task four more times.

Running Speech Task.

1. This task uses the same setting as the IPIP (Voice Eff.) task.
2. Select **Running Speech** from the menu.

   Instructions: *"Again, place this tube centrally on top of your tongue, but do not bite it. Hold the face mask over your nose and mouth. Say aloud the sentence 'A baby boy' with your most comfortable pitch and loudness level."*

3. Press **ENTER** to start the recording.
4. Press **END** to finish the recording.
5. Repeat the task four more times.

DATA ANALYSIS

1. Press the **R** key for **Replay old data** and retrieve the file for analysis.
2. Select the section of voice sample for analysis. Move the cursor on the screen using the **left arrow** and **right arrow** keys and mark the onset of the signal by pressing the **Insert** key.

3. Move the cursor to the offset of the signal and mark the offset by pressing the **Insert** key.
4. The selected section between the two marks will be highlighted automatically by the program.
5. Press the **C** key to start the calculation process.

NORMATIVE DATA

Table 3–1 lists the means and standard deviations of airflow and air pressure measures in 153 native speakers of Cantonese (128 females and 25 males). These figures were taken from a previous study by the author (Ma, 2003). More normative aerodynamic data are reported in Chapter 2 by Stemple, Weinrich, and Brehm; and Chapter 4 by Solomon.

CASE STUDY

Patient K. L. (ventricular dysphonia)
K. L., a 45-year-old male, was referred to a speech pathologist by an otolaryngologist with the diagnosis of ventricular dysphonia. He reported that his voice had deteriorated significantly since he took up the position as the chief executive officer of an international finance firm. K. L. reported that he had to make overseas business trips frequently and that he now spent much less time with his family. K. L. had been very stressed by the excessive workload demands. He also worried seriously about his job performance. He reported a loss of appetite, aching muscles, and getting bad tempered very easily. Initial voice assessment revealed that his upper body and clavicu-

Table 3–1. Normative Data of Mean Airflow Rate and Estimated Subglottal Pressure Reported in Ma (2003)

| Aerodynamic voice measures | Female (n = 128) | | | | Male (n = 25) | | | |
| | Dysphonic (n = 93) | | Vocally healthy (n = 35) | | Dysphonic (n = 19) | | Vocally healthy (n = 6) | |
	Mean	(SD)	Mean	(SD)	Mean	(SD)	Mean	(SD)
Mean airflow rate (L/sec)								
Most comfortable /a/ phonation	0.16	(0.07)	0.13	(0.04)	0.23	(0.13)	0.15	(0.07)
Maximum sustained /a/ phonation	0.14	(0.07)	0.11	(0.04)	0.19	(0.12)	0.11	(0.05)
Maximum sustained /i/ phonation	0.13	(0.06)	0.11	(0.04)	0.20	(0.14)	0.13	(0.03)
Maximum sustained /u/ phonation	0.15	(0.06)	0.13	(0.05)	0.24	(0.15)	0.11	(0.04)
Peak intraoral pressure (cm H_2O)								
/pi/ string production	17.30	(5.30)	10.06	(1.79)	15.28	(5.98)	7.97	(1.02)
Sentence production	12.51	(3.85)	7.90	(1.76)	11.40	(5.33)	6.59	(0.94)

lar breathing was noticeably tense during speech. Videostroboscopic examination of the larynx revealed marked adduction of the ventricular folds (false vocal folds) during phonation. The true vocal folds were not visible during phonation due to the squeezing of the ventricular folds. Perceptually, his voice in conversations was described as low-pitched, moderately rough and moderately-to-severe strained-strangled. Pretreament assessment results indicated that K. L. demonstrated:

■ An increased subglottal pressure—This is consistent with the perceptual signs of strained-strangled voice and the clinical observation of effortful speech.

Table 3–2. Performance of K.L.

Parameter	Pretreatment	Posttreatment
Mean airflow rate		
Most comfortable /a/ phonation	0.09 L/s	0.18 L/s
Maximum sustained /a/ phonation	0.06 L/s	0.15 L/s
Estimated subglottal pressure		
/pi/ string production	16.82 cm H_2O	8.20 cm H_2O
Sentence production	15.26 cm H_2O	6.89 cm H_2O

■ A significantly reduced mean airflow rate—This is consistent with the videostroboscopic results of marked adduction of the ventricular folds.

Inhalation phonation was introduced to K. L. with the aim to facilitate true vocal fold adduction during phonation. K. L. received 10 sessions of voice therapy over the course of 3 months. He also received counseling sessions on stress management. Posttreatment aerodynamic data (Table 3–2) suggested that K. L. benefited from the voice therapy by showing an increase in the mean phonatory airflow together with a decrease in the subglottal pressure.

REFERENCES

Colton, R. H., Casper, J. K., & Leonard, R. (2006). *Understanding voice problems: A physiological perspective for diagnosis and treatment* (3rd ed.). Philadelphia, PA: Lippincott Williams & Wilkins.

Giovanni, A., Heim, C., Demolin, D., & Triglia, J.-M. (2000). Estimated subglottic pressure in normal and dysphonic subjects. *Annals of Otology, Rhinology, and Laryngology, 109,* 500-504.

Hertegard, S., Gauffin, J., & Lindestad, P. A. (1995). A comparison of subglottal and intraoral pressure measurements during phonation. *Journal of Voice, 9*(2), 149-155.

Higgins, M. B., Netsell, R., & Schulte, L. (1994). Aerodynamic and electroglottographic measures of normal voice production: Intrasubject variability within and across sessions. *Journal of Speech and Hearing Research, 37*(1), 38-45.

Hillman, R. E., Holmberg, E. B., Perkell, J. S., Walsh, M., & Vaughan, C. (1989). Objective assessment of vocal hyperfunction: An experimental framework and initial results. *Journal of Speech and Hearing Research, 32,* 373-392.

Hillman, R. E., Holmberg, E. B., Perkell, J. S., Walsh, M., & Vaughan, C. (1990). Phonatory function associated with hyperfunctionally related vocal fold lesions. *Journal of Voice, 4*(1), 52-63.

Hirano, M. (1989). Objective evaluation of the human voice: Clinical aspects. *Folia Phoniatrica, 41*(1), 89-144.

Iwata, S., von Leden, H., & Williams, D. (1972). Airflow measurement during phonation. *Journal of Communication Disorders, 5,* 67-79.

Kitajima, K., & Fujita, F. (1990). Estimation of subglottal pressure with intraoral pressure. *Acta Otolaryngology (Stockh.), 109,* 473-478.

Leeper, H. A., & Graves, D. K. (1984). Consistency of laryngeal airway resistance in adult women. *Journal of Communication Disorders, 17*, 153-163.

Löfqvist, A., Carlborg, B., & Kitzing, P. (1982). Initial validation of an indirect measure of subglottal pressure during vowels. *Journal of Acoustical Society of America, 72*, 633-635.

Ma, E. P.-M. (2003). *Impairment, activity limitation and participation restriction issues in assessing dysphonia.* Unpublished doctoral thesis, The University of Hong Kong, Hong Kong.

Ng, M. L., Gilbert, H. R., & Lerman, J. W. (1997). Some aerodynamic and acoustic characteristics of acute laryngitis. *Journal of Voice, 11*(3), 356-363.

Plant, R. L., & Younger, R. M. (2000). The interrelationship of subglottic air pressure, fundamental frequency, and vocal intensity during speech. *Journal of Voice, 14*(2), 170-177.

Rosen, C. A., Lombard, L. E., & Murry, T. (2000). Acoustic, aerodynamic, and videostroboscopic features of bilateral vocal fold lesions. *Annals of Otology, Rhinology, and Laryngology, 109*(9), 823-828.

Schutte, H. K. (1992). Integrated aerodynamic measurements. *Journal of Voice, 6*(2), 127-134.

Smitheran, J. R., & Hixon, T. J. (1981). A clinical method for estimating laryngeal airway resistance during vowel production. *Journal of Speech and Hearing Disorders, 46*(2), 138-146.

Tanaka, S., & Gould, W. J. (1985). Vocal efficiency and aerodynamic aspects in voice disorders. *Annals of Otology, Rhinology and Laryngology, 94*, 29-33.

Yiu, E. M.-L., Yuen, Y.-M., Whitehill, T., & Winkworth, A. (2004). Reliability and applicability of aerodynamic measures in dysphonia assessment. *Clinical Linguistics and Phonetics, 18*(6-8), 463-478.

CHAPTER 4

Assessment of Laryngeal Airway Resistance and Phonation Threshold Pressure: Glottal Enterprises

NANCY PEARL SOLOMON[1]

PURPOSES

- To assess vocal function by determining:
  - airflow through the larynx during phonation.
  - an estimate of air pressure delivered from the lungs to the larynx for phonation.
- To calculate the resistance provided by the laryngeal airway during phonation.
- To determine the minimum subglottal pressure needed to phonate.

INTRODUCTION

Aerodynamic analysis of speech and voice has been a mainstay of speech laboratories for decades. Early studies of aerodynamic properties of speech addressed the dysar-thria of cerebral palsy (Hardy, 1961, 1967), the velopharyngeal function of children with cleft palate (Dickson, Barron, & Mc-Glone, 1978; Honjow, Isshiki, & Morimoto, 1968; Warren, 1975; Warren & Dubois, 1964), the aerodynamic characteristics of skilled singing (Large & Iwata, 1971;

---

[1]Disclaimer: This chapter expresses the views of the author which do not necessarily reflect the official policy of the Department of the Army, Department of Defense, or U.S. Government.

Large, Iwata, & von Leden, 1970), as well as aerodynamic aspects of normal speech (Koike, Hirano, & von Leden, 1967).

The properties of air as it flows from the lungs through the larynx and upper airways provide a glimpse into the physical and physiologic production of speech. In the classic movie, *My Fair Lady* (1964), Professor Higgins (Rex Harrison) instructed Eliza Doolittle (Audrey Hepburn) to pronounce "h" at the beginning of words that were dialectically cropped, by using her breath to fan the flame of a candle with each production (see movie clip at http://www.glottal.com). This illustration of speech aerodynamics brought the importance of speech-related airflow to the consciousness of consumers of popular entertainment.

One of the most influential scientists for the understanding of airflow for speech and voice is Martin Rothenberg, Ph.D., Professor Emeritus of electrical engineering at Syracuse University (Syracuse, NY, USA). He developed an instrument to study speech aerodynamics. Dr. Rothenberg described airflow during stop-plosive consonant productions in his 1968 monograph, during the glottal fricative /h/ in the proceedings of an international congress in 1971 (published 1972), and during phonation using inverse filtering starting in 1973. These original principles and methods were incorporated into the commercial products marketed as Glottal Enterprises system, and have influenced the study of speech and voice production to this day.

Based on principles of aerodynamics, including biomechanical properties of airflow and air pressure, researchers have developed clinical procedures for assessing laryngeal function. The most widely used of these in current research and clinical practice are the noninvasive assessment of laryngeal airway resistance (R_{law}) and phonation threshold pressure (PTP). The original and most complete account of the theoretical basis and methodological details for the clinical determination of R_{law} was provided by Smitheran and Hixon (1981). PTP as an indicator of phonatory function was developed and described by Titze (1988). Many studies have been conducted that refine and elaborate upon these measures, some by the original authors (Lucero, Van Hirtum, Ruty, Cisonni, & Pelorson, 2009; McHenry, Kuna, Minton, & Vanoye, 1996; Solomon, Ramanathan, & Makashay, 2007; Titze, 1992); their basic principles and procedural methods are remarkably intact.

It should be noted that other types of clinically relevant aerodynamic assessment also have been developed using the Glottal Enterprises system. These include the measurement of inverse-filtered airflow during sustained vowels and connected speech, determination of velopharyngeal valve functioning during nasal and non-nasal consonant production in connected speech, and measures of airflow through the lower and upper airways for connected speech purposes. These methods are not reviewed in this chapter, but are available elsewhere (cf. Baken & Orlikoff, 2000).

Laryngeal Airway Resistance (R_{law})

A simple resistance calculation can reveal the degree to which the vocal folds and surrounding tissues impede air from flowing from the lungs, through the laryngeal airway, and to the mouth. Aerodynamic resistance is calculated as air pressure divided by airflow. In the speech-production system, the air pressure of interest is the change in pressure across the larynx, or translaryngeal pressure. Comparably, airflow is that which passes through the larynx, or "translaryngeal airflow." The task Smitheran and Hixon (1981) described to determine these quantities was designed to be easy enough to be performed by children as well as by individuals with movement disorders. Data collection is straightforward, brief, and comfortable for the speaker.

Translaryngeal pressure is calculated as the difference between sublaryngeal (or tracheal) pressure and supralaryngeal (or pharyngeal) pressure. For most voices, pharyngeal pressure during phonation is often close to nil (i.e., atmospheric pressure), in which case it can be ignored. However, pharyngeal pressure should be monitored and can be estimated as pressure in the oral cavity during vowel production. Tracheal pressure can be estimated from the mouth rather than from the trachea under certain conditions, a finding that has allowed this assessment to become common in clinical practice as well as in research.

Oral pressure is equivalent to alveolar (lung) pressure and everywhere in between (trachea, pharynx) when the airway mimics a closed hollow tube. That is, the airway is unobstructed, closed at either end, and does not leak. It is important to note that no air can leak through the velopharynx or between the lips, or the pressure in the mouth will be an underestimate of lung pressure. Note also that the vocal folds must be separated and the tongue must not occlude or substantially constrict the oral airway to achieve oral-to-lung pressure equivalency. It is for these reasons that the voiceless bilabial stop-consonant /p/ is used to estimate tracheal pressure from the oral cavity.

Although a voiceless stop consonant is used for this purpose, one must remember that the measure of interest is R_{law} *during phonation*. Theoretically, it would be preferable to assess tracheal pressure directly, that is, by inserting a needle coupled with a pressure sensor into the trachea while the individual is phonating. Of course, this usually is impractical. Therefore, an estimation of tracheal pressure is obtained from the mouth during moments when phonation stops (i.e., during the voiceless portion of /pi/). Peak oral pressure during the closed (voiceless) phase of /pi/ provides a momentary "snapshot" of the tracheal pressure that is most present during phonation. This is sometimes referred to as a "shutter" technique where the lips act as the shutter. External shutters have been designed as well (Jiang, O'Mara, Conley, & Hanson, 1999). The validity of these techniques is based on the fact that pressure generation during speech generally is steady, consistent with the perception of relatively constant loudness. Pharyngeal pressure, estimated as oral pressure during vowel production, should be subtracted from the estimate of tracheal pressure to derive translaryngeal pressure.

Translaryngeal flow is easily determined as the air that leaves the mouth and nose during exhalation. This value is the same whether it is measured just above the vocal folds or just outside of the mouth and nose. Therefore, airflow can be measured with a pneumotachograph positioned near the face, coupled with a face mask that covers both the mouth and the nose, and placed such that there is an airtight seal with the skin. Average airflow is determined during vowel production. The choice of the specific vowel is not critical, but Smitheran and Hixon (1981) selected /i/. The most important reason is that /i/ is associated with a highly elevated velum, an important consideration for the likelihood of airtight velopharyngeal closure during the surrounding consonants. However, some researchers use the vowel /æ/ instead of /i/ because they wish to have greater separation between the acoustic fundamental frequency and the first formant (Milenkovic & Mo, 1988). This becomes important if the signal is to be used for inverse filtering for the determination of glottal pulsing during phonation. The vowel /a/ has also been suggested, but is problematic in that it encourages greater jaw excursion, which can affect the seal between the mask to the face.

Phonation Threshold Pressure (PTP)

An additional assessment of subglottal pressure is commonly conducted while the speaker phonates as quietly as possible without whispering. This is termed *phonation threshold pressure* (PTP; Titze, 1988, 1992). This measure has proven sensitive to changes in the voice as a result of inherent and superficial hydration (Roy, Tanner, Gray, Blomgren, & Fisher, 2003; Sivasankar & Fisher, 2002; Verdolini et al., 1994), vocal loading (Chang & Karnell, 2004; Milbrath & Solomon, 2003; Solomon & DiMattia, 2000; Solomon, Glaze, Arnold, & van Mersbergen, 2003), and diseases, including Parkinson's disease (Jiang et al., 1999), end-stage renal disease (Fisher et al., 2001), and mass lesions of the vocal folds (Verdolini et al., 1994).

PTP is the smallest amount of air pressure needed to just barely vocalize. Titze (1988) hypothesized that PTP is determined by static, vibratory, and viscous properties of the vocal folds. Static

properties include glottal half-width, or half the distance between the vocal processes of the arytenoid cartilages just before vocalization begins, and vocal-fold cross-sectional thickness. Representing the vibratory component is a variable for mucosal wave velocity. Finally, a damping coefficient represents the viscous properties of the tissue. PTP seems to be particularly sensitive to vocal function at high pitches, as it increases as the vocal folds are stretched and thinned, making them stiffer (Solomon, Ramanathan, & Makashay, 2007; Titze, 1992). PTP also reflects phonatory ease, and has been shown to correlate to some degree to self-perceived phonatory effort (Chang & Karnell, 2004; Solomon et al., 2003).

Determining PTP relies on the same principles described above for estimating tracheal pressure. That is, pressure is sensed in the mouth while the lips act as a shutter to close the airway during the voiceless stop consonant /p/. The speaking task is slow, legato (connected) repetitions of /pi/, produced just barely above a whisper. Confirming the stoppage of airflow during the closed phase of /p/ is especially important for this task, because velopharyngeal and interlabial leakage is not unusual during very quiet speaking tasks. Therefore, although airflow is not a required variable for measuring PTP, it is essential as a monitoring device to ensure that the pressure values are valid. Airflow, recorded at relatively high sampling rate, is also useful to confirm that phonation is steady (witnessed as oscillating airflow). It is easy to detect whispering from the airflow signal. A new method, relying on thin tubing inserted through the lips, has been introduced in the literature to assess subglottal pressure from the mouth during sustained phonation rather than during a shutter technique; this method is described as using a "semi-occluded vocal tract" (Titze, 2009). It is promising as a simpler and more straightforward measurement procedure for PTP, but requires additional validation and refinement before it is ready for clinical application.

EQUIPMENT AND MATERIALS

Glottal Enterprises MS-110 system with calibrator. The latest models of the primary components are illustrated in Figures 4–1 and 4–2. The primary components are:

- A circumferentially vented (CV) face mask with two holes within which the nipples of the two pressure transducers are inserted. An advantage of the CV face mask over standard face masks is that it does not distort or attenuate sound appreciably (Rothenberg, 1973; http://www.glottal.com/products/soundsamples.htm). Furthermore, the presence of the mask does not change speech-breathing patterns (Huber, Stathopoulos, Bormann, & Johnson, 1998).

- A handle with a rubber or plastic cork that is inserted into the open end of the face mask;

- Two pressure transducers:
  - Low-frequency response (PTL-1 transducer, 30 Hz low-pass filter) for pressure signal. A short length of tubing (inside diameter = 3 mm) is attached to the nipple of the transducer, passed through the lips, and the open end, placed in the mouth; take care not to occlude the tubing with the tongue.
  - High-frequency response (PT-2E pressure transducer, 3-kHz low-pass filter (previous model PTW-1) for flow signal (allows for detection of individual glottal pulses).

- Transducer and Analog Data Computer Interface (Model MS-110; previous model MS-100). This is the electronic system that inputs and outputs the data

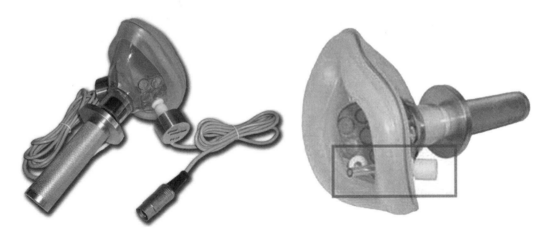

Figure 4–1. *Left:* Circumferentially vented pneumotachographic face mask, transducers, and handle by Glottal Enterprises. *Right:* mask with tubing for sensing oral pressure (box drawn around adapter plug and tubing). (Reprinted with permission from http://www.glottal.com)

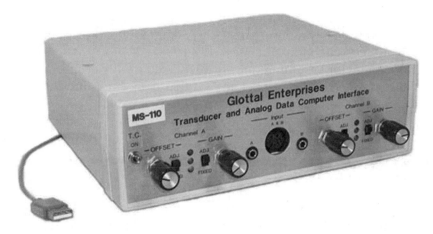

Figure 4–2. Glottal Enterprises Transducer and Analog Data Computer Interface (MS-110). (Reprinted with permission from http://www.glottal.com)

signals. A splitter cable receives signals from both transducers and is plugged into the "Input" jack in the center of the unit.

In addition, the user needs:

- Computerized external data recording and viewing system. Glottal Enterprises markets its own software to accompany the system (Aeroview). The author uses DATAQ hardware (DI-205 and DI-720) and WINDAQ/PRO software (Akron, OH) for this purpose. The DATAQ company offers low-cost multichannel A-to-D converters and free browser software, which can be accessed from its Web site (http://www.windaq.com). Figure 4-3 illustrates airflow and air pressure signals recorded and displayed with Aeroview. Figure 4-4 illustrates signals displayed with WINDAQ.
- Calibration unit (MCU-4). This microprocessor-driven 2-L bellows calibrator was designed for this system. Figure 4-5

illustrates the MCU-4 set up for flow calibration. Figure 4-6 shows the setup for pressure calibration.

TEST PROCEDURES

Calibration

Calibration is needed so that the signal generated by the MC-110 is compared to known values (e.g., flow signal is set to 0.5 L/s or 1.0 L/s; pressure signal is set to 5 cm H_2O or 10 cm H_2O). Once the known value of is selected, other values can be tested for comparison purposes. The equipment should be calibrated at least once per day because aerodynamic signals can be affected by temperature, humidity, and barometric pressure.

1. Turn on the equipment at least 10 minutes before collecting data to stabilize the electronics.

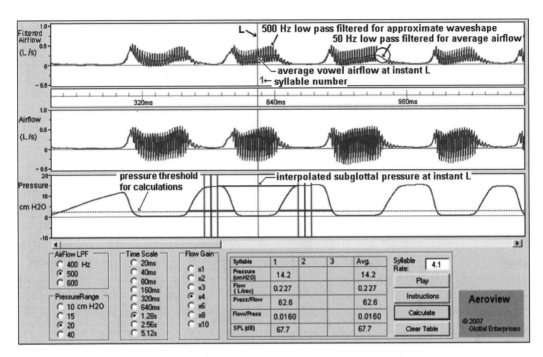

Figure 4–3. Screenshot of Aeroview software illustrating airflow and air pressure waveforms for a series of /pæ/ syllable repetitions at 4.1 syllables/second. *Top window:* linearly low-pass filtered airflow at 50 Hz (*black line*) to illustrate a smoothed, average airflow signal, and at 500 Hz (*gray line overlaid*) to illustrate the presence of vocal fold oscillation (vibration). *Middle window:* Raw airflow signal. *Bottom window:* Oral pressure signal. Tracheal (subglottal) pressure is taken as the interpolation of two adjacent pressure peaks, as noted. The line, L, is automatically inserted by the software to note the midpoint between the pressure peaks. The horizontal line ("pressure threshold for calculations") is set as a fixed value for the software algorithm to detect the presence of a consonant-related increase in pressure. (Figure provided by M. Rothenberg, Glottal Enterprises, May 21, 2010)

   a. Set offset to zero. This is verified by observing the output display and turning the **offset** knob on the MS-110 until the baseline signals are shown at 0 V (0 flow should generate 0 V, atmospheric pressure should generate 0 V). Verify after the equipment is warmed up.
2. Calibrate airflow (see Figure 4-5 for setup)

   a. Remove the cork from the airflow outlet at the top of the calibrator. THIS IS IMPORTANT! If the flow calibration is run with the cork inserted, it could damage the bellows.
   b. Plug the hole in the mask where the pressure transducer for pressure usually goes with a small cork.
   c. Using the handle, firmly press the mask over the top of the

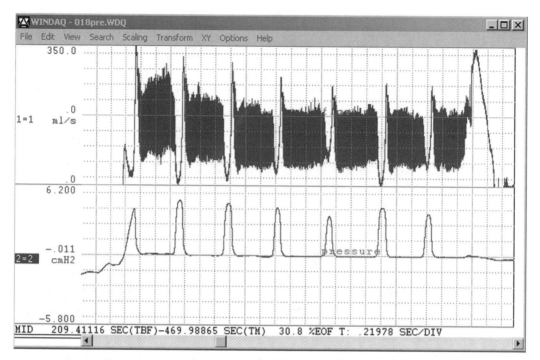

Figure 4–4. Airflow (channel 1) and air pressure (channel 2) signals collected during assessment of R_{law} at typical pitch and loudness displayed with WINDAQ software. Note that the flow signal does not reach baseline at the beginning of the 4th, 5th, and 7th syllables, and that there is a reduction in the corresponding pressure peaks associated with these "air leaks." This illustrates the underestimation of subglottal pressure from oral pressure when the velopharynx or lips do not completely stop airflow during the closed phase of /p/.

airflow opening using the facemask mold provided. DO NOT HOLD THE MASK ITSELF because this may occlude the screens.

d. Set the calibrator on **flow** and select 0.5 L/s. Press **apply** while recording the output. The clinician may wish to complete this procedure with the 1 L/s setting if one expects high airflow values for the client.

3. Calibrate air pressure (see Figure 4-6 for setup)

a. Plug the airflow outlet at the top of the MCU-4 calibration system

with the black rubber cork provided or another tight-fitting cork.

b. Plug the pressure transducer being used for the pressure signal (PTL-1) into the pressure port on the front face of the MCU-4.

c. Select **pressure**.

d. Use the toggle switch to set pressure exactly on the "0" line. Press the **apply** button and record result on computerized data collection system.

e. Set pressure on several more values and press **apply** each time. For assessing PTP, 3 cm

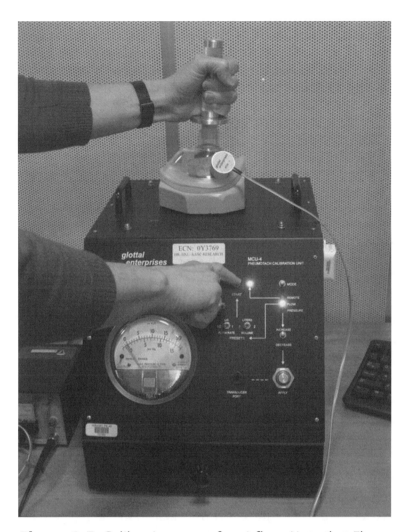

Figure 4–5. Calibration setup for airflow. Note that Flow is selected (*lit buttons*), the flow toggle switch is set to 0.5 L/s for 1 liter, and the mask is firmly held atop the face mold which covers the opening of the bellows. The flow transducer is inserted into the face mask; the opening in the mask for the other pressure transducer (not visible here) is plugged tightly. The examiner presses the "Start" toggle switch when ready.

H_2O and 5 cm H_2O are recommended values. For assessing R_{law} at normal loudness, values 7 cm H_2O and 10 cm H_2O are recommended.

4. Set baselines and calibration levels.

a. After recording and saving calibration signals, open the file with the WINDAQ playback software. Place the cursor on the portion of the data that represents "0" (zero) flow and pressure

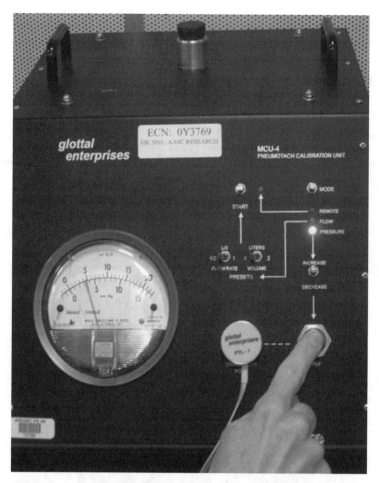

Figure 4–6. Calibration setup for air pressure. Pressure is selected ("red light"), a cork is placed in the top of the bellows, the pressure transducer is inserted into the pressure port, and the pressure gauge is set at 5 cm H_2O (distorted slightly by camera angle). The examiner presses the "apply" button to deliver the prescribed pressure to the transducer. Pressure calibration should also be conducted at 0 cm H_2O to set the baseline level.

and set the baselines ("low calibration" from the **Edit** menu) to match.

b. Position the cursor on the data at the various values, and set a "high calibration," usually using the 5 cm H_2O signal for pressure and the 0.5 L/s signal for flow. Check the other calibration levels just for consistency.

c. At the end of the session, the baselines should be the same. If they shifted, it will be necessary to determine when that happened during the session by examining the data file and adjusting the offset accordingly.

Preparing the Client for Data Collection: Precautions

1. The face mask does not fit every face. The most troublesome part is the bridge of the nose. For wide, flat noses, the clinician may need to pad the gap at the top of the mask. To do this, the clinician can cut a piece of dense foam rubber and use double-sided tape to stick it in place.

2. Some clients' faces are rather short in the vertical dimension, usually related to a small chin. For these clients, a small (pediatric) mask is recommended. This works well, but it is a bit crowded if nose clips are also needed (see below).

3. Be careful not to place the hand on or too close to the mask because it can block the screens. Use the handle!

4. Some clients may prefer to hold the mask in place him- or herself. This is acceptable, but avoid it when possible, because the client will need to use neck muscles to stabilize the head against the backward pressure of the mask, which could contribute to vocal strain. The correct position of the examiner stabilizing the client's head and pressing the mask on the client's face is shown in Figure 4–7.

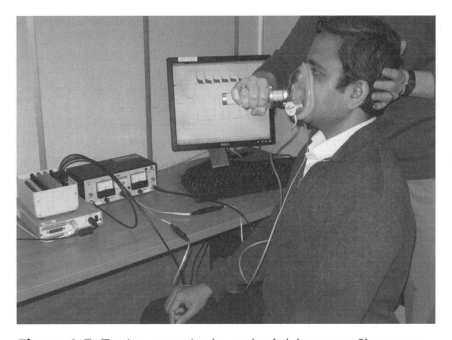

Figure 4–7. Testing setup in the author's laboratory. Shown are the Glottal Enterprises MS-100 connected by cables with BNC connectors from Channels A (flow) and B (pressure) to Channels 1 and 2 of the DATAQ DI-205 via double-banana plugs. The box under the DI-205 is the DI-720 which serves as a USB adapter. The examiner stabilizes the client's head with one hand while applying counter pressure with the other hand by holding the handle and firmly applying the face mask so that it seals around the mouth and nose. The tube placed in the mouth for pressure assessment is inside the mask and is not visible here.

Instructions to the Client

1. "I am going to push this mask on your face firmly. I don't want you to strain, so I am going to brace your head with my other hand behind you. Let me know if it's uncomfortable."

2. Determine pitch and loudness requirements, and cue these parameters appropriately. For conversational pitch, ask the client to count to 5 or 10 and then, when repeating the sequence, to hold out the /i/ in "three" or the /a/ in "five." This should provide a pitch that is typical of the client's speech. For R_{law}, loudness should be "typical" or "comfortable." For PTP, loudness should be "as quiet as possible; just barely above a whisper."

3. "Say /pi:pi:pi:pi:pi:pi:pi:/ at the rate of 1.5 syllables per second (demonstrate or play metronome at 1.5 syllables per second, while connecting the syllables in legato fashion). When you say /pi/, your lips should touch the tube." R_{law} can vary with lung volume (Solomon, Garlitz, & Milbrath, 2000), so make sure that the client does not take a deep breath before beginning this task; the instruction, "Take a medium-sized breath" may be used.

4. Usually, a demonstration is enough. If it's not, some of the additional instructions/procedures listed below can be used. When extra cues are used, it is imperative to take care that the client's productions sound natural.
   a. "Connect the vowels to the consonants, keeping it even/smooth/legato."
   b. "Make sure your lips close around the tube."
   c. "Think of the lips as a shutter on a camera—keep the vowel going and just use the lips to interrupt the vowel."
   d. "Watch the signal on the computer—make sure this line touches the bottom every time your lips come together (indicate the baseline for flow)."
   e. If flow still does not touch the baseline for the closed phase of /p/ (as in Figure 4–4), it will be necessary to use nose plugs. Cut the handles off of standard pulmonary nose plugs, place them across the nares, confirm that the client cannot breathe through the nose (ask him or her to try to sniff), and place the mask back onto the face. *Note:* before placing the nose clips, instruct the client to swallow. This will prevent the need to swallow after the clips are on, which could build uncomfortable pressure in the middle ear.

5. Collect at least 3 strings of 7 syllables each that meet measurement criteria. It is recommended that at least 5 to 7 strings are collected so that there are enough productions to choose from. Acceptable trials have the following features:
   a. Pressure peaks that are relatively even and are well shaped (single peak, reaches a peak after a quick rise followed by a slight rise or flat plateau)
   b. Pressure signal returns to zero or near zero throughout the vowel
   c. Flow signal that indicates phonation is relatively steady during the vowels
   d. Flow signal that returns to baseline during or just prior to the pressure peak

e. Voice that sounds natural and typical for the client

6. Repeat procedure at other desired pitches or loudness levels.

7. It may be desirable to record the speech signal along with the air pressure and airflow signals for auditory confirmation of the task.

DATA ANALYSIS

Data signals for pressure and flow should be viewed on the computer monitor. If calibration was not adjusted and saved during data collection, it should be done before starting data analysis. Quickly skim through the file to confirm that the baselines stayed constant and that they are set at zero.

Examples of data analysis are provided with the case studies. Figure 4–8 shows a trial collected for R_{law} analysis (comfortable loudness) and Figure 4–9 shows a PTP trial (quietest phonation). Examine the first set of syllables. The 3rd, 4th, 5th, and 6th pressure peaks from the /p/ closure are selected and marked if they are of a relatively consistent height (within ~1 cm H_2O) and well shaped, as defined above. In addition, the flow signal that coincides with, or occurs just prior to, each pressure peak should be at or very close to baseline (zero). This confirms that no air was leaking through the lips or nose during the closed phase of /p/ (see Figure 4-4, which shows the consequences of air leaks). Record these peak pressure values.

For R_{law}, determine average flow for a midportion of the vowel segments that occur between the selected pressure peaks. In WINDAQ, this involves highlighting a central segment of the airflow signal during vowel phonation, and setting time markers around it. The "Statistics" function of WINDAQ provides statistical results for the signal. For this purpose, select the average (mean) and record it in L/s (will most likely require a conversion from mL/s). Similarly, determine the average pressure during this same vowel segment to be used as the estimate of pharyngeal pressure (in cm H_2O).

Each syllable now has two pressure peak values (these are generated during the closed phase of /p/ which surround the vowel) and the average flow and pressure values for the intervening vowel. Average the peak pressure values, subtract the average pharyngeal pressure, and then divide this result by average flow. Repeat this procedure for at least 2 more trials, so that a total of approximately 9 syllables are analyzed. Markers were inserted manually for the pressure peaks selected for data analysis shown in Figures 4-8 and 4-9.

For PTP, only the pressure peaks are needed; the flow signals are used only to monitor the presence of phonation during the vowels and the absence of airflow during the closed phase of /p/. Select three or four pressure peaks from each syllable string and average them. Because the goal of determining PTP is to assess the smallest pressure possible to phonate, take care to select the lowest pressure peaks that meet measurement criteria. Average approximately nine of these pressure peaks to determine PTP.

Results Interpretation

R_{law} reflects the amount of constriction that the larynx applies to air that is traveling through it. During phonation, this

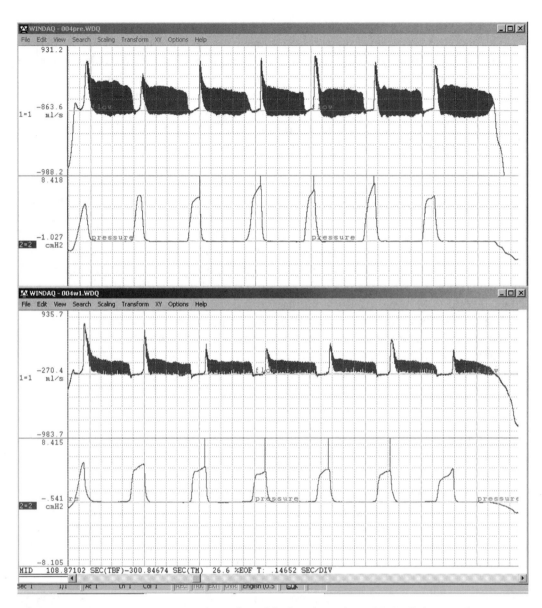

Figure 4–8. R_{law} assessment (comfortable loudness) at 30% of the pitch range before (*top*) and after (*bottom*) recurrent laryngeal nerve resection during thyroid surgery. Note lower pressure peaks and average flows during phonation after thyroidectomy. The pressure peaks are marked for analysis. Pressure during the vowels is at the baseline level (atmospheric pressure), so no correction for pharyngeal pressure is needed for these productions.

resistance is optimal when the amount of effort required to phonate is minimized and when voice is produced efficiently. Typically, R_{law} for voice produced by normally phonating adults at comfortable pitch and loudness levels approximates 30 to 45 cm H_2O/L/s for men and 35 to 55 cm H_2O/L/s for women; expected

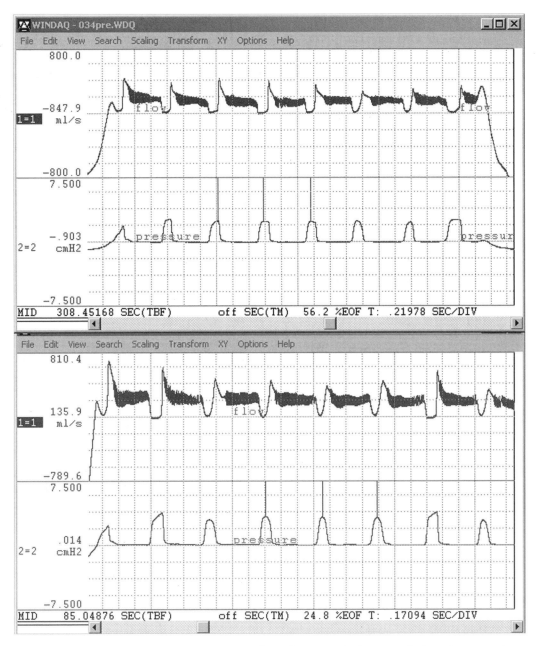

Figure 4–9. PTP assessment at 30% of pitch range before and after laryngeal and sublaryngeal edema resulting from thyroid surgery. Note higher pressure peaks after thyroidectomy. Also, the pressure peaks before the 4th, 5th, and 6th vowels were selected rather than the typical 3rd, 4th, and 5th syllables because the patient had some difficulty initiating voicing (seen as a delay between the peak flow and onset of voicing) for the 3rd syllable.

values are approximately 5 to 7 cm H_2O for lung pressure and 0.15 L/s for airflow (Hoit & Hixon, 1992; Melcon, Hoit, & Hixon, 1989; Smitheran & Hixon, 1981; Stathopoulos, Hoit, Hixon, Watson, & Solomon, 1991).

- When R_{law} is lower than normal, this implies that constriction, or "valving," of the air by the larynx is insufficient or inadequate. The voice may sound breathy, and airflow is not efficiently used by the vocal folds to generate sound pressure. If low air pressure is the primary contributor to low R_{law}, then expiratory muscle weakness may be implicated. It also is plausible that incomplete laryngeal closure may prevent pressure from building adequately below the vocal folds. Higher than normal airflow may also contribute to a finding of low R_{law}. In this case, it is most likely that the vocal folds are not valving the air adequately, although strong expiratory muscle force could also lead to this situation.

- When R_{law} is higher than normal, the most likely interpretations are that the larynx is adducting too firmly and/or the vocal folds are too stiff. Increased adduction will lead to low airflow through the larynx. Additionally, the expiratory muscles may be generating greater than necessary air pressure. The voice may sound too loud, and pressed or strained, and the client may perceive greater than normal effort to phonate.

PTP reflects the ease with which the vocal folds can vibrate once they are in the proper position for phonation (slightly separated vocal folds; Lucero, 1998). PTP is low when the vocal fold mucosa is healthy and well lubricated. Extra mass on the vocal folds or dry tissues will elevate PTP, because greater lung pressure is needed to effectively cause the vocal folds to oscillate. Normative data for PTP are not readily available in the literature. Table 4–1 summarizes PTP data of vocally normal young adults from baseline sessions (no experimental manipulations) derived from three studies by this author (Solomon & DiMattia, 2000; Solomon et al., 2003; Solomon et al., 2007). PTP values generally are lowest in the lower half of the pitch range (determined in semitones, ST). The amount of increase in PTP as pitch increases varies across persons, as exhibited by the much larger SDs at 80% of the pitch range (Solomon et al., 2007).

CASE STUDIES

As part of a large study examining voice outcomes before and after surgery to remove the thyroid gland, aerodynamic measures are collected before and 2 weeks after surgery and again several months after surgery (Solomon, Helou, Makashay, & Stojadinovic, in press). Two cases are presented here to illustrate the correspondence between voice disorders and aerodynamic assessment.

Case 1. A 53-year-old woman sustained a unilateral recurrent laryngeal nerve resection during the removal of the thyroid gland. This iatrogenic injury resulted in unilateral vocal fold paralysis, consequent severe dysphonia, and nearly a 60% reduction in pitch range. Figure 4–8 illustrates her production of a string of /pi/ syllables produced at comfortable loudness and at 30% of her pitch range before and after surgery. Translaryngeal (tracheal–

Table 4–1. Phonation Threshold Pressure Values (Mean and SD, in cm H_2O)*

	Percentage of the Pitch Range			
Gender	*10%*	*30%*	*50%*	*80%*
Female				
Mean	3.6	3.5	4.3	7.3
SD	0.5	0.5	0.7	1.5
Male				
Mean	3.8	3.4	4.5	6.9
SD	0.8	0.3	0.8	2.3

*Data from 9 females and 7 males (exception: 3 males for 30% of pitch range) with normal voices at approximately (±5%) 10%, 30%, 50%, and 80% of their pitch ranges. Data at 30% of the pitch range include values from 4 females who produced PTP at habitual conversational pitch.

(Source: Data derived from baseline conditions in Solomon and DiMattia, 2000; Solomon et al., 2003; Solomon et al., 2007).

pharyngeal) pressure estimates decreased from 6.4 cm H_2O to 4.7 cm H_2O, and airflow during phonation increased from 134 mL/s to 724 mL/s; consequently, R_{law} decreased from 47.7 cm H_2O/L/s to 33.8 cm H_2O/L/s. The decrease in R_{law} indicates that the laryngeal valve was working less effectively than before the nerve injury.

Case 2. Laryngeal examination (videostroboscopy) after a total thyroidectomy in a 69-year-old woman revealed marked postsurgical laryngeal and sublaryngeal edema. Her voice was rough and low-pitched. Pitch range decreased 40%. Figure 4–9 illustrates PTP assessment (repetitions of /pi/ as quietly as possible) at 30% of her pitch range. Peak pressures during this task increased from 2.8 cm H_2O to 3.4 cm H_2O. This indicates that slightly greater lung pressure was required to move the edematous vocal folds into vibration.

Additional Observations from the Case Studies

1. Pre- and postoperative values presented for both cases were all within normal limits. Difficulties were revealed only by comparing each patient's performance to his or her own over time.

2. Changes in pitch range because of laryngeal pathology can impact results. In both cases, pitch range was significantly reduced after thyroidectomy, so that the pitches used before and after surgery were not the same. In the first case, a high pitch tested (80% of pitch range) was not even within her postoperative pitch range. In these cases, it is better to rely on the low, or comfortable, pitch, because aerodynamic measures are relatively stable within the lower half of the pitch range.

REFERENCES

Baken, R. J., & Orlikoff, R. J. (2000). *Clinical measurement of speech and voice* (2nd ed.). San Diego, CA: Singular.

Chang, A., & Karnell, M. P. (2004). Perceived phonatory effort and phonation threshold pressure across a prolonged voice loading task: A study of vocal fatigue. *Journal of Voice, 18*, 454–466.

Dickson, S., Barron, S., & McGlone, R. E. (1978). Aerodynamic studies of cleft-palate speech. *Journal of Speech and Hearing Disorders, 43*(2), 160–167.

Fisher, K. V., Ligon, J., Sobecks, J. L., & Roxe, D. M. (2001). Phonatory effects of body fluid removal. *Journal of Speech, Language, and Hearing Research, 44*, 354–367.

Hardy, J. C. (1961). Intraoral breath pressure in cerebral palsy. *Journal of Speech and Hearing Disorders, 26*, 309–319.

Hardy, J. C. (1967). Suggestions for physiological research in dysarthria. *Cortex, 3*, 128–156.

Hoit, J. D., & Hixon, T. J. (1992). Age and laryngeal airway resistance during vowel production in women. *Journal of Speech and Hearing Research, 35*, 309–313.

Honjow, I., Isshiki, N., & Morimoto, M. (1968). Aerodynamic pattern of cleft palate speech. *Plastic and Reconstructive Surgery, 42*, 465–471.

Huber, J. E., Stathopoulos, E. T., Bormann, L. A., & Johnson, K. (1998). Effects of a circumferentially vented mask on breathing patterns of women as measured by respiratory kinematic techniques. *Journal of Speech, Language, and Hearing Research, 41*, 472–478.

Jiang, J., O'Mara, T., Chen, H. J., Stern, J. I., Vlagos, D., & Hanson, D. (1999). Aerodynamic measurements of patients with Parkinson's disease. *Journal of Voice, 13*, 583–591.

Jiang, J., O'Mara, T., Conley, D., & Hanson, D. (1999). Phonation threshold pressure measurements during phonation by airflow interruption. *Laryngoscope, 109*, 425–432.

Koike, Y., Hirano, M., & von Leden, H. (1967). Vocal initiation: Acoustic and aerodynamic investigations of normal subjects. *Folia Phoniatrica (Basel), 19*(3), 173–182.

Large, J., & Iwata, S. (1971). Aerodynamic study of vibrato and voluntary 'straight tone' pairs in singing. *Journal of the Acoustical Society of America, 49*(1A), 137.

Large, J., Iwata, S., & von Leden, H. (1970). The primary female register transition in singing: Aerodynamic study. *Folia Phoniatrica (Basel), 22*(6), 385–396.

Lucero, J. C. (1998). Optimal glottal configuration for ease of phonation. *Journal of Voice, 12*, 151–158.

Lucero, J. C., Van Hirtum, A., Ruty, N., Cisonni, J., & Pelorson, X. (2009). Validation of theoretical models of phonation threshold pressure with data from a vocal fold mechanical replica. *Journal of the Acoustical Society of America, 125*(2), 632–635.

McHenry, M. A., Kuna, S. T., Minton, J. T., & Vanoye, C. R. (1996). Comparison of direct and indirect calculations of laryngeal airway resistance in connected speech. *Journal of Voice, 10*(3), 236–244.

Melcon, M. C., Hoit, J. D., & Hixon, T. J. (1989). Age and laryngeal airway resistance during vowel production. *Journal of Speech and Hearing Disorders, 54*, 282–286.

Milbrath, R. L., & Solomon, N. P. (2003). Do vocal warm-up exercises alleviate vocal fatigue? *Journal of Speech, Language, and Hearing Research, 46*, 422–436.

Milenkovic, P., & Mo, F. (1988). Effect of the vocal tract yielding sidewall on inverse filter analysis of the glottal waveform. *Journal of Voice, 2*, 271–278.

Rothenberg, M. (1968). The breath-stream dynamics of simple-released plosive production. *Bibliotheca Phonetica, No. 6*, New York, NY: S. Karger.

Rothenberg, M. (1972). The glottal volume velocity waveform during loose and tight voiced glottal adjustments. *Proceedings of the Seventh International Congress of Phonetic Sciences* (pp. 380–388). Paris, France: Mouton.

Rothenberg, M. (1973). A new inverse-filtering technique for deriving the glottal air flow waveform during voicing. *Journal of the Acoustical Society of America, 53,* 1632-1645.

Roy, N., Tanner, K., Gray, S. D., Blomgren, M., & Fisher, K. V. (2003). An evaluation of the effects of three laryngeal lubricants on phonation threshold pressure (PTP). *Journal of Voice, 17,* 331-342.

Sivasankar, M., & Fisher, K. V. (2002). Oral breathing increases Pth and vocal effort by superficial drying of vocal fold mucosa. *Journal of Voice, 16,* 172-181.

Smitheran, J. R., & Hixon, T. J. (1981). A clinical method for estimating laryngeal airway resistance during vowel production. *Journal of Speech and Hearing Disorders, 46,* 138-146.

Solomon, N. P., & DiMattia, M. S. (2000). Effects of a vocally fatiguing task and systemic hydration on phonation threshold pressure. *Journal of Voice, 14,* 341-362.

Solomon, N. P., Garlitz, S. J., & Milbrath, R. L. (2000). Respiratory and laryngeal contributions to maximum phonation duration. *Journal of Voice, 14,* 331-340.

Solomon, N. P., Glaze, L. E., Arnold, R. R., & van Mersbergen, M. (2003). Effects of a vocally fatiguing task and systemic hydration on men's voices. *Journal of Voice, 17,* 31-46.

Solomon, N. P., Helou, L. B., Makashay, M. J., & Stojadinovic, A. (in press). Aerodynamic evaluation of the post-thyroidectomy voice. *Journal of Voice.*

Solomon, N. P., Ramanathan, P., & Makashay, M. J. (2007). Phonation threshold pressure across the pitch range: Preliminary test of a model. *Journal of Voice, 21,* 541-550.

Stathopoulos, E. T., Hoit, J. D., Hixon, T. J., Watson, P. J., & Solomon, N. P. (1991). Respiratory and laryngeal function during whispering. *Journal of Speech and Hearing Research, 34,* 761-767.

Titze, I. R. (1988). The physics of small-amplitude oscillation of the vocal folds. *Journal of the Acoustical Society of America, 83,* 1536-1552.

Titze, I. R. (1992). Phonation threshold pressure: A missing link in glottal aerodynamics. *Journal of the Acoustical Society of America, 91,* 2926-2935.

Titze, I. R. (2009). Phonation threshold pressure measurement with a semi-occluded vocal tract. *Journal of Speech, Language, and Hearing Research, 52,* 1062-1072.

Verdolini, K., Titze, I. R., & Fennell, A. (1994). Dependence of phonatory effort on hydration level. *Journal of Speech and Hearing Research, 37,* 1001-1007.

Warren, D. W. (1975). The determination of velopharyngeal incompetence by aerodynamic and acoustical techniques. *Clinics in Plastic Surgery, 2,* 299-304.

Warren, D. W., & Dubois, A. B. (1964). A pressure-flow technique for measuring velopharyngeal orifice area during continuous speech. *Cleft Palate Journal, 16,* 52-71.

CHAPTER 5

Kinematic Respiratory Analysis: Respiratory Inductance Plethysmography

PETREA CORNWELL

PURPOSES

- To observe the behaviors of the respiratory system in terms of chest wall kinematics during both quiet and speech breathing.
- To assess net changes in lung volume during speech breathing, and identify the lung volumes at which speech is initiated and terminated relative to tidal volumes and vital capacity.
- To assess the timing of respiratory behaviors relative to voice production.
- To provide a visual representation of an individual's respiratory patterns during a range of speech production tasks.

THEORETICAL BACKGROUND

Normal speech production involves a complex interplay between the four components of the speech mechanism (respiration, phonation, resonance, and articulation), with respiration and phonation serving as foundation stones. Understanding the mechanics of speech breathing (respiration) is important in evaluating an individual's voice disorder presentation as vocal fold vibration for phonation is dependent on respiratory forces as the basic energy source. The mechanics of speech breathing can be examined in two ways. The first involves evaluating features related to the airstream used for speech including pressure, flow, and volume expenditure (covered in Chapters 2, 3, and 4), whereas the second (the focus of this chapter) entails measurement of chest wall movements or kinematics. Kinematic assessment of breathing involves taking measurements that provide estimates of changes in chest wall size (where the chest wall is a two-part system: rib cage and diaphragm-abdomen) via measurement of one of three variables: (1) circumference, (2) anteroposterior diameter, and (3) cross-sectional area (Hixon & Hoit, 2005). There are three types of devices that respectively measure each of these variables and that are reflective of changes in body surface area: (1) bellows pneumographs, (2) respiratory magnetometers, and (3) respiratory inductance plethysmography. Although each device measures a different aspect of chest wall function, they all are based around the same theoretical concept, which is that movement in each of the chest wall components individually displaces a volume and their collective movement displaces a volume equal to that of the lungs due to the close anatomic and physiological relationship between the chest wall and lungs (Baken & Orlikoff, 2000). Specifically, the lungs are anatomically encased by the rib cage and diaphragm, while physiologically external forces that arise from movements of the diaphragm, rib cage wall, and abdominal wall change the shape and therefore volume of the lungs (Hixon & Hoit, 2005). Consequently, kinematic devices can be used to mathematically summate net changes in lung volume from changes in the rib cage and abdomen displacement (Mazeika & Swanson, 2007), as well as to determine the relative contributions of each component of the chest wall to

these net volume changes. A range of other observations also can be extrapolated from the data including respiratory rate, syllables produced per breath, relative timing of the inspiratory-expiratory cycle, and lung volumes at which speech is initiated and terminated relative to tidal volumes and vital capacity.

The configuration of the chest wall changes as we breathe either for physiologic need or speech production. The normal pattern of movement in the two-part chest wall has been documented in healthy speakers. During inspiration, the rib cage expands with active muscular contraction allowing for lung inflation, while in unison the diaphragm contracts resulting in increased volume displacement of the abdomen (Hixon & Hoit, 2005). Innate elasticity and recoil of thoracic structures on cessation of inspiration decreases rib cage size and expiration results. Simultaneously, diaphragm relaxation reduces the size of the abdomen. Further reduction in the cross-sectional area of the abdomen can occur with active contraction of the abdominal musculature to increase expiratory drive if required (Baken & Orlikoff, 2000). For speech production, the expiratory airstream utilized for phonation is sufficient to activate vocal fold vibration. Increased vocal loudness, however, is an example where the air pressure required may exceed that created by passive forces resulting in the recruitment of the abdominal musculature to increase the expiratory drive (Boone & McFarlane, 2000).

The relative timing of chest wall movements occurs in keeping with the requirements of the inspiratory-expiratory cycles for quiet breathing to meet physiologic life needs which differs for speech breathing (Figure 5–1). Quiet breathing involves the volume of air inspired and expired during each respiratory cycle with approximately equal time attributed

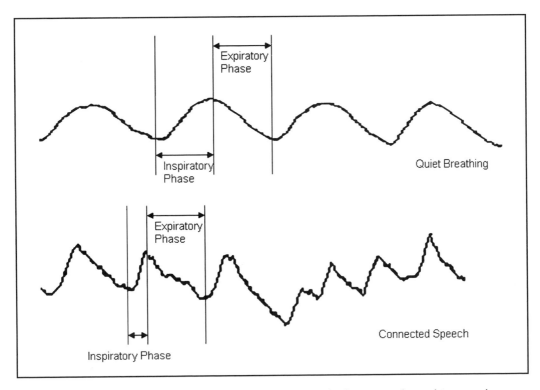

Figure 5–1. Timing of inspiratory-expiratory cycle for quiet breathing and speech breathing during connected speech.

to each phase. In contrast, the respiratory cycles associated with speech often involve a shortened inspiratory period followed by a sustained expiration upon which phonation and speech production occur (McFarland, 2001). This change in the timing of respiratory patterns in normal speakers does not seem to interfere with obtaining adequate lung volumes for speech production but instead requires adjustments to be made to the neuromuscular control of the respiratory mechanism (e.g., using greater muscular effort during inspiration, and controlled release of expiratory airflow including laryngeal valving).

Movements of the chest wall, as discussed previously, correlate with changes in lung volumes. The lung volumes required for speech production have been found to fall well within a person's vital capacity (i.e., total amount of air that can be expired following a maximum inspiration), with speech often produced within the midrange of a person's vital capacity (Hixon & Putnam, 1983; Kalliakosta, Mandros, & Tzelepis, 2007). Specifically, the initiation of breath groups for connected speech (e.g., conversation) has been found to occur at lung volumes larger than tidal volume and finish around the level of resting tidal end-expiratory level (Hixon, 1982; Hixon & Hoit, 2005).

Kinematic assessment of speech breathing has been used to examine the respiratory behaviors evident in people with dysphonic voices, although less frequently used than other modes of assessment. The complex interplay between respiration and phonation must be remembered when assessing respiratory and laryngeal events in people with voice disorder as respiratory impairment may either be the cause, or the result of a voice disorder (Aronson, 1990). Vocal hyperfunction has been allied with atypical speech breathing for some time (Hixon & Putnam, 1983; Sapienza & Stathopoulos, 1994). Boone and McFarlane (2000) suggested that increased muscle tension during speech production can be the result of trying to speak on inadequate expiratory airflow. Contributing to this reduced expiratory flow could be an ineffective inspiratory phase leading to reduced lung volumes for speech, the improper use of expiratory air (e.g., initiation of speech after some volume of air has been expired), or chest wall paradoxical movements. Alternatively, disordered respiratory behaviors may arise as a compensatory strategy to optimize phonation in the presence of vocal pathology (Bahr, Biedess, & Ridley, 2007). Therefore, it is important to determine if observed respiratory behaviors are a symptom of dysphonia or a compensatory strategy (Sapienza, Stathopoulos, & Brown, 1997).

In individuals with a voice disorder, there may be:

■ Use of larger lung volume excursions in individuals with vocal nodules, with initiation of speech at higher lung volumes (Sapienza et al., 1997) and termination of utterances at lower lung volumes the primary facilitators (Sapienza & Stathopoulos, 1994; Sapienza et al., 1997). As vocal nodules can prevent complete vocal fold adduction, there can be breathiness and air wastage during phonation (Boone, McFarlane, & von Berg, 2005). The use of larger lung volumes in dysphonic speakers due to vocal nodules may suggest this is a compensatory strategy that develops to manage air wastage through incomplete vocal fold adduction (Sapienza

et al., 1997). Increased lung volume excursion expired in a controlled way may allow the speaker to maintain the required subglottal pressure and counteract higher than normal glottal airflow.

■ Use of lung volume excursions at a magnitude similar to those of normal speakers, but with speech production occurring at lower lung volumes within an individual's vital capacity and terminating below the resting expiratory level (Hixon & Putnam, 1983; Lowell, Barmeier-Kraemer, Hoit & Story, 2008; Schaeffer, Cavallo, Wall, & Diakow, 2002; Sperry, Hillman, & Perkell, 1994). Normal speakers have been found to produce speech between 40 and 60% of vital capacity. However, individuals with dysphonic voices may produce speech at lower levels (Hixon & Putnam, 1983; Schaeffer et al., 2002), for example, between 10 and 45% vital capacity lung volume. The use of lower lung volumes within an individual's vital capacity for speech production requires greater expiratory effort to maintain phonation throughout an utterance. This involves increased muscle tension at the laryngeal level to valve lower air pressures available for speech, particularly if initiated after a volume of air has been expired (Boone & McFarlane, 2000). This may result in vocal hyperfunction with dysphonia of phonotraumatic origins. Additionally, greater expiratory drive can be achieved through the recruitment of abdominal musculature, which could contribute to the fatigue levels often reported by individuals with dysphonia during extended periods of speaking (Sapienza et al., 1997).

■ Suboptimal use of the respiratory system to facilitate increased vocal loudness, with initiation and termination of breath groups at lower lung volumes (Lowell et al., 2008; Sperry et al., 1994). Increased vocal loudness can be achieved most effectively by increasing the air pressure supplied to the laryngeal mechanism by the respiratory system. Consequently, speakers without dysphonia tend to initiate loud speech at lung volumes 10 to 20% greater than when speaking at normal loudness, and finish breath groups at similar lung volumes (around the level of functional residual capacity). In contrast, speakers with dysphonia do not initiate loud speech at higher lung volumes than speech at normal loudness but rather use lung volumes well into the expiratory reserve volume to complete loud speaking tasks (Lowell et al., 2008; Sperry et al., 1994). The implications of producing speech well into the expiratory reserve volume is that airflow is being driven initially by passive forces (elastic recoil) and then needs to recruit active forces (expiratory muscular pressure from the abdominal muscles) to complete the breath group. Sperry and colleagues (1994) noted that the recruitment of abdominal musculature to achieve vocal loudness contributed to the observation of paradoxical abdominal movements during the expiratory phase coinciding with the onset of phonation. Additionally, the need to utilize expiratory muscular pressure to produce loud speech may contribute to higher levels of fatigue with prolonged speaking.

▪ Different patterns of rib cage and abdomen movement used to achieve net lung volume changes. It generally is held that the rib cage and abdomen work in synchrony during respiration to achieve the required net lung volume changes. In normal speakers, Hixon (1982) suggested that the mean

equal volume contribution of the abdomen and rib cage is similar and results in constant slopes on trace recordings on respiratory inductance plethysmography. However, as stated above, Sperry et al.'s (1994) case study of a speaker with vocal nodules identified paradoxical abdominal movements during the expiratory phase of speech that appeared to coincide with the onset of phonation. The role of abdominal musculature in increasing expiratory effort where speech encroaches on the expiratory residual volume may relate to this observation. In addition, greater abdominal contribution to speech breathing during expiratory phases than the rib cage has been found in individuals with adductor spasmodic dysphonia (Bahr et al., 2007) and Parkinson disease (Bunton, 2005).

▪ Other aspects of speech breathing behaviors (speaking rate, appropriateness of inspiratory boundaries, and frequency of inspirations) that can be assessed with respiratory inductance plethysmography. A few studies have shown that syllables per breath (Sperry et al., 1994) and syllables per second (Bahr et al., 2007) are reduced for individuals with voice disorders, and that inhalation occurs more frequently (Schaeffer et al., 2002; Sperry et al., 1994). In opposition to these findings, Sapienza et al. (1997) found that during reading, speakers with vocal nodules paused and inhaled at expected phrasal boundaries. Schaeffer and colleagues' (2002) study, however, highlights the importance of testing stimuli as their findings suggested that a reading task using 10-syllable sentences did not compromise speech breathing patterns, but those with longer sentences (60-syllable) resulted in the aforementioned changes to inspiratory and speaking rate. This highlights the importance both in research and clinical practice to choose assessment tasks representative of daily speech requirements.

DESCRIPTION

Several commercial systems are available for recording speech breathing kinematics using a respiratory inductance plethymography approach. These systems include the Inductotrace (formerly known as Respitrace) from Ambulatory Monitoring, Inc. (http://www.ambulatory-monitoring.com), the Respitrace Plus from Viasys

Healthcare (http://www.viasyshealthcare.com), and SummitIP from Compumedics (http://www.compumedics.com) that all have data acquisition software available to capture and analyze data, as well as others, which will connect with standard electroencephalography (EEG) or Polygraphy units (e.g., RIPmate™, Ambu Sleepmate; TRIPS Respiratory Inductive Plethysmography System, TEMEC; zRIP Inductive Respiratory Effort Sensors, Pro-Tech). This chapter uses the Inductotrace system to illustrate how to assess speech breathing, although the data acquisition program utilized for capturing and analysis is not the Inductoview software currently available from Ambulatory Monitoring Inc. Figure 5–2 provides

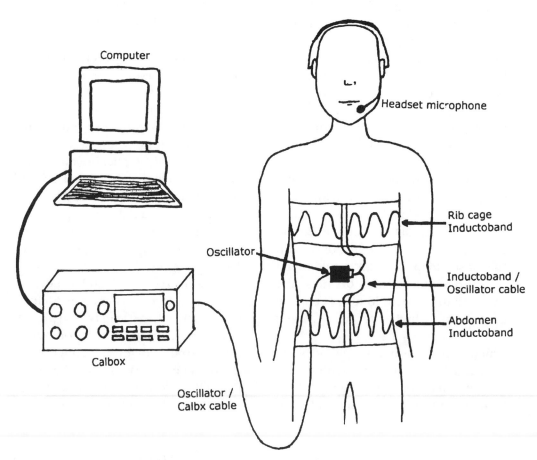

Figure 5–2. Schematic representation of the Inductotrace System.

a schematic representation of the equipment setup and Figure 5–3 is the main display of a MATLAB based acquisition program developed for research purposes (**Note:** This is not the commercially available Inductoview software).

EQUIPMENT AND MATERIALS

The Inductotrace system is composed of four basic components:

- Inductotrace calibrator/demodulator
- Transducer oscillator
- Transducers (include Inductobands, Retainers, and Cables)
- Recording and analysis software (Inductoview Software is available from Ambulatory Monitoring Inc., or lab specific software can be developed)

Other equipment and materials required:

- Accessories for calibration: spirobag or spirometer, and nasal clip (to prevent nasal escape of air during calibration procedure)
- Accessories for recording: head-set microphone (e.g., AKG C420), straight-backed chair (if using seated position for recordings), standard passage such as The Rainbow Passage (Fairbanks, 1960) or The Grandfather Passage (Darley, Aronson, & Brown, 1975)

TEST PROCEDURES

General Guidelines

- **Recording environment.** There are no specific requirements with regard

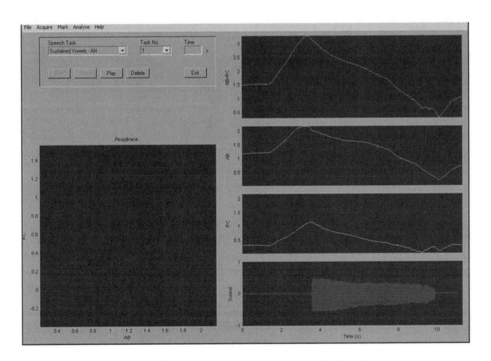

Figure 5–3. Main display of MATLAB program during Inductotrace data acquisition.

to the acoustic environment required for assessment using respiratory inductance plethysmography. If, however, voice recordings made as a component of this kinematic assessment are also to be analyzed for vocal quality, guidelines pertaining to recording environment for those perceptual or acoustic analyses should be followed (see Chapters 17, 18, and 19 by Ma; Madill and McCabe; and Vogel in this book for details).

- **Recording time-of-day.** There is no documented reason to suggest that time-of-day impacts on speech breathing behavior. However, deteriorating vocal function (e.g., reduced pitch range and flexibility, reduced vocal projection or power, reduced control of vocal quality) over the course of a day frequently has been reported in populations with vocal hyperfunction (Solomon, 2008). Consequently, given the close interplay between speech breathing and voice production, and in the interest of holding as many variables constant as possible when seeking to measure change over time, it probably would be best for assessments before, during and after treatment to be conducted at the same time of day.

- **Positioning for recording.** Changes in body position are known to influence speech breathing mechanics due to the influence of gravity, such that each time body orientation changes there is an alteration in the mechanical processes used to achieve the required respiratory load (Hixon & Hoit, 2005). The greatest changes in speech breathing mechanics will occur when an individual moves from a supine to upright position. Therefore, when assessing speech breathing using kinematic analysis, it is important that the client remain in similar position throughout the assessment (usu-

ally sitting in a straight-backed chair or standing). Throughout the recording, the clinician should monitor the client's position and reposition when necessary.

- **Inductoband placement.** Two inductobands are placed around the chest wall system, fastened at the front with Velcro, and can be further secured in place using the retainers (see Figure 5–2). One inductoband is placed around the rib cage under the axilla, positioned about halfway between the sternal notch and the xiphoid process. The coil pins should be pointed in a downward direction toward the umbilicus. The second inductoband is placed around the abdomen with the top of the band at the level of the umbilicus and ensuring that this is below the level of the last rib. Coil pins on this transducer band should be pointed in an upward direction toward the rib cage. If the bands are positioned while the client is in a standing position and recordings be taken in a seated position, the clinician will need to check the placement of both bands once the client is seated. The clinician should monitor the positioning of the transducer bands throughout the assessment to ensure slippage does not occur.

Calibration

The Inductotrace system detects changes in the cross-sectional areas of a client's rib cage and abdomen through the inductobands positioned as described above during the act of breathing. This changes the shape of magnetic field generated by the bands, which induces a change in electrical current within the Inductotrace system that can be measured. Key to capturing these changes in electrical current are the oscillator and Calbox; therefore, the first calibration procedures required apply to the Inductotrace system itself. Calibration should be completed prior to each recording session. Prior to the calibration procedures for the Calbox and transducer oscillator, the system should be turned on for approximately 30 minutes for "warm-up." Calibration of the Calbox and oscilloscope are necessary to ensure that all channels used during the assessment display equal deflection for equivalent input voltages (i.e., a 1-volt change due to rib cage movement is represented as 4-unit change on the relative motion chart, with the same degree of deflection occurring for a 1-volt change due to abdominal

movement). There are two stages to the calibration of the system: (1) adjustment of zero line on the Calbox for the rib cage and abdomen channels, and (2) setting gain for Calbox channels to 1 volt. Calibration of the system occurs prior to the client being connected to the system via the inductobands.

Step 1: Adjust zero line on Calbox for Rib Cage and Abdomen Channels
Start by pressing in the **Calibrate** button (Figure 5–4) and then the **Rib Cage** button. Check that the digital display reads 0.00, if any other value is displayed, use the **Rib Cage** zero dial (bottom row of dials—the **Zero** dials

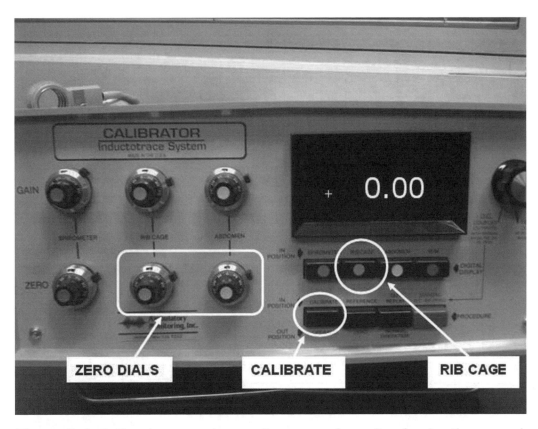

Figure 5–4. Calibration procedures: adjustment of zero line for the rib cage and abdomen channels.

on lower left of the Calbox) to return the display to 0.00. Then repeat the same procedure for the **Abdomen** button and its respective zero dial.

Step 2: Set gain for Calbox channels to 1 volt

Depress the **Calibrate** and **Reference** buttons and push in the **Rib Cage** button (Figure 5–5). The digital display should read 1.00. If any other value is shown, then use the **Rib Cage** gain dial (upper row) to return the displayed value to 1.00. The same procedure should be followed with the **Abdomen** button and gain dial. The final step is to press in the **Sum** button and check the digital display.

It should display a value of 2.00 volts if both the **Rib Cage** and **Abdomen** gains have been correctly set at 1.00 volts. This finishes the calibration process.

Recording of Speech Breathing

Prior to recording speech breathing tasks to acquire lung volume data, it is necessary to define specific kinematic landmarks through a number of respiratory maneuvers (tidal breathing and maximal lung capacity maneuvers). The data generated from these maneuvers allow for con-

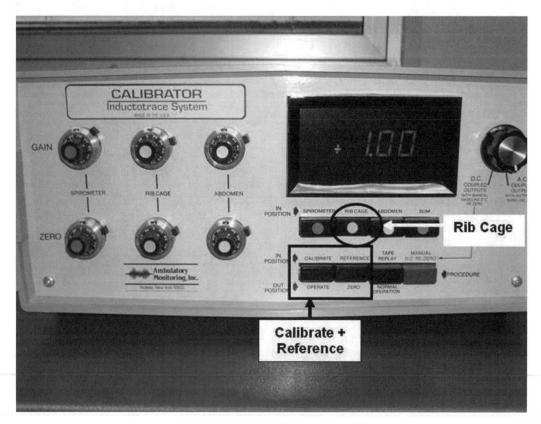

Figure 5–5. Calibration procedures: setting gain on Calbox.

struction of a volume-volume chart that represent rib cage, abdominal and lung capacities (Figure 5-6), and can be used to interpret changes in lung volumes and the relative contribution of the rib cage and abdomen to these volume changes.

1. Once the client is fitted with the inductobands and seated in position for the recording, begin by taking recordings of tidal (or quiet) breathing. Tidal (quiet) breathing refers to the breath pattern used when a person is at rest, that is, not participating in an active movement, which includes the absence of speech pro-

duction. Recordings of tidal breathing (i.e., quiet breathing) should be taken to determine the tidal volume and resting-end expiratory level (REL). Tidal volume equates to volume of air inspired and expired during a typical respiratory cycle, with the lung volume at the end of expiration during tidal breathing referred to as REL. Under this procedure, the client is instructed to sit quietly for a few minutes while the recordings are being taken, and the clinician can monitor the graphic display representing the changes in rib cage and abdominal cross-sectional area, as well as their sum.

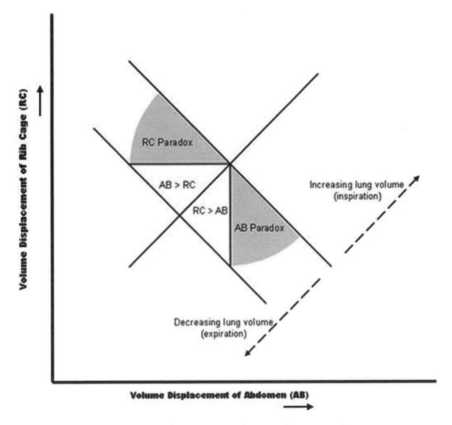

Figure 5-6. Example of volume-volume chart used to interpret changes in lung volumes and the relative contribution of the rib cage and abdomen to these volume changes.

Instructions: *"We are going to assess your breathing during talking as the air you breathe in and out provides the source for producing your voice. First we need to see what your breathing patterns are while you are resting and not talking. You don't need to do anything at this point, just sit quietly and relax for a few minutes while I take some recordings. I will tell you when we have finished taking these recordings."*

2. The clinician then obtains estimations of the maximal capacity of the lungs, rib cage, and abdomen through a vital capacity (VC) task. The VC tasks will provide estimations of minimum and maximum rib cage volumes generated, and similarly can provide estimation of minimum and maximum abdominal volumes (Murdoch, Theodoros, Stokes, & Chenery, 1993). During the VC task, the client is asked to take a deep breath and then let out all of the air until the lungs are empty. Simultaneously, a spirometer is used to measure the vital capacity in liters. Verbal encouragement can be provided to the client if required to ensure that she or he completes the task accurately. Between each VC maneuver, the client should be allowed to rest and the clinician should observe that the breathing has returned to tidal breathing patterns. Abdominal capacity tasks also can be completed if the clinician believes that the client has not demonstrated maximal range of movement in the abdomen during the VC task (Huber & Spruill, 2008). If this task is completed, the clinician will require the client to make movements

that represent the maximum and minimum displacements of the abdomen.

Instructions (Vital Capacity): *"We now want to look at how much air it is possible for you to breathe in and out, and how your rib cage and abdomen move while you are breathing in this way. At the same time I am going to measure the amount of air breathed out using a spirometer. To do this, I am going to place a nose clip over your nostrils to stop air from escaping through your nose as you breathe out through your mouth. I will place the spirometer just inside your mouth and you need to close your lips around the tube. You can breathe in and out through this tube. Now I want you to take as deep a breath in as you can, and then let it out until there is nothing left in your lungs."* (The clinician should model the deep breathe in and out, ensuring that there is no upper torso movement during the out breathe.) *"We will repeat this task three times."*

Instructions (Abdominal Capacity): *"I want to see how much you can increase and decrease the size of your tummy. To complete this task, you will have to breathe out all the air in your lungs, then you need to hold your breath while pushing your tummy out so that it becomes bigger and then pull it in as far as you can. You should not take a breath in during these movements of your tummy."* (The clinician should model the process required.) *"We will repeat this task three times."*

3. Once recordings have been taken that allow for kinematic landmarks to be measured for later analysis procedures, the clinician should move on to record speech breathing behaviors during speechlike or speech tasks. Before proceeding to the next task, the client should be given some time to relax, with the clinician initiating the next task only when tidal breathing has stabilized. As vowel prolongation (speech-like task) is a common assessment task used to evaluate respiratory-phonatory control (Kent, Vorperian, & Duffy, 1999) and subsequently a therapy task (Holmberg, Hillman, Hammarberg, Sodersten, & Doyle, 2001). It is important to assess speech breathing behaviors in this context. The client is asked to produce the vowel "ah" for as long as she or he can after taking in a deep breath. The instructions below should be given to the client, the task can be modeled by the clinician if necessary, and tidal breathing observed between each repetition.

Instructions: *"I want you to take in a deep breath, and as you let the air out say the sound "ah" at a comfortable pitch and loudness until you run out of breath. We will repeat this task three times."*

4. The specific speech tasks used to evaluate speech breathing then can be designed based on the needs of the clinician and/or client. Generally, tasks can be divided into two groups; extended steady utterances (e.g., counting, sentence recitation), and running speech (e.g., reading or conversation). Decisions regarding the type and number of speech stimuli used in assessing speech breathing behaviors should base on client's and clinician's need. Using a combination of extended steady utterance and running speech tasks is highly recommended to ensure that the clinician gains an understanding of speech breathing behaviors in activities that mirror both therapy tasks and naturalistic communication. In the first instance, the client should be asked to complete the speech tasks using his or her normal vocal loudness. Some examples of speech stimuli used and instructions for the client are provided. Ensure that tidal breathing has stabilized between each repetition of a task, and when moving between tasks.

Instructions (Counting): *"I want you to take a breath in, and then count from 1 to 20, or as many as you can on one breath. Speak at a comfortable pitch and loudness. We will repeat this task three times."*

Instructions (Sentence recitation): *"I want you to repeat the sentence: 'Combine all the ingredients in a large bowl' aloud at a comfortable pitch and loudness, as if talking to a friend. We will repeat this sentence three times."*

Instructions (Reading, the Grandfather Passage): *"I have a reading passage here that I would like you read through and familiarize yourself with the content. When you're ready, let me know. Then I want you to read this passage out loud in a conversational manner, at a comfortable pitch and loudness level, as if you are reading out something to a friend."*

Instructions (Conversation sample): *"We need to have a sample of how you would talk when in a conversation with someone. There are a couple of topics you could choose to tell me about, you can choose the one you're the happiest to talk about. You can choose to tell me about your last holiday, your family, or your work/hobbies. We will talk just as you would in a daily conversation."*

5. As mentioned previously, different clinical needs will arise for different clients, and so the assessment protocol for speech tasks may be altered dependent on these requirements. Specific dimensions that the clinician may want to assess with respect to speech breathing behaviors during speech tasks include increased/decreased vocal loudness or higher/lower pitch. Therefore, assessment tasks might require the client to increase his or her vocal loudness during a sentence recitation or reading task. If increasing vocal loudness is the targeted dimension, the clinician will need to obtain a baseline sound pressure level on which to base the subsequent "loud" condition. An increase of 10 dB above baseline sound pressure level should be the volume required of the client during this condition (Huber & Spruill, 2008; Lowell et al., 2008). The clinician should provide the client with a situational cue to increase in vocal loudness, for example, *"as if you are speaking to a friend across the table in a noisy restaurant and you need to increase your volume."* Prior to beginning recordings, the clinician should ensure that tidal breathing has stabilized.

Instructions (Sentence recitation): *"You are in a noisy restaurant and you need to speak with your friend across the table. Repeat the sentence: 'Combine all the ingredients in a large bowl' in a loud voice so that your friend can hear you clearly."*

Data Analysis

1. Kinematic data recorded can be used to evaluate the size of lung volume excursions with respect to the client's vital capacity (VC), and where these excursions occur with respect to total VC. The range of lung volume excursions used by a client should be defined using the VC maneuvers as the first step in analysis. Start by reviewing the VC traces and identify the one that represents the largest volume expired. This should be taken as the client's vital capacity, and used to evaluate the range of lung volume excursions for that client. Then determine the full range of rib cage, abdomen, and lung volume excursions during this VC maneuver by identifying the maximum and minimum values for each. Use the graphic displays available in the data acquisition program (the examples provided in this chapter use the MATLAB program detailed previously). Replay the recorded VC maneuver observing both the X-Y plot (relative motion chart) and the Y-T oscillographic channels to determine the point at which the expiratory phase begins (Figure 5–7). This point should be marked using the purple cursor, then determine the point at which expiration ceases and mark with a second cursor. Marking

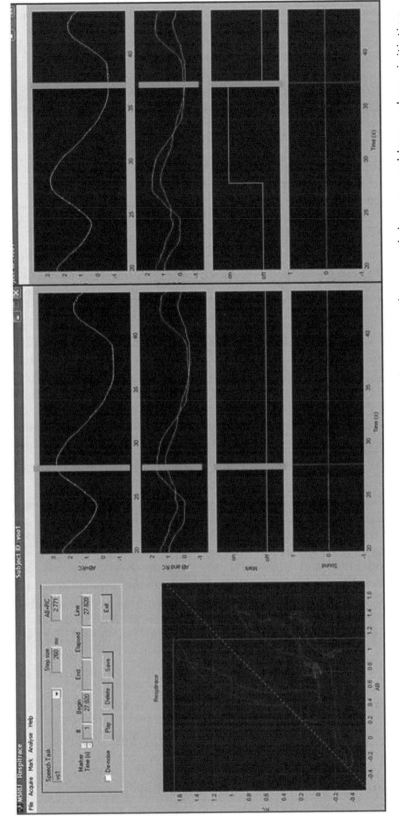

Figure 5–7. Analysis procedure using a Matlab-based program to determine rib cage, abdomen, and lung volume initiation and termination points.

these two points allows the analysis program to compute the limits of the client's vital capacity (VC), rib cage capacity (RCC), and abdominal capacity (ABC). The lowest termination points recorded for the rib cage, abdomen, and lung capacity axes therefore represent the 0% limit, and the highest initiation points represent 100% capacity. A data chart then can be constructed that represents percent rib cage (%RCC) on the *y*-axis increasing upward, percent abdomen (%ABC) on the *x*-axis increasing to the right, and percent vital capacity (%VC) on the diagonal. All subsequent measures of lung volume excursions across speech and speechlike tasks can be made in comparison to these values, and referred to as speech production measures referenced to the 0% limit.

For each speechlike task such as sustained vowel prolongation, measurements can be taken from each trial of a task and an average calculated. For speech tasks, however, the number of speech breath cycles analyzed and averaged will be dependent on the nature of the task. Breath groups for sentence recitation, reading, and conversational tasks first should be identified by replaying the recording with the acoustic signal used to identify the onset and offset of breath groupings. Then, using all available graphic displays (X-Y plot, Y-T oscillographic channels, and acoustic signal), the expiratory limb for each breath group should be identified and marked using the procedure previously outlined for marking initiation and termination points. The computerized data acquisition and analysis program utilizes the same procedure for identifying and marking the expi-

ratory portions of speech breathing cycles with respect to initiation and termination points as detailed above. Nine measures of chest-wall (lung volume) excursions can be calculated and provide initiations, termination, and excursions of the rib cage, abdomen, and lung volume axes with respect to the 0% limits (Table 5–1). Using this information, the clinician can determine if speech is being produced using large lung volumes, or lower or higher lung volumes within VC.

2. Speech breathing behaviors also can be analyzed with reference to resting-end expiratory level (REL). Analysis seeking to interpret kinematic findings in this way first must identify the client's REL. This is achieved by identifying the average termination point of the expiratory limbs recording during quiet (tidal) breathing with measurements taken on at least three consecutive breaths. The same procedure used for identifying termination points on the VC maneuvers should be followed when seeking to identify the REL point. Six measures of volume initiations and terminations in relation to REL can be made (see Table 5–1 for a summary). These data can be used to determine if the client is initiating or terminating speech at lung volumes higher or lower than REL.

3. Further kinematic analysis of speech breathing can address the relative contributions of the rib cage and abdomen. Relative volume contribution of the rib cage (%RC) over the entire expiration represents the slope of the line that links the initiation and termination points of an expiratory limb within a speech breathing cycle (Hoit & Hixon, 1987). The formula used to calculated the slope of this line:

Table 5–1. Rib cage, Abdomen, and Lung Volume Calculations to Measure Initiation, Termination, and Excursion Values in Relation to the 0% Limit and Resting-end Expiratory Level (REL)

Excursion Relative to the 0% Limit		Excursion Relative to the 0% REL	
LVI	lung volume initiation (in %VC)	**LVI–R**	lung volume initiation in relation to lung volume (in %VC)
LVT	lung volume termination (in %VC)	**LVT–R**	lung volume termination in relation to lung volume (in %VC)
LVE	lung volume excursion (in %VC)	**LVE-R**	lung volume excursion in relation to lung volume (in %VC)
RCVI	rib cage volume initiation (in %RCC)	**RCVI-R**	rib cage volume initiation in relation to rib cage volume (in %RCC)
RCVT	rib cage volume termination (in %RCC)	**RCVT-R**	rib cage volume termination in relation to rib cage volume (in %RCC)
RCVE	rib cage volume excursion (in %RCC)	**RCVE-R**	rib cage volume excursion in relation to rib cage volume (in %RCC)
ABVI	abdominal volume initiation (in %ABC)	**ABVI-R**	abdominal volume initiation in relation to abdominal volume (in %ABC)
ABVT	abdominal volume termination (in %ABC)	**ABVT-R**	abdominal volume termination in relation to abdominal volume (in %ABC)
ABVE	abdominal volume excursion (in %ABC)	**ABVE-R**	abdominal volume excursion in relation to abdominal volume (in %ABC)

$$\frac{\dfrac{(RCVI - RCVT) \times RC/AB}{(ABVI - ABVT)} \times 100}{\dfrac{(RCVI - RCVT) \times RC/AB}{(ABVI - ABVT)} + 1}$$

where:

RCVI = rib cage volume initiation (in %RCC)

RCVT = rib cage volume termination (in %RCC)

ABVI = abdominal volume initiation (in %ABC)

ABVT = abdominal volume termination (in %ABC)

RC/AB = rib cage capacity/ abdominal capacity

4. Although the relative volume contribution of the rib cage and abdomen to lung volume displacement can be calculated mathematically, analysis of the volume-volume charts also can be used more generally to interpret the relative volume displacements of the rib cage and abdomen, as well as presence or absence of paradoxic movements. Speech breathing traces consistent with an expiratory phase are reflected on a volume-volume chart as decreased lung volume in the presence of decreased rib cage and/or abdominal displacement (refer to Figure 5–6). Different combinations of rib cage and abdominal displacement can be used to achieve expiration. Normal speech breathing patterns are represented by decreasing lung volumes resultant from expiratory volume displacements for both the rib cage and abdomen, and the pathway direction is dependent which provides the greater contribution. Paradoxic movements occur when the expiratory volume displacement of one chest wall component (e.g., abdomen) exceeds that of the expiratory volume displacement of the lungs equal to the inspiratory volume displacement of the other chest wall component (e.g., rib cage) and this example reflects rib cage paradoxing. See Figure 5–6 for a visual representation of rib cage and abdominal paradoxical movements.

NORMATIVE DATA

There are several key points to consider when evaluating the findings of kinematic analyses of speech breathing:

■ Lung volumes expired during speech production usually fall between 10 to 20% of a client's vital capacity, and midrange lung volumes (between 60 to 40%) within a client's vital capacity are used for speech production (Hixon, Goldman, & Mead, 1973).

■ Speech production tends to finish around lung volume levels equivalent to REL (Hixon & Hoit, 2005).

■ During speech production, equal volume contributions from the rib cage and abdomen are observed in changes to lung volume with constant slopes on expiratory traces. However, in running speech, the relative volume contribution of the rib cage wall may exceed that of the abdomen (Hixon, 1982).

■ The rib cage and abdomen usually work in synchrony, so paradoxical movements are not commonly seen in normal speakers (Schaeffer et al., 2002; Sperry et al., 1994).

CASE STUDY

Patient M.J. (Unilateral Right Vocal Fold Palsy)

M.J., a 32-year-old male mechanical engineer, was referred to speech pathology by an otolaryngologist following resection of a right hypoglossal schwannoma. He had been diagnosed with right vocal fold palsy with central glottic gap, with pooling of secretions due to poor opening of the upper esophageal sphincter. At this time, his voice was described as severely dysphonic with a breathy and rough quality. A Gore-Tex thyroplasty of the right vocal fold and Botox injection to the cricopharyngeal muscle were undertaken. Following the thyroplasty, he reported that his dysphonia was continuing to interfere with both his work and social lives. In particular, he was finding it difficult to make himself understood over background noise. Perceptually, his voice in daily conversations was characterized by a mild degree of breathiness, and moderate levels of roughness and strain. His voice was low-pitched with occasional pitch breaks and his habitual volume was soft. Signs of increased jaw, neck, and shoulder tension were evident during conversation. Upper thoracic breathing was also observed. Prior to commencing therapy, a kinematic assessment of speech breathing patterns was conducted to determine how respiratory patterns might be contributing to his dysphonia. The assessment results indicated that M.J. demonstrated (Table 5–2):

■ Lung volumes expired during running speech at a conversational volume were around 10% of his vital capacity, and fell within the midrange of his vital capacity.

■ Lung volumes expired during running speech at a loud volume did not reflect the expected increase of 10%, but also recorded at around 10% of vital capacity within the mid-range of his vital capacity. This suggested that he was not using increased respiratory drive to increase vocal loudness, and was consistent with his complaint that speaking in "noisy environments" was difficult. It also might suggest that the development of vocal strain as a characteristic of M.J.'s dysphonia came from the use of increased muscular tension

Table 5–2. Pretreatment Assessment Results for M.J.

Tasks	LVE	%VC LV Range (LVI–LVT)	%VC LV Range ref to REL (LVI-R–LVT-R)	%RC
Quiet Breathing	20.36	56.67–36.30	—	68.00
Maximal Effort Speech				
Sustained phonation	81.34	89.67–8.33	—	53.68
Counting	91.96	94.89–2.93	—	57.59
Running Speech				
Sentence Recitation (NV)	9.96	59.18–49.23	↑22.88–↑2.93	43.87
Sentence Recitation (LV)	10.43	60.26–49.83	↑23.97–↑9.77	31.40

LVE—lung volume excursion; %VC LV Range—lung volume initiation and termination points within individuals vital capacity with reference to 0% limit; %VC LV Range ref to REL—lung volume initiation and termination points within individuals vital capacity with reference to resting-end expiratory level; %RC—relative contribution of rib cage in percent; ↑ = above REL.

in the neck and laryngeal region to produce a loud voice.

- Lung volumes expired during running speech at both loudness levels volumes were compared to REL, with comparisons revealing that speech was initiated just above the level of his tidal inspiratory volume and terminated.
- Relative rib cage and abdomen contributions to speech breathing patterns varied across tasks with:
  - Equal contributions of the rib cage and abdomen observed during extended utterance (maximal effort speech tasks). This suggested that M.J. could use standard speech breathing patterns when focusing on the inspiratory phase.
  - During running speech the relative contribution of the abdomen to expiration was found to be greater than rib cage contribution. This pattern was more noticeable for the "loud" condition and might suggest that M.J. was using active abdominal muscle movements to control expiratory airflow during these tasks, or paradoxical movements occurred during the expiratory phase. The latter hypothesis might be consistent with observations of thoracic breathing during conversation speech, with closer inspection of the expiratory limbs of the volume-volume charts required.

- Paradoxic movements of the rib cage were noted on the expiratory limbs of both maximum effort speech but were most evident during serial counting (Figures 5–8A and 5–8B) and sentence recitation at loud volume task (Figure 5–8D), but not during sentence recitation at normal volume (Figure 5–8C). This was consistent with the use of thoracic breathing observed during conversational speech.

The findings of the kinematic assessment for M.J. suggested that, although his speech was being produced on appropriate lung volumes expired and within the optimal midrange vital capacities, the speech breathing patterns used to achieve this differ from those of speakers without dysphonia. The clinical observation of thoracic breathing was supported by the kinematic analyses. Additionally, M.J. did not utilize increased lung volumes to produce loud speech, which was likely to contribute to the rough and strained vocal qualities. Therefore, his voice therapy program should include respiratory training alongside other resonant voice therapy (Boone, 1997). The combination of these two approaches aimed at improving M.J.'s respiratory control and resonance, as well as transfer the mental focus of phonation away from the larynx to the activator and resonator (respiration and resonance respectively).

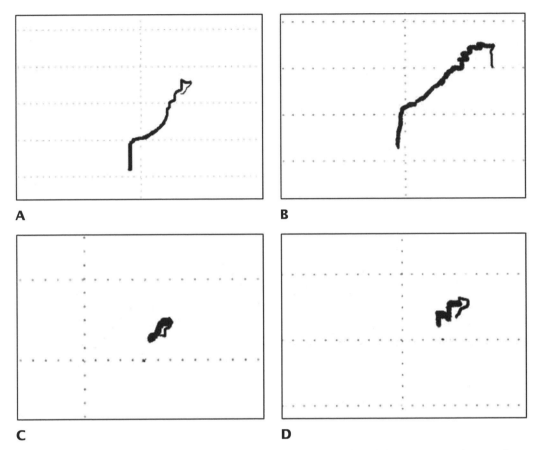

A

B

C

D

Figure 5–8. Expiratory limbs produced during sustained phonation (A), serial counting (B), sentence recitation at normal voice (C), and sentence recitation at loud volume (D) with rib cage paradoxing evident in A, B, and D.

REFERENCES

Aronson, A. E. (1990). *Clinical voice disorders* (3rd ed.). New York, NY: Thieme.

Bahr, R. H., Biedess, K., & Ridley, M. B. (2007). *Speech breathing in patients with adductor spasmodic dysphonia.* 16th International Congress of Phonetic Sciences, Saarbrucken, Germany (conference presentation available at http://www.icphs2007. de Book of abstracts ID1547).

Baken, R. J., & Orlikoff, R. F. (2000). *Clinical measurement of speech and voice* (2nd ed.). San Diego, CA: Singular.

Boone, D. R. (1997). *Is your voice telling on you?* (2nd ed.). San Diego, CA: Singular.

Boone, D. R., & McFarlane, S. C. (2000). *The voice and voice therapy* (6th ed.). Boston, MA: Allyn & Bacon.

Boone, D. R., McFarlane, S. C., & von Berg, S. L. (2005). *The voice and voice therapy* (7th ed.). Boston, MA: Allyn & Bacon.

Bunton, K. (2005). Patterns of lung volume use during an extemporaneous speech task in persons with Parkinson disease. *Journal of Communication Disorders, 38,* 331-348.

Darley, F. L., Aronson, A. E., & Brown, J. R. (1975). *Motor speech disorders.* Philadephia, PA: W. B. Saunders.

Fairbanks, G. (1960). *Voice and articulation drillbook*. New York, NY: Harper and Row.

Hixon, T. J. (1982). Speech breathing kinematics and mechanism inferences therefrom. In S. Grillner, B. Lindblom, J. Lubker, & A. Persson (Eds.), *Speech motor control*. New York, NY: Pergamon Press.

Hixon, T. J., & Hoit, J. D. (2005). *Evaluation and management of speech breathing disorders*. Tuscon, AZ: Reddington Brown LLC.

Hixon, T. J., Goldman, M. D., & Mead, J. (1973). Kinematics of the chest wall during speech production: Volume displacement of the rib cage, abdomen, and lung. *Journal of Speech and Hearing Research, 16*, 78–115.

Hixon, T. J., & Putnam, H. B. (1983). Voice disorders in relation to respiratory kinematics. *Seminars in Speech and Language, 4*, 217–231.

Hoit, J. D., & Hixon, T. J. (1987). Age and speech breathing. *Journal of Speech and Hearing Research, 30*, 351–366.

Holmberg, E. B., Hillman, R. E., Hammarberg, B., Sodersten, M., & Doyle, P. (2001). Efficacy of a behaviorally based voice therapy protocol for vocal nodules. *Journal of Voice, 15*(3), 395–412.

Huber, J. E., & Spruill, J. (2008). Age-related changes to speech breathing with increased vocal loudness. *Journal of Speech, Language, and Hearing Research, 51*, 651–668.

Kalliakosta, G., Mandros, C., & Tzelepis, G. E. (2007). Chest wall motion during speech production in patients with advanced ankylosing spondylitis. *Journal of Speech, Language, and Hearing Research, 50*, 109–118.

Kent, R. D., Vorperian, H. K., & Duffy, J. R. (1999). Reliability of the Multi-dimensional Voice Program for the analysis of voice samples in subjects with dysarthria. *American Journal of Speech-Language Pathology, 8*, 129–136.

Lowell, S. Y., Barkmeier-Kraemer, J. M., Hoit, J. D.,

& Story, B. H. (2008). Respiratory and laryngeal function during spontaneous speaking in teachers with voice disorders. *Journal of Speech, Language and Hearing Research, 51*, 333–349.

Mazeika, G. G., & Swanson, R. (2007). Respiratory inductance plethysmography: An introduction [Technical brochure]. Retrieved from http://www.ptservices.com/downloads/misc/pdf/RIP_Intro.pdf

McFarland, D. H. (2001). Respiratory markers of conversational interaction. *Journal of Speech Language and Hearing Research, 44*(1), 128–143.

Murdoch, B. E., Theodoros, D. G., Stokes, P. D., & Chenery, H. J. (1983). Abnormal patterns of speech breathing in dysarthric speakers following severe closed head injury. *Brain Injury, 7*, 295–308.

Sapienza, C. M., & Stathopoulos, E. T. (1994). Respiratory and laryngeal measures of children and women with bilateral vocal fold nodules. *Journal of Speech and Hearing Research, 37*, 1229–1243.

Sapienza, C. M., Stathopoulos, E. T., & Brown, W. S. (1997). Speech breathing during reading in women with vocal nodules. *Journal of Voice, 11*, 195–201.

Schaeffer, N., Cavallo, S. A., Wall, M., & Diakow, C. (2002). Speech breathing behavior in normal and moderately to severely dysphonic subjects during connected speech. *Journal of Medical Speech-Language Pathology, 10*, 1–18.

Solomon, N. P. (2008). Vocal fatigue and its relation to vocal hyperfunction. *International Journal of Speech-Language Pathology, 10*, 254–266.

Sperry, E. E., Hillman, R. E., & Perkell, J. S. (1994). The use of inductance plethysmography to assess respiratory function in a patient with vocal nodules. *Journal of Medical Speech-Language Pathology, 2*, 137–145.

CHAPTER 6

Maximum Phonation Performance

EDWIN M.-L. YIU

PURPOSE

■ To assess how an individual manages the air supply efficiently during sustained phonation by noting the maximum sustained phonation time.

THEORETICAL BACKGROUND

Maximum phonation performance often is assessed in tasks such as voice range profile (for loudness and pitch) and maximum phonation time. This assessment protocol provides information related to vocal fold functions, as well as respiratory support, and is useful before and after voice therapy. The assessment of voice range profile is covered in this handbook in Chapter 19 by Ma. This chapter focuses on the assessment of maximum phonation time (MPT). Alternative terms that have been used in the literature include "maximum sustained phonation time," "maximum phonation duration" (e.g., Kent, Kent, &

Rosenbek, 1987; Treole & Trudeau, 1997), "maximum duration of phonation" (e.g., Ptacek & Sander, 1963), and "maximum phoneme duration" (e.g., Soman, 1997). Maximum phonation time or maximum sustained phonation time refers to the longest duration that an individual can sustain a tone after a deep inhalation (Colton, Casper, & Leonard, 2006). It is one of the clinical tools most commonly used for voice assessment (Beckett, 1971; Finnegan, 1985; Ptacek & Sander, 1963). MPT is considered useful to examine the phonatory and respiratory coordination (Solomon, Garlitz, & Milbrath, 2000; Treole & Trudeau, 1997). It correlates well with oral airflow rate (Yu, Ouaknine, Revis, & Giovanni, 2001) but not with the respiratory vital capacity (Solomon et al., 2000).

There is, however, controversy in the use of MPT in clinical voice assessment due to the great variability of the procedural aspects and the normative data obtained in various studies (Larson, Mueller, & Summers, 1991; Neiman & Edeson, 1981; Reich, Mason, & Polen, 1986; Soman, 1997; Sorensen & Parker, 1992). It should be noted that the assessment of the MPT does not make any diagnosis of laryngeal disease, but merely indicates the degree of vocal function (Hirano, Koike, & von Leden, 1968).

Variability in Maximum Phonation Time

The normative data of MPT varies greatly across and within studies. Reported MPT values of male adults ranged from 9.3 to 62.3 seconds (Hirano et al., 1968; Ptacek & Sander, 1963; Yanagihara & Koike, 1967) and those of females varied from 6.2 to 40.4 seconds (Hirano et al., 1968; Ptacek & Sander, 1963; Yanagihara & Koike, 1967).

A number of procedural factors may have contributed to the large variability of the normative data. These factors include the methods of elicitation, data collection, and analysis (Lee, Stemple, & Kizer, 1999). For methods of elicitation, it has been found that the provision of modeling, verbal instructions, and coaching, can affect the MPT performances (Soman, 1997). The number of trials used for elicitation of MPT also affects the MPT performance. Clinically, it has been common to find the recommendation of using three to five trials of sustained phonation (Prathanee, Soew, Ponganyakul, & Sae-Heng, 2003; Yanagihara & Koike, 1967; Yanagihara & von Leden, 1967). However, it has long been observed that many speakers were not able to achieve the longest MPT by the third trial (Neiman & Edeson, 1981). Some speakers may require up to 10 (Neiman & Edeson, 1981) or 15 trials (Stone, 1983) to achieve the maximum performance. This may be interpreted as practice effect (Kent et al., 1987) and one would argue that requiring a speaker to repeat as many as 10 to 15 trials of sustained phonation may lead to vocal fatigue (Kent et al., 1987). More recently, Speyer et al. (2010) have shown that the MPT procedure showed a higher reliability (interclass correlation coefficient >0.98) when the number of trials increased from one to five. Intensity and frequency of the sustained tones is another major factor causing the variability in MPT performance (Lee et al., 1999; Neiman & Edeson, 1981).

The methods in determining or calculating the MPT also contribute to the variability in MPT performance. Some suggested the use of the average of the two longest trials (Eckel & Boone, 1981) or the average of five trials (Rastatter & Hyman, 1982); whereas others recommended the use of the longest of three trials (Eckel & Boone, 1981; Fendler & Shearer, 1988; Hufnagle & Hufnagle, 1988; Soman, 1997; Tait, Michel, & Carpenter, 1980).

EQUIPMENT AND MATERIALS

MPT can be assessed using the simplest method by employing a stopwatch (or a watch with a second hand) or a more sophisticated method using a microphone connected to a computer with any software program (e.g., Audacity) that shows the duration of the recording. When a microphone is used, a constant mouth-to-microphone distance (e.g., 15 cm) should be used.

TEST PROCEDURES

Following the recommendation of Neiman and Edeson (1981), clients should be given a standardized verbal instruction and visual demonstration of the task before the actual recording. The examiner should demonstrate the MPT task with the maximum effort following a maximum inspiration. A minimum of three trials of maximum phonation time is required. The client is instructed to take a deep breath and sustain the vowel (/a/, /i/, or /u/ can be used) at a comfortable pitch and loudness level for as long as possible. Remind the client that the pitch and loudness should be kept at about similar levels across all three trials during assessment. If a software program with instantaneous fundamental frequency and intensity extraction function is used, these two measures should be kept within ±10% range across the three recordings. Of the three trials, the one with the longest duration is to be taken as the MPT for the client.

Verbal Instructions

■ *"Take a deep breath, and then say /a/ (/i/ or /u/) using your most comfortable pitch and loudness for as long as you possibly can until you run out of breath completely. While you are producing the sound, try to keep your pitch and loudness levels constant each time. Now I will demonstrate the task once."* (The examiner then gives a complete and full model of the MPT with the most comfortable pitch and loudness of his or her own.)

(**OPTIONAL:** If available, a sound level meter may be used to monitor the intensity of the phonation. The intensity should be constant during the phonation. The sound level meter can be placed at a distance of 10 cm from the speaker's mouth to monitor the sound pressure level of the phonation. Normally, a comfortable loudness would be around 50 to 60 dB SPL.)

■ *"Now you have to do this a second time, try to prolong the /a/ (/i/ or /u/) longer this time. Remember to keep your pitch and loudness similar to those at the first time. Okay, you can start now."*

■ *"Now do it one more time, try to prolong the /a/ (/i/ or /u/) even longer this time. Okay, you can start now."*

NORMATIVE DATA

A number of reports of normative data for MPT are available in the literature (Hirano et al., 1968; Ma & Yiu, 2006; Neiman & Edeson, 1981; Ptacek & Sander, 1963; Yanagihara & Koike, 1967). Baken and Orlikoff (2000) provide an overview of these data. As mentioned earlier, these normative data are highly varied. The reported MPT values of male adults ranged from 9.3 to 62.3 seconds (Hirano et al., 1968; Ptacek & Sander, 1963 Yanagihara & Koike, 1967), and those of female adults ranged from 6.2 to 40.4 seconds (Hirano et al., 1968; Ptacek & Sander, 1963; Yanagihara & Koike, 1967). Table 6–1 summarizes the normative data from these investigators.

As the vital capacity, vocal function and the general compliance behavior of children are different from those of the adults, one would expect the MPT normative data for children to be different from those of the adults. Finnegan (1984)

Table 6–1. Some Normative Data of Mean (Range) Maximum Phonation Time (MPT)

Investigators	Mean (range) MPT in Seconds			
	Males	Females	Combined Males + Females	Remarks
Ptacek and Sander (1963)	22.6 (9.3–43.3)	15.2 (6.2–28.6)		Young adults
Hirano et al. (1968)	34.6 (15.0–62.3)	25.7 (14.3–40.4)		Adults
Yanagihara and Koike (1967)	27.4 (23.7–30.2)	20.3 (16.4–22.5)		Mean age of Male = 26 years Female = 28 years
Finnegan (1984)	18.23	15.79		Children age 3;6–17; 11
Cielo and Cappellari (2008)			5.77* 7.16# 10.32^	* For 4-year-old # For 5-year-old ^ For 6-year-old

reported a mean of 18.23 seconds of MPT for boys and 15.79 seconds for girls (see Table 6-1). Cielo and Cappellari (2008) reported the mean MPT for Brazilian children to vary from 5.77 seconds (4-year-old) to 7.16 seconds (5-year-old) and 10.32 seconds (6-year-old).

A number of studies have shown that dysphonic individuals demonstrated significant shorter MPT than vocally healthy individuals (e.g., Ma & Yiu, 2006; Schindler, Mozzanica, Vedrody, Maruzzi, & Ottaviani, 2009; Xu, Han, Hou, Hu, & Wang, 2009).

CASE EXAMPLE

Patient A. X. complained of a severe breathy voice and frequent vocal fatigue shortly after talking for a while. He consulted a laryn-gologist and a left vocal polyp was diagnosed. Behavioral voice therapy and surgery to remove the polyp were planned. Prior to voice therapy and surgery, the longest MPT for a sustained /a/ among three trials was 8 seconds (the three trials were 6 seconds, 7 seconds, and 8 seconds). Four sessions of voice therapy was given and another MPT assessment was carried out before the surgery. The longest MPT was 10 seconds (the three trials were 6 seconds, 9 seconds, and 10 seconds). After the surgery, a third MPT assessment found the longest duration to be 17 seconds (the three trials were 17 seconds, 12 seconds, and 16 seconds).

Interpretation

Table 6-2 lists the MPT data of dysphonic and normal speakers reported by Ma and

Table 6–2. Mean and Standard Deviation (SD) of Maximum Phonation Time as Reported by Ma and Yiu (2006)

Maximum Phonation Time (Seconds)	Dysphonic Group (Male = 19, Female = 93) (N = 112)		Vocally Healthy Group (Male = 6, Female = 35) (N = 41)	
	Mean	SD	Mean	SD
/a/	15.29	7.79	22.90	8.86
/i/	16.45	7.64	24.45	8.79
/u/	15.40	6.67	23.06	9.05

Yiu (2006). It can be seen that the dysphonic and normal speakers demonstrated overlapping MPT values. The MPT achieved by A.X. improved following surgery (17 seconds). This was above the mean of the dysphonic group but also below the mean of the normal group. This value also is within one standard deviation of both the mean dysphonic and normal group data. Therefore, the MPT alone cannot be used to determine whether A.X.'s performance is within normal limits or not. One can only say that it has improved when compared to the presurgery condition. As for the behavioral therapy, the MPT was 11 seconds, which is below the mean of the dysphonic group, thus indicating the behavioral therapy did not bring about any significant improvement. It also should be noted that practice effect might have happened within the prebehavioral therapy and presurgery recording, but no such effect was noted in the postsurgery recording.

REFERENCES

Baken, R. J., & Orlikoff, R. F. (2000). *Clinical measurement of speech and voice.* (2nd ed.) San Diego, CA: Singular Publishing Group.

Beckett, R. L. (1971). The respirometer as a diagnostic and clinical tool in the speech clinic. *Journal of Speech and Hearing Disorders, 4,* 235-241.

Cielo, C. A., & Cappellari, V. M. (2008). Maximum phonation time in pre-school children. *Brazilian Journal of Otorhinolaryngology, 74*(4), 552-560.

Colton, R. H., Casper, K. J., & Leonard, R. (2006). *Understanding voice problems: A physiological perspective for diagnosis and treatment* (3rd ed.). Philadelphia, PA: Lippincott Williams & Wilkins.

Eckel, F., & Boone, D. R. (1981). The s/z ratio as an indicator of laryngeal pathology. *Journal of Speech and Hearing Disorders, 46,* 147-149.

Fendler, M., & Shearer, W. M. (1988). Reliability of s/z ratio in normal children's voices. *Language, Speech and Hearing Services in Schools, 19,* 2-4.

Finnegan, D. E. (1985). Maximum phonation time for children with normal voices. *Folia Phoniatrica, 37,* 209-215.

Hirano, M., Koike, Y., & von Leden, H. (1968). Maximum phonation time and air usage during phonation: Clinical study. *Folia Phoniatrica, 20,* 185-201.

Hufnagle, J., & Hufnagle, K. K. (1988). S/z ratio in dysphonic children with and without vocal cord nodules. *Language, Speech, and Hearing Services in Schools, 19,* 418-422.

Kent, R. D., Kent, J. F., & Rosenbek, J. C. (1987). Maximum performance tests of speech production. *Journal of Speech and Hearing Disorders, 52*, 367-387.

Larson, G. W., Mueller, P. B., & Summers, P. A. (1991). The effect of procedural variations on the s/z ratio of adults. *Journal of Communication Disorders, 24*, 135-140.

Lee, L., Stemple, J. C., & Kizer, M. (1999). Consistency of acoustic and aerodynamic measures of voice production over 28 days under various testing conditions. *Journal of Voice, 13*, 477-483.

Ma, E. P.-M., & Yiu, E. M.-L. (2006). Multiparametric evaluation of dysphonic severity. *Journal of Voice, 20*, 380-390.

Neiman, G. S., & Edeson, B. (1981). Procedural aspects of eliciting maximum phonation time. *Folia Phoniatrica, 33*, 285-293.

Ptacek, P. H., & Sander, E. K. (1963). Maximum duration of phonation. *Journal of Speech and Hearing Disorders, 28*, 171-182.

Prathanee, B., Soew, P. S., Ponganyakul, A., & Sae-Heng, S. (2003). Time and frequency of maximum phonation of normal Thai children in Khon Kaen. *Journal of Multilingual Communication Disorders, 24*, 71-78.

Rastatter, M. P., & Hyman, M. (1982). Maximum phoneme duration of /s/ and /z/ by children with vocal nodules. *Language, Speech, and Hearing Services in Schools, 13*, 197-199.

Reich, A. R., Mason, J. A., & Polen, S. B. (1986). Task administration variables affecting phonation-time measures in third-grade girls with normal voice quality. *Language, Speech, and Hearing Services in Schools, 17*, 262-269.

Schindler, A., Mozzanica, F., Vedrody, M., Maruzzi, P., & Ottaviani, F. (2009). Correlation between the Voice Handicap Index and voice measurements in four groups of patients with dysphonia. *Otolaryngology-Head and Neck Surgery, 141*(6), 762-769.

Solomon, N. P., Garlitz, S. J., & Milbrath, R. L. (2000). Respiratory and laryngeal contributions to maximum phonation duration. *Journal of Voice, 14*, 331-340.

Soman, B. (1997). The effect of variations in method of elicitation on maximum phoneme duration. *Journal of Voice, 11*, 285-294.

Sorensen, D. N., & Parker P. A. (1992). The voiced or voiceless phonation time in children with and without laryngeal pathology. *Language, Speech and Hearing Services in Schools, 23*, 163-168.

Speyer, R., Bogaardt, H. C. A., Passos, V. L., Roodenburg, N., Zumach, A., Heijnen, M. A. M., . . . Brunings, J. W. (2010). Maximum phonation time: Variability and reliability. *Journal of Voice, 24*(3), 281-284.

Stone, R. E. (1983). Issues in clinical assessment of laryngeal function: Contraindications for subscribing to maximum phonation time and optimum fundamental frequency. In D. M. Bless & J. H. Abbs (Eds.), *Vocal fold physiology: Contemporary research and clinical issues* (pp. 410-424). San Diego, CA: College-Hill.

Tait, N. A., Michel, J. F., & Carpenter, M. A. (1980). Maximum duration of sustained /s/ and /z/ in children. *Journal of Speech and Hearing Disorders, 45*, 239-246.

Treole, K., & Trudeau, M. D. (1997). Changes in sustained production tasks among women with bilateral vocal nodules before and after voice therapy. *Journal of Voice, 11*, 462-469.

Xu, W., Han, D., Hou, L., Hu, R., & Wang, L. (2009). Clinical and electrophysiological characteristics of larynx in myasthenia gravis. *Annals of Otology, Rhinology, and Laryngology, 118*(9), 656-661.

Yanagihara, N., & Koike, Y. (1967). The regulation of sustained phonation. *Folia Phoniatrica, 19*, 1-18.

Yanagihara, N., & von Leden, H. (1967). Respiration and phonation: The functional examination of laryngeal disease. *Folia Phoniatrica, 19*, 153-166.

Yu, P., Ouaknine, M., Revis, J., & Giovanni, A. (2001). Objective voice analysis for dysphonic patients: A multiparametric protocol including acoustic and aerodynamic measurements. *Journal of Voice, 15*, 529-542.

SECTION II

Vocal Fold Movements

CHAPTER 7

Stroboscopy in the Clinical Setting: Sweden Perspective

PER-ÅKE LINDESTAD

PURPOSES

The overall purpose of the examination is to get a plausible explanation for the cause of voice problem. Stroboscopy aims to:

- Obtain a sharp image of the vocal fold edges during phonation.
- Assess the presence and the extent of vocal fold lesion.
- Judge the degree of closure, localization of an insufficiency or to estimate the time that the vocal folds are closed and open respectively.
- Study phase differences in anteroposterior direction as well as side differences in vibration amplitude.

THEORETICAL BACKGROUND

Vocal Fold Vibrations

The membranous portion of the vocal folds vibrates with a certain *amplitude*, which is the difference between maxi-

mum lateral extent of the vibration and the maximum closure. When the vocal fold edges are in the closing phase during vibration, the lower part of the edges will get in contact first, before the middle, and finally the superior part of the edges. During the moment of closure, a deformation of the superficial layers of the fold is created. This will travel cranially and laterally across the upper surface of the vocal fold. Each normal vibratory cycle creates such a *mucosal wave* (Hirano, 1974; Smith, 1954; Sundberg, 1987). The mucosal wave as well as the amplitude and the closure of the vocal folds during vibration can be studied with stroboscopy (Hirano, 1981; Kitzing, 1985; Schönhärl, 1960). It is important to know that normal variation in the voice source will create changes in mucosal wave, amplitude, and closure of the vocal folds. For example, with increasing phonatory pitch, both the amplitude and the mucosal wave will decrease and the closed time in the vibratory cycle will get shorter (Hirano, 1974; Smith, 1954). Females usually have a small posterior glottic chink even at comfortable phonatory pitch, whereas males as a rule have complete glottal closure during the same conditions (Hirano & Bless, 1993; Södersten, 1994). The findings also vary with vocal registers. In falsetto phonation, the closure is short or absent, with the mucosal wave and the amplitude much less pronounced compared to modal register (Lindestad & Södersten, 1987). However, falsetto phonation sometimes can be quite useful for diagnostic purposes, which are described in the following sections.

Why Stroboscopy?

Stroboscopy is a very common clinical tool in the practice of an otolaryngologist. Although it is a very useful tool in the diagnostic work, not all otolaryngologists are familiar enough with the technique to be able to perform an examination. This could be because it takes a significant number of examinations to master the technique and be able to interpret the results. Moreover, it is much easier to perform strobos-

copy if an examiner has a sensitive ear, some musical talent, or at least is a good voice user. This is because it is a definite advantage if the examiner can elicit good phonation from the patient with the examiner's own voice as prompts. This helps to facilitate the production of the patient's voice through conscious or unconscious mirroring.

There are some obvious advantages that make stroboscopy invaluable for the voice clinician:

1. Sharp images of abducted vocal fold edges are visualized best during breathing. During phonatory adduction, the contour of the vocal fold edges will be blurred and diffuse because the folds are vibrating with a certain amplitude. With the use of stroboscopy, the vocal fold edges will appear sharp also during phonation. Any pathology on the vocal fold, such as a polyp, an edema, or nodules also will appear with much greater clarity, enabling the examiner to see its anterior and posterior borders.

2. The mechanical or elastic properties of the vocal folds as such or of any lesion on them can be estimated using stroboscopy. This may give an indication if mass lesions like polyps or nodules are likely to heal with conservative therapy or will require surgery. Although there is no scientific evidence for such a statement, in the author's experience, a lesion that is changing shape during the vibration and even, as is sometimes the case, almost is assimilated or "disappears" in the mucosal wave during the closed phase is more likely to be resolved by the tissue over time than a lesion that retains its shape.

3. Vocal fold closure can be estimated during laryngoscopic examination without stroboscopy, but to judge the degree of closure, to locate an insufficiency, and/or to estimate the time that the vocal folds are closed and open, respectively, one needs the stroboscopic image. Even with stroboscopy, this kind of estimation is more difficult than with methods such as videokymography or high-speed imaging (Larsson, Hertegard, Lindestad, & Hammarberg, 2000; Svec & Schutte, 1996).

4. Vibratory regularity cannot be judged directly with stroboscopy. However, if the voice is rough and irregular, the microphone signal will not be able to trigger a regular series of light flashes from the light source and no vocal fold vibrations will be depicted. From this finding, one can infer that the voice is irregular. It is not possible to observe how the vocal folds vibrate with different frequency between the sides but it is possible to study phase differences in anteroposterior direction and side differences in amplitude.

DESCRIPTION

The sound signal during phonation (or actually the vibrations of air in the pharynx) is picked up with the help of a neck microphone and fed into the light source. In addition, some stroboscopes are equipped with a microphone for airborne sound that can be used as an option if the local anatomy on the neck makes it difficult to achieve good triggering with the contact microphone. It is tricky to use the air microphone because it also will pick up the sound from the examiner's

voice. As the examiner gives continuous instructions, this may be a problem. The light source in turn emits flashes that are used to illuminate the vibrating vocal folds. By varying the degree of delay of the light flashes, one gets a visual illusion of slowly vibrating vocal folds. When the fundamental frequency of the vibration is too irregular, the stroboscopic images will appear as random fluttering such that neither the amplitude, the closure nor the mucosal wave can be assessed.

EQUIPMENT AND MATERIALS

Stroboscopy can be performed with one of the three principally different ways of laryngoscopic examination in a patient.

■ *Nasolaryngoscopy* with a flexible fiberoptic endoscope is perhaps the easiest and most widely used technique (Figures 7-1 and 7-2). The most modern instruments today are not even fiberscopes but videoscopes that look like fiberscopes and with part of the camera system placed at the tip of the instrument, which allows for much better resolution in the images. Videoscopes cannot be used other than with video systems. Thus, it is not possible to look with your eye directly in the instrument as in the case of fiberscope. In all other respects, the examination routine in the clinic will be the same as when a fiberscope is used. Fiberscopes and videoscopes are provided by a wide range of firms. The availability of the products differ a bit over the world but the most common are Olympus, Wolf, Storz, Atmos, Nagashima, and KayPENTAX.

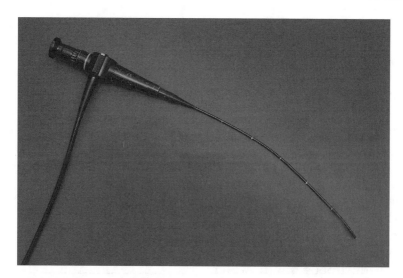

Figure 7–1. Flexible fiberscope.

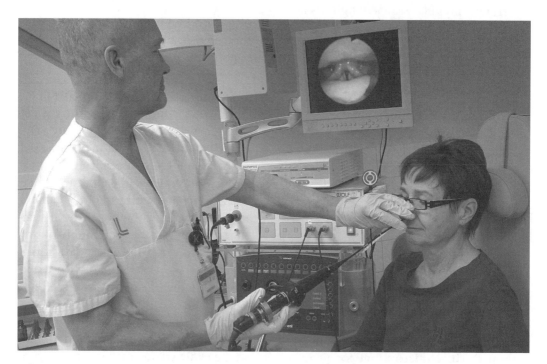

Figure 7–2. Flexible endoscopy.

■ *Rigid endoscopes* are light conductors with a 70- or 90-degree angle mirror at the tip (Figures 7-3, 7-4, and 7-5). These are introduced through the mouth to the back of the pharynx. Light is reflected to the vocal fold level and reflected back through the scope to the eye of the examiner or the attached

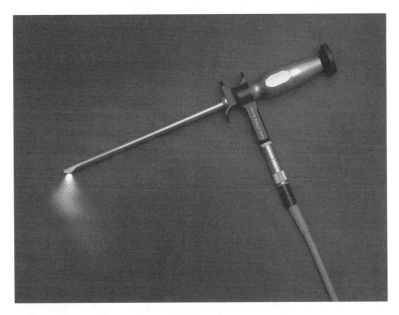

Figure 7–3. 70-degree rigid endoscope.

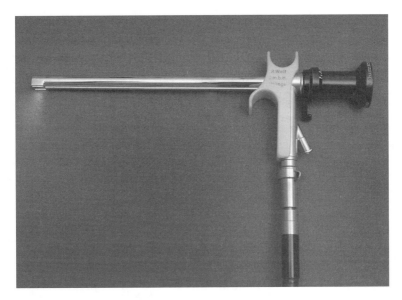

Figure 7–4. 90-degree rigid endoscope.

video camera. Different brands of rigid scopes are available, the most popular in Europe being Storz and Wolf, but they all work similarly and are discussed as one and the same in the following.

■ A *microscope* like the one usually used for ear examination can be used for 3D stroboscopic examination (Figure 7–6). The focal distance has to be adjusted from 20 to 25 cm (used for

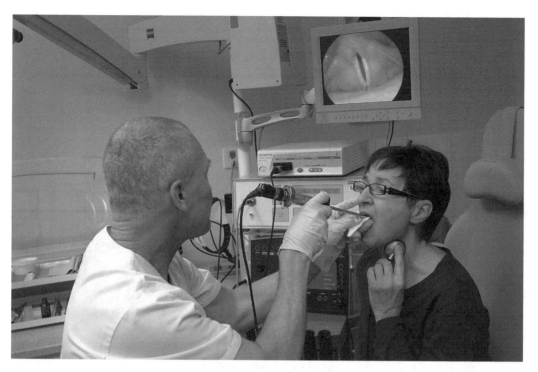

Figure 7–5. Rigid endoscopy with 70-degree endoscope.

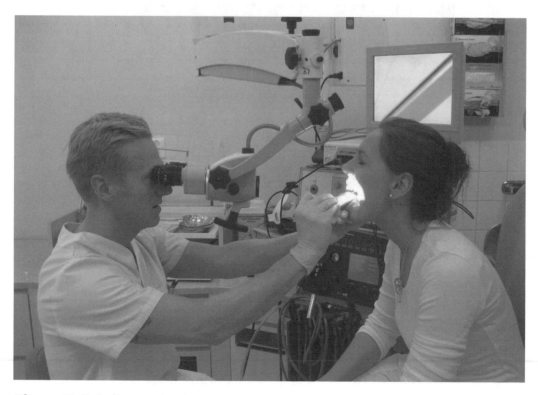

Figure 7–6. Indirect microlaryngoscopy requires a lens that uses 35- to 40-mm focal distance and gives a three-dimensional image.

the ear) to 35 to 40 cm. Then the light of the microscope is shed on an ordinary laryngeal mirror. This technique requires more practice than nasolaryngoscopy and rigid endoscopy but it gives a fascinating resolution and a three dimensional image of the vocal folds. Indirect microlaryngoscopy is not very common today and is not commented on further in this chapter.

Both nasofiberscopy and rigid laryngoscopy can easily be combined with video equipment for documentation. This has in fact become a valuable diagnostic tool because it allows: (1) for comparisons over time and (2) for consulting other colleagues at a later time without the patient present. Moreover, video recordings of laryngeal examinations have become a useful tool for the education of any student in the field. It takes some time to get used to looking at a video screen during examination instead of looking directly through the endoscope. Otherwise, the only disadvantage seems to be a slightly lower resolution of the image. There are many different video recording systems around and the best way to handle this fact is to test systematically which one suits the examiner best.

TEST PROCEDURES

Stroboscopy requires good cooperation from the patient; hence, thorough information about what is going to take place is essential for a successful examination. The patient deserves to know about the inconveniences of the examination as well as what is required from him or her in terms of cooperation. In fact, it is necessary if one wants to achieve good results. There-

fore, a good routine for patient information is most important. The way of instructing the patient differs somewhat between fiberscopy and rigid endoscopy. A common feature is that the importance of the neck microphone has to be explained. The patient should be shown how it should be applied tightly on the neck and told that it must stay in place during the whole examination (Figure 7–7). For both fiberscopy and rigid endoscopy, it is crucial that the patient's body position is upright with the torso slightly leaning forward with the cheek in front of the body axis. This adjustment has to be done before examination starts. Phonations most suitable for stroboscopy are prolonged /i/ sounds. This is because the larynx is elevated and the epiglottis tilted forward during production of this vowel.

Nasolaryngoscopy

Although most people do not find flexible endoscopy difficult to endure, some individuals find even the thought of someone putting an instrument through their nose almost unbearable. It is important to show

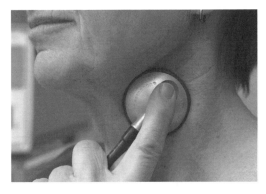

Figure 7–7. Correct placement and grip of the contact microphone during stroboscopy.

patients the instrument and demonstrate how it is handled, describe how far it is going to be inserted, and so on. Before the examination starts, a simple direct nasendoscopy with a speculum should be performed. Any problems with nose bleeds on one side or the other should be identified. Otherwise, what can be seen in terms of narrow passages deviations or spines will decide which nostril to choose. However, if the nostrils seem to be equally good and it is known on beforehand which vocal fold has a lesion, it may be advantageous to choose the nostril opposite to the lesion to get a better angle when the vocal folds are approached. Topical anesthesia with spray and/or lubricant in the nose is recommended. This also requires explanation to the patients as to why this is applied. Inform the patient that the spray will spread to the tongue and pharynx to some extent and may cause some discomfort. Tell the patient to breathe calmly through the nose throughout the examination unless other direct instructions are given. Once the tip of the instrument has been introduced in the pharynx, the real stroboscopy can start.

The instructions given before and during a typical examination could be as follows:

Instructions: *"I'm going to have a look at your vocal folds while they are producing sound. This little device is basically a microphone that you should hold firm and tight to your neck here at the level just above the vocal folds. Please do not press the microphone hard because then everything may dislocate inside and it may also hamper your voice. The microphone picks up the sound from your voice and transfers that to this light source on the table. This in turn gives twinkling light that enables me to see how the vibrating folds work. Try to remember to hold it in place at all times during the examination. (Patient phonates and the triggering is tested as well as the position of the microphone.) This narrow instrument is going to pass gently through your nose cavity and into the pharynx (showing the fiberoptic). You will feel some discomfort during the passage but once we're in place you won't feel very much. Most people tend to produce too short phonations so some time during the examination I may ask you to take a deep breath and to sustain a vowel /i/ for as long as you can. Now please sit in an upright position with you back straight and lean forward toward me (I usually grip the shoulders of the patient and show physically what I mean). Now hold out your cheek a bit and lift the nose. That's the perfect position. During the examination, if you think it is unpleasant you might pull your head and maybe also the body back. Then I will remind you to reposition to this posture. Remember that I can see all the time where the instrument is positioned and even if there is some discomfort I will not harm you!"*

Rigid Endoscopy

Before the examination starts, inform the patient that you are going to hold the tongue during the examination. Also explain that you will ask for a phonation as close to /i:/ as possible but that this will be impossible to perform with the mouth open and the tongue out. Otherwise the patient will stop the examination and tell you. Instead of an /i/, the patient invariably will produce a neutral sound, but the more intensely he thinks of an /i/ the more the epiglottis will tilt forward in favor of a good insight in the larynx. It is seldom necessary to pull on the tongue, but you hold on to it gently to keep it from slipping back into the mouth. This is what you should tell the patient to avoid unnecessary worries. If you let the patient stretch the tongue out maximally and then take your grip and pull, this will hurt and the patient will not be able to endure the intended voice examination. Your examination will be interrupted by rightful complaints.

Instructions: (***Note:*** About stroboscopy in general and microphone, see instructions for fiberoptic examination above.) *"This metal instrument is actually a mirror that I will place in your mouth over the tongue to view the vocal folds. It is by no means going all the way down in the throat (which is what the patient immediately suspects). While doing this, I will ask you to keep your mouth open and to phonate with as steady voice as possible, imitating my voice. I will ask you to stretch your tongue out and I will hold on to it to prevent you from pulling it back, I will not pull on it hard. Now, let's test once without the instrument. Please stretch your tongue out, I hold on to it, now phonate. Did it feel OK? Well, the rest of the examination should not be much worse, because if I do this properly, you won't feel much of the instrument. Most people tend to produce too short phonations so some time during the examination I may ask you to take a deep breath and to sustain a tone /i/ for as long as you can. Now sit in an upright position with you back*

straight and lean forward toward me (I usually grip the shoulders of the patient and show physically what I mean). *Now hold out your cheek a bit. That's the perfect position. During the examination, if you think it is unpleasant you might pull your head and perhaps also the body back. Then I will remind you to reposition to this posture. Remember that I see all the time where the instrument is positioned and even if there is some discomfort I will not harm you!"*

If the patient has sensitive gag reflexes it often is worthwhile to try to introduce the endoscope in the pharynx during sustained phonation and then ask the patient to breathe for a second to see the larynx at rest. The first stroboscopic sequence can be recorded during that introductory phonation. Ask the patient to phonate a note as long as possible and then breathe in for you to inspect the vocal fold edges during abduction. Sometimes you will need to apply a topical anesthetic to the pharynx to be able to perform rigid laryngoscopy. Beware that this may even increase the tendency to gag. The patient must be informed that anesthesia is going to be used in case there is risk for allergic reactions.

REMARKS ON ERGONOMICS

Because the clinician may perform 10 to 15 examinations or more in a day, it is important to use a technique that saves energy and that does not cause problems like back or shoulder pain. It is important for the patient's as well as the examiner's chair to be adjustable in height. In the case of fiberoptic examination, the instrument should come from a position lower than the nose and with the 70-degree rigid scope, the angle must be from above. Figure 7–5 shows the proper examiner's position sitting down performing rigid endoscopy. For some patients, it is preferable to do the examination in a standing posture. This is definitely the case during fiberoptic examination. Many examiners prefer to have the lever for bending the tip of the instrument so that it is placed on the upper side and to work it with the index finger. The author prefers to hold it with the handle facing down and to work it with the third finger which allows for a very comfortable arm position and less muscular problems. The camera head rests on the wrist (see Figure 7–2).

PRECAUTIONS, TRICKS, AND PITFALLS

As stated above all results are dependent on the instructions and on how well the examiner can cooperate with the patient. All examinations start with a simple perceptual voice quality assessment to find out what to expect during the laryngoscopy. An estimation of the habitual pitch is useful. At least part of the examinations should be performed on phonations at or close to habitual pitch. From there, variation in pitch and intensity during examination often give useful information. Much can be said about stroboscopy of different vocal fold lesions such as nodules, cysts, or pareses and this is touched on below. The following sections list the tricks and pitfalls concentrating on certain general phenomena that may occur during examination. Video clips demonstrating various techniques are available at the Web site http://www.hku.hk/speech/voice-handbook.

Nasolaryngoscopy

Rotation or Obliqueness in the Image

1. Camera is rotated or the fiberscope is not held right in front of the nose. If the fiberscope is bent sideways there will be a rotation of the scope itself that will cause a rotation in the image or at least an excentric image.
2. The patient turns his or her head. This will rotate the posterior opening of the nasal passage to the other side, thus moving the tip of the fiberscope in an oblique angle to the larynx. Adjusting the head will solve the problem.
3. The patient presses microphone too hard on the neck, dislocating the larynx.
4. An otherwise straight image becomes rotated during phonation. This is most often due to the action of the velum which lifts and dislocates the fiberoptic instrument to the lateral aspect of the nasopharynx. This problem is easily solved by having the patient phonate on a nasal sound during which the velum will drop. The easiest way is to use closed lips and say /m/.

Problems to Get Close Enough to See Details

This is a problem inherent with the fiberoptic technique. If the tip of the fiberscope goes past the tip of the epiglottis during silent breathing, the result often will be a gag reflex as it may be difficult to avoid contact with the epiglottis. However, it is much easier to get close to the vocal folds during phonation. The trick is to assume a resting position for the scope just above the tip of the epiglottis and then approach the vocal folds to get a close up as the phonation starts, and to withdraw before phonation ends.

Triggering Problems

Sometimes the voice signal does not elicit regular light flashes from the stroboscope. The most common cause is that the microphone is held in the wrong place or is not in full contact with the skin of the neck. Patients often concentrate so heavily on what is happening in the mouth or nose that they forget to hold the microphone tight. Figure 7–7 shows the correct placement and grip of the microphone whereas Figure 7–8 shows incorrect placements and grips. If the voice signal is too weak or irregular, the examiner has to manipulate a bit with the voice. Asking the patient to phonate with closed lips often works. The resulting nasalization elongates the resonating tube (adds the nose), which stabilizes phonation. Another way is to have the patient phonate on a voiced fricative sound like /z/.

Ventricular Fold Adduction

Often, when the vocal folds have some difficulty in vibrating, compensatory ventricular fold adduction may close the view of the vocal folds. It may be possible to avoid this by nasalizing or using voiced fricative sounds. If this does not work, pitch manipulation may help. Often, if one tries a higher phonatory pitch, the laryngeal inlet will open as the vocal folds are elongated, especially if there was an element of anteroposterior narrowing present.

Arytenoids in the Way for a Good View of the Posterior Parts of the Glottis

In children, this can be a problem. The key is that the instrument "looks at" the larynx too much from behind. Some fiberoptic instruments are so stiff that they do not follow the curvature of the velum entering the pharynx in the free space, but rather are pressed against the posterior pharyngeal wall, which makes the angle to the larynx unfavorable. Aside from choosing a soft and pliable instrument for examination, some maneuvers can be tested. First, check that the patient really is sitting with the head extended forward in front of the body. This moves the nose forward and makes the angle better. Second, to avoid contact with the epiglottis and to tip the larynx forward, the vowel /i/ is most often used. In this situation, however, it may work to make a compromise and have the patient phonate a more open vowel like /æ/ for the stroboscopy. This will tilt the larynx a bit more backward and thus possibly move the arytenoids out of the

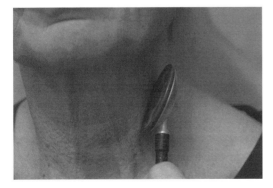
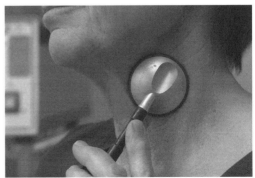

Figure 7–8. Incorrect grip and positioning of the contact microphone.

way a little bit. In this case, a higher pitch also may help.

Irregular Voice

Hoarseness is the result of irregular vocal fold vibration. On the other hand, stroboscopy is not very useful if the signal is irregular, which means that any examiner has to work hard to make the patient phonate with regular or smooth voice during examination. Phonation with closed lips and the use of voiced fricatives were mentioned above. Soft, breathy phonation or variation in pitch often works.

Pain in the Nose

The most common reason for nose pain is that the instrument presses on the bony part of the septum or the bottom of the nose, less often the chonchae. This in turn is caused mostly by a rotation or "twisted" bent position of the scope in the nose. The solution is make sure that the fiberscope is held in a straight line in front of the nostril, not to the side, and furthermore that the hand that holds the instrument is placed lower than the nose (see Figure 7–2). A similar situation may arise if the hand that holds the instrument is too high. It is practical to use the middle meatus for the entry of the fiberscope, unless the anatomy is abnormal. This way, the angle for the view of the epipharynx gets better and it is neither better nor worse for laryngeal examination. The same kind of problems with pain arises if the patient places the head in an awkward position, rotated or bent backward. Gentle repositioning will solve the problem.

Rigid Endoscopy

Compared to fiberoptic examination, examination with the rigid endoscope is more difficult both for the patient and the examiner. However, with a good technique and some training, it really gives good value for the work in terms of higher resolution and hence a detailed image.

Epiglottis Is in the Way of a Good View of the Folds

Body position may have to be adjusted, the torso leaning slightly forward, chin out. The patient should be instructed to think of an /i/ during phonation. This may be difficult to achieve so it is necessary for the examiner to be persistent with this instruction.

Triggering Problems

The strobe will not produce regular light flashes. The microphone may have to be adjusted. A contact microphone works best if the whole surface is in contact with the neck. If the microphone is correctly adjusted, it often works to ask the patient to try to close the lips on the endoscope during phonation, which results in a nasal tone. One would think that this is impossible when the patient has an open mouth and the tongue is stretched out. What happens when the patient tries to close the mouth is that the resonating tube is elongated as the velum is lowered and thus the nose is added to the resonating cavities. This results in a more stable voice production. It also may be helpful to ask the patient to start phonation in a breathy sighlike manner and then increase the intensity.

Lively Gag Reflexes Can Make Rigid Endoscopy Difficult

This can be solved by a short training session with the patient who is instructed to phonate while the examiner pulls the tongue without any instrument in the mouth. The procedure is then repeated while the laryngoscope is inserted during phonation. Sometimes it is indeed possible for the patient to tolerate the instrument better once it is in place. It is always necessary to hold the endoscope firmly with a steady hand. Waving the tip of the instrument around in the throat easily elicits a gag reflex.

GENERAL REMARK ON LESIONS ON THE LOW EDGE OF THE FOLDS

If a lesion below the edge of either vocal fold is suspected, one might instruct the patient to deliberately produce a very breathy sound at low pitch. The vocal fold edges close from below during phonation seen in the frontal plane and when they are seen from above, as is the case during laryngoscopy. What can be seen at the medial edge when closure starts is actually the lower surface of the fold. With breathy phonation, the amplitude increases and this movement is exaggerated. Thus, the lesions on the lower border such as edemas or cysts present themselves nicely.

REMARKS AND ADVICE CONCERNING SPECIFIC DIAGNOSES

Functional Voice Disorders

Patients with functional voice disorders essentially have normal vocal folds but a functional disturbance causing hoarseness, vocal fatigue, or symptoms of vocal tension. To be successful with the stro-

boscopic evaluation, one must be aware that the endoscopic examination may compromise voice function even more. Therefore, most of the time it is easiest to use the fiberoptic rather than the rigid endoscope. The goal must be to help the patient relax and phonate close to habitual pitch. If hyperfunctional phonation is a problem, relaxation is best achieved by phonation with closed lips or in a lax sigh-like manner.

Vocal Fold Nodules, Marginal Edemas, and Reinke Edema

In these patient groups, stroboscopy is mainly a tool for evaluation of the mechanical properties of the lesion. Generally, one can say that, when nodules or edemas are soft and pliable and it is possible to have the patient phonate with well-supported and stable voice, the lesion often is incorporated in the mucosal wave in a way that the vibrations become almost normal. If the lesions are more solid and elastic or even hard, they will not change their shape during vibration and therefore affect both glottal closure, mucosal wave, and vibratory amplitude much more than the soft lesions. In the author's subjective view, soft lesions that change shape during phonation are more likely to diminish and be resolved over time with conservative treatment than solid lesions. Thus, stroboscopy can be used as a prognostic evaluation and guide the examiner concerning the need for surgery. A Reinke edema sometimes becomes organized with fibrous degeneration of the tissue. In such a case, the vocal folds may become stiff and it will be difficult to achieve regular vocal fold vibration that will trigger a good stroboscopy. It usually is possible to evaluate if portions of the folds have a softer consistency. Stroboscopy also is a valuable tool when it comes to differential diagnosis between nodules, polyps, and cysts, partly because it is possible to see and judge features of the surface of the lesion in detail and partly because of differences in vibratory findings (see sections on polyps and cysts).

Polyps

For small polyps, the use of stroboscopy has many similarities to that for nodules and edemas, especially concerning softness and pliability. It is unusual for a polyp to become totally integrated in the mucosal wave during vibration. Most of the time, it is more like a little boat that sits on the vocal fold surface. To disclose a little polypoid lesion on the lower margin of the fold, it is most useful to try to have the patient phonate in a breathy manner at low pitch, which will create a large vibratory amplitude. The lesion will be seen best during the closing phase when the vocal fold edges are approaching each other from below. Bigger polyps often interfere considerably with vocal fold closure and vibration amplitude because of their volume and also increase vocal fold mass and decrease elasticity.

Sulci

When there is a longitudinal thinning of the superficial layer of the vocal fold, it may indicate a vocal fold sulcus. Sometimes the sulcus forms a pocketlike excavation (Bouchayer, Cornut, Loire, Roch, Witzig, & Bastian, 1985). For discussions about the origin and the treatment of sulcus, see textbooks on voice disorders (e.g., Merati & Bielamowicz, 2007). In stroboscopy, there will be a decreased amplitude

and mucosal wave on the affected side. Moreover, phonation almost invariably results in a spindle-shaped glottal insufficiency and a breathy voice character. A sulcus may be difficult to detect and as the rigid endoscope gives a better resolution of the image, it is more likely that rigid endoscopy will reveal the lesion. However, it is not impossible with the fiberoptic (Lindestad, 1994). It is necessary to get close to the vocal fold edges during phonation as described in previous sections.

Cysts

Cysts are common in the larynx, more so in the supraglottal parts than in the true vocal folds. The cysts in the true vocal folds are of two principally different kinds, inclusion cysts probably derived from small glands, and epidermal cysts that are probably inborn. These two kinds of cysts cannot be distinguished by stroboscopy with any certainty although it seems that the epidermal type often sits deeper in the superficial layer, sometimes partly affecting also the ligament. During stroboscopy, the structure of the cyst wall will appear more clearly than with white light. The affected vocal fold will vibrate with a decreased mucosal wave and a decreased amplitude and the cyst will behave like a reef in the water surface, the mucosal wave often passing by on each side (Bouchayer et al., 1985).

Chronic Laryngitis and Cancer

This is the clinical area in which stroboscopy probably is most invaluable. In chronic laryngitis, generally there is an increased thickness of the superficial layer of the lamina propria but if there is a free movement of the surface in relation to the underlying ligament the mucosal wave is only decreased to a minor degree. Even superficial keratosis of the epithelium will cause minor changes in the mucosal wave. A thicker keratosis may affect closure and vibration in the same way as a polyp would. When there is an epithelial lesion that becomes infiltrating and connects the epithelium with the ligament across the superficial lamina propria, the mucosal wave will be severely affected as will the amplitude of vibration. Thus, stroboscopy allows for early detection of infiltrative growth of glottal cancer. A larger cancer is always hard, solid, and nonvibrating (Hirano, 1981; Merati & Bielamowicz, 2007; Schönhärl, 1960).

Aging Voice, Spindle-Shaped Insufficiency, and Glottal Atrophy (Bowing)

The most common finding in individuals with a voice disorder due to aging is an insufficient vocal fold closure, most often a spindle-shaped glottal insufficiency. The reason for this may be vocal fold atrophy of the mucosa, the vocal muscle, or both, but quite often vocal inactivity in the elderly may lead to weakness in the thyroarytenoid muscles or problems with muscle activation. Voice tremor is another rather common symptom, especially in elderly females (Ramig et al., 2001).

During examination, most often performed with fiberoptic instruments, the examiner may try to manipulate the patient's breathy and unstable voice to achieve vocal fold vibrations regular enough to produce a regular stroboscopic image. It often is possible to improve vocal fold closure and vocal timbre during laryngos-copy by the use of phonation with closed lips or a narrowed vocal tract at the mouth opening using voiced fricative sounds. If the vocal fold vibrations indeed get much better during this procedure, it may indicate that the voice disorder is functional to a significant extent and thus possible to change with behavioral therapy. If the vocal folds appear atrophic and there is no way to achieve even a short closure, it may be wise to discuss some surgical procedures to help the patient.

Voice tremor causes a fluctuation in fundamental frequency that follows the tremor. This causes problems with the triggering of the stroboscopic light flashes as there is no stable phonatory pitch but rather a constant change in pitch. Sometimes exaggerated breathy phonation or the use of voiced fricative sounds may stabilize the phonation enough to solve the problem for a few seconds.

Vocal Fold Paresis

In vocal fold paresis, the voice disorder may vary a lot between individuals. The degree of possible vocal fold closure is determined by the abductory and adductory movements on the paretic side and the extent of compensatory adduction on the unaffected side. Moreover, the quality of vocal fold vibrations in terms of amplitude, mucosal wave and regularity is dependent on the bulk and tone of the affected vocal muscle. Thus, during the clinical course of the paresis, gradual reinnervation of the vocal muscle most often takes place. While a denervated fold vibrates with flaccid movements without mucosal wave, a gradual restitution of amplitude and mucosal wave is a reliable sign of reinnervation (Fex, 1970). An important factor during examination is the phonation time, which is often reduced in these patients. Before the actual examination, it is advisable to train the patient to extend sustained phonations for as long as possible. As there is a slight delay between voicing and triggering of the light flashes of the stroboscope, short phonations for may cause problems. Also, as voice production is problematic in the first place, it is difficult for the patient to concentrate on other things than just voicing. Thus, thinking of an /i/, especially if the rigid endoscope is used to allow for better inspection may need extra instructions before the actual laryngoscopy. It often is easy to create stable phonation and optimal vocal fold closure if phonation with closed lips can be produced.

To some extent, the degree of vocal fold closure is dependent on pitch. Also, if one of the vocal folds lacks tone, the voice often becomes unstable or even diplophonic at low fundamental frequencies. In those cases, it may be useful to ask the patient to produce a high-pitched note, which most of the time will allow for stable vibrations. One can still see a difference in vibratory quality between the sides.

CASE STUDY

An actress of 35 years presented with a persistent hoarseness and vocal fatigue of a few months duration. It occurred after a period of intense work in the theater. The referral from a colleague in private practice, who did not use stroboscopy, talked about normal vocal folds at examination. She was a nonsmoker, was well-trained vocally, and did regular workouts at the local gymnasium. The voice was breathy and unstable.

Considering the unstable voice, it might be difficult to examine her with stroboscopy. In examining the mouth, everything looked normal and it seems that there was plenty of room for an endoscopy with the rigid instrument. Before introducing this, you checked for excessive gag reflexes by pulling on the patient's tongue gently while she had her mouth wide open. You also checked that the contact microphone was held in a good place and that light flashes were triggered at phonation. If everything seemed fine, the rigid endoscope was introduced while the patient sat in a position with the torso slightly leaning forward and the head slightly in front of the body, with face lifted. There were no problems viewing the vocal folds from posterior glottis to the anterior commissure. The abductory and adductory movements appeared normal but at phonation, there was a problem as expected. The voice was too unstable and the vibrations apparently were too irregular to achieve regular stroboscopic vibrations that were possible to interpret. By asking the patient to try to close the lips on the instrument, although the tongue was actually pulled by the hand, the patient was able to produce a breathy but smooth and stable phonation at a pitch close to the habitual level. The vocal folds were found to be pale and without signs of irritation. The left fold had a very subtle thickening at the middle of the membranous portion. The vibrations on the right side showed a normal amplitude and mucosal wave, whereas the amplitude was slightly decreased on the left side and the mucosal wave was present anteriorly and posteriorly but significantly decreased at the middle of the membranous portion.

It was suspected that the patient had an intracordal cyst in the left fold so we planned for a direct laryngoscopy in general anesthesia for this patient who was eager to get better fast. Preoperative voice assessment by a speech pathologist also was planned. A cordotomy eventually revealed a small retention cyst in the superficial layer. After cyst removal, the patient was seen 4 weeks later. She now had a stable voice with normal timbre.

Acknowledgments. The pictures in this chapter were produced by Johan Garsten, HS media, Stockholm.

REFERENCES

Bouchayer, M., Cornut, G., Loire, R., Roch, J. B., Witzig, E., & Bastian, R. W. (1985). Epidermoid cysts, sulci, and mucosal bridges of the true vocal cord: A report of 157 cases. *Laryngoscope, 95,* 1087–1094.

Fex, S. (1970). Judging the movements of vocal cords in larynx paralysis. *Acta Oto-Laryngologica (Stockh.), 263,* 82–83.

Hirano, M. (1974). Morphological structure of the vocal cord as a vibrator and its variations. *Folia Phoniatrica, 26,* 89–94.

Hirano, M. (1981). *Clinical examination of voice.* Wien, Germany: Springer-Verlag.

Hirano, M., & Bless, D. M. (1993). *Videostroboscopic examination of the larynx.* San Diego, CA: Singular.

Kitzing, P. (1985). Stroboscopy: A pertinent laryngological examination. *Journal of Otolaryngology, 14,* 151–157.

Larsson, H., Hertegard, S., Lindestad, P. Å., & Hammarberg, B. (2000). Vocal fold vibrations: High-speed video imaging, kymography and acoustic analysis. *Laryngoscope, 110,* 2117–2122.

Lindestad, P. Å. (1994). *Electromyographic and laryngoscopic studies of normal and disturbed voice function.* Doctoral dissertation, Stockholm, Sweden: Karolinska Institute.

Lindestad, P. Å., & Södersten, M. (1987). Vocal fold vibrations in counter tenor singing. *Acta Phoniatrica Latina, 18*(Suppl.), 19–22.

Merati, A. L., & Bielamowicz, S. A. (2007). *Textbook of voice disorders.* San Diego, CA, Plural Publishing. (pp. 37–57).

Ramig, L. O., Gray, S., Baker, K., Corbin-Lewis, K., Buder, E., Luschei, E., ... Smith, M. (2001). The aging voice: A review, treatment data and familial and genetic perspectives. *Folia Phoniatrica et Logopedica, 53,* 252–265.

Schönhärl, E. (1960). *Die Stroboskopie in der praktischen Laryngologie.* Stuttgart, Germany: Georg Thieme-Verlag.

Smith, S. (1954). Remarks on the physiology of the vibrations of the vocal cords. *Folia Phoniatrica, 6,* 166–178.

Södersten, M. (1994). *Vocal fold closure during phonation: Physiological, perceptual and acoustical studies.* Dissertation, Stockholm, Sweden: Karolinska Institute.

Sundberg, J. (1987). *The science of the singing voice.* DeKalb, IL: Northern Illinois University Press.

Svec, J. G., & Schutte, H. K. (1996). Videokymography: High-speed scanning of vocal fold vibration. *Journal of Voice, 10,* 201–205.

Titze, I. R. (1994). *Principles of voice production.* Englewood Cliffs, NJ: Prentice-Hall.

CHAPTER 8

Videostroboscopy: USA Perspective

VYVY N. YOUNG AND CLARK A. ROSEN

PURPOSES

- To provide the clinician with a detailed view of vocal fold structure, especially during vibration.
- To provide the clinician with information on a variety of aspects of the vocal folds including closure pattern and duration, as well as vocal fold tension, tone, and mucosal pliability.
- To provide the clinician with vital information on the nature and degree of vocal pathology, especially structural and neurogenic pathology, as it pertains to the client's vocal fold-related dysphonia.

THEORETICAL BACKGROUND

Production of the human voice is a complex phenomenon, dependent not only on the inherent characteristics of the vocal folds but also on a host of aspects involving the entire vocal tract, the respiratory system, and the upper aerodigestive tract (Postma, Courey & Ossoff, 2005). Knowledge of how voice production occurs is essential to evaluating the nature of a voice disorder. A thorough review of normal vocal fold physiology is beyond the scope of this chapter. Briefly, the production of voice depends fundamentally on the vibration of the vocal folds. In the prephonatory phase, the vocal folds adduct and the glottis (space between the vocal folds) is closed or nearly closed. Subglottic pressure then builds beneath the adducted vocal folds due to air expired from the lungs via the bronchi and trachea. When the pressure is sufficiently high, the vocal folds are pushed apart, from an inferior to superior direction, releasing air into the vocal tract. The now decreased subglottic pressure then contributes to the vocal folds coming to a closed or near-closed position again due to the Bernoulli effect. Subglottic pressure again increases due to persistent tracheal airflow and vocal fold adduction, and the cycle repeats (Duflo & Thibeault, 2007; Woo & Yanagisawa, 2003). A single sequence of vocal fold closure, opening and then closing again, is called a vibratory cycle.

The human vocal folds vibrate at rates of 100 to 300 times per second during normal conversational speech (Connor & Bless, 2007), although rates of 60 to 1500 times per second have been reported (Kaszuba & Garret, 2007). Vocal fold vibration occurs too quickly to be seen with the naked eye, as the retina cannot distinguish more than five distinct images per second (as described by Talbot's law). When presented with more than five images per second, the eye perceives an apparent smooth and fluid motion (Carroll, Nunez, & Rosen, 2008; Kaszuba & Garret, 2007; Postma et al., 2005).

Stroboscopy utilizes flashes of light to take snapshot images of various aspects of many vocal fold vibratory cycles. When more than five images are presented to the eye, these images are then streamed together to give the illusion of a "single" cycle, shown in "slow motion." Although each individual image originates from a different vibratory cycle, stroboscopy pieces these images together to provide a "moving montage" or representation of the client's glottic cycle. This technique essentially tricks the eye into "seeing" slow motion of the vocal folds vibrating. In reality, no one vibratory cycle is ever visualized in its

entirety by stroboscopy (Carroll et al., 2008; Connor & Bless, 2007; Postma et al., 2005; Samlan, Gartner-Schmidt, & Kunduk, 2010). The subsequent "pseudo-slow motion" video of the vocal fold vibrations allows the reviewer to evaluate the vocal folds, specifically tension, tone, closure pattern, duration of closure, and the mucosal wave and its pliability, during vibration. High-speed laryngoscopy, which is described in Chapter 12, can provide real slow-motion pictures of a single vibratory cycle.

EQUIPMENT AND MATERIALS

To perform stroboscopy, the following equipment is required:

■ A vocal fold vibration source trigger (either a microphone or electro-glottograph).
■ Endoscope (either flexible or rigid).
■ A light source.
■ Videostroboscopy requires the addition of a camera and video monitor with recording system. (**Note:** Recording of videostroboscopic examinations for review and comparison is an indispensable tool in the management of voice patients, especially in the long term.)

Several stroboscopic systems are available. These include KayPENTAX Model 9295 (KayPENTAX, Lincoln Park, NJ), StroboCAM® II (JedMed, St. Louis, MO), ATMOS Endo-stroboscope-L (ATMOS MedizinTechnik GmbH & Co., Germany), ENT-5000 Video Endoscopy System (Medtronic ENT, Jacksonville, FL), and STROBE VIEW 5570 (Richard Wolf Medical Instruments Corp., Vernon Hills, IL). The various systems produce the videostroboscopic image via slightly different mechanisms. Each system uses a xenon light source, although the ATMOS system also offers an alternative LED source. Specifications can be found in the Web sites of manufacturers. The KayPENTAX Stroboscope, Model 9100B and the ATMOS Endo-stroboscope-L device provide "pulsed" light timed to vocal fold vibration. In contrast, the StroboCAM (JedMed) utilizes a continuous light source while electronically shuttering the camera to provide the "pulsed" imaging of the vocal folds. Advocates of a "pulsed" light source argue for an improved image quality and clarity, whereas those favoring shuttering from the camera believe that the constant light source on the vocal folds contributes to a better image.

Rigid endoscopes (70-degree or 90-degree) are more commonly used, due to the higher degree of magnification obtained (Connor & Bless, 2007; Heman-Ackah, 2004) as well as improved contrast and availability of various viewing angles (Samlan et al., 2010). A 70-degree endoscope is preferred by most examiners. For flexible endoscopy, newer technology such as distal chip-tip endoscopy provides an improved image over the traditional fiberoptic flexible endoscope The distal chip-tip endoscope utilizes a camera chip at the end of the endoscope to capture images that are then transmitted back electronically, resulting in a higher quality image (Rosen, et al., 2009). Videostroboscopy done via a flexible endoscope can be advantageous in the examination of difficult clients (e.g., client with a strong gag reflex and children). The disadvantages associated with flexible endoscopy are the need for anesthetic spray as well as the lower level of magnification and image resolution (Connor & Bless, 2007).

PROCEDURES

Setting

The examiner should position him- or herself directly in front of, or slightly to the side of the client. The monitor should be positioned for easy viewing by the examiner (Figure 8–1). A second monitor may be used for observation by the client during the examination.

Client Positioning

1. The client should be seated comfortably.
   a. The client should sit back in the chair as far as possible, with legs uncrossed.
   b. The client should then lean forward at the waist, maintaining a straight back.
   c. The hands should be placed on the knees, and the shoulders should be relaxed.
   d. The chin should be protruded forward. This is the so-called "sniffing" position (Figure 8–2).
2. Raise the chair to a level that is comfortable for the examiner, allowing the arms to remain relaxed at the side during the procedure.
3. A liquid defogging agent should be applied to the tip of the rigid endoscope to maintain image clarity. Alternatively, warm water may be used to prevent fogging of the image.

Instructions:
- *"Please uncross your legs."*
- *"Sit with your hips in the back of the chair."*
- *"Lean forward at the waist."*

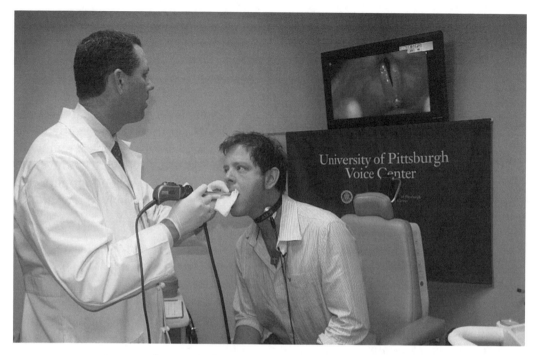

Figure 8–1. Endoscopic procedure.

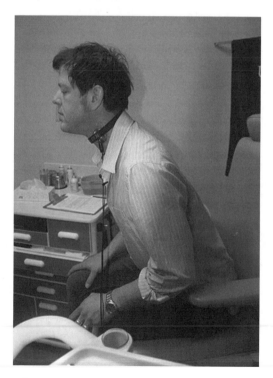

Figure 8–2. Client positioning.

■ *"Put one hand on each knee."*
■ *"Put your chin out."*
■ *"Relax your shoulders."*

Rigid Peroral Videostroboscopy

1. Ask the client to protrude the tongue.
2. The examiner uses a piece of gauze to grasp the anterior portion of the client's tongue between the thumb and index finger of his/her non-dominant hand, with the thumb below the tongue. Gentle traction is applied to maintain the tongue's protruded position throughout the examination. Care should be taken not to squeeze the tongue too tightly or to pull the tongue downward. The latter will cause pain from the ventral surface of the tongue pressing against the lower teeth.

3. The middle through last fingers of the non-dominant hand rest against the client's upper lip and cheek for stability (Figure 8–3).
4. Alternatively, the client's tongue may be grasped between the thumb and middle finger of the examiner's non-dominant hand. The index finger is then placed against the upper lip or in the upper gingivobuccal sulcus for stability (Figure 8–4).
5. An additional alternative is to have the client hold his or her tongue using a piece of gauze. This is best performed

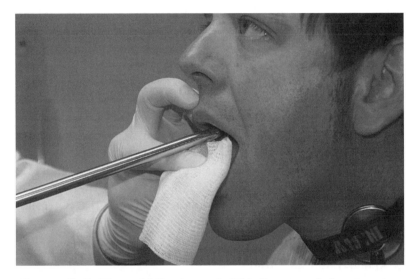

Figure 8–3. The middle through fifth fingers of the examiner's nondominant hand rest against the client's upper lip and cheek for stability.

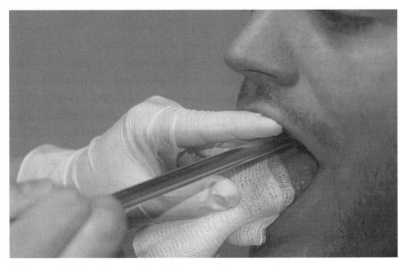

Figure 8–4. Alternative fingers placement.

with only one finger (typically the index finger) on top of the tongue to minimize interference with the examiner's manipulation of the endoscope.

6. A rigid endoscope is then passed perorally. The endoscope should rest on the examiner's finger that is overlying the dorsum of the tongue for stability. Alternatively, the endoscope may be gently braced against the client's maxillary central incisors. It is important to keep the endoscope centered for optimal view of the vocal folds.

7. Phonatory tasks
   - Have the client phonate "ee" (/i/)
     - Evaluate modal pitch, low pitch, and high pitch.
     - Evaluate loud phonation and soft phonation.
     - Ask the client to produce a low-pitched "ee." Glide up to a higher pitch in a single breath. This can be done both from low to high pitch, and from high down to low pitch.

Instructions:
- *"Stick your tongue out."*
- *"Say 'ee.'"*
- *"Say a high-pitched 'ee.'"*
- *"Say a low-pitched 'ee.'"*
- *"Say 'ee' and glide from a low pitch up to a high pitch."*
- *"Say 'ee' and glide from a high pitch down to a low pitch."*

Flexible Transnasal Videostroboscopy

1. Phonatory tasks
   - Have the client phonate "ee"
     - Evaluate modal pitch versus low pitch versus high pitch.
     - Evaluate loud phonation versus soft phonation.

- Ask the client to produce a low-pitched "ee" and then without taking a breath, glide up to a higher pitch. This can be done both from low to high pitch, and from high down to low pitch.

After completion of all tasks, the recorded examination is played back for review and discussion of the findings with the client.

Dynamic Voice Assessment with Flexible Laryngoscopy

A dynamic voice assessment consists of various modifications to the standard flexible laryngoscopic examination, including evaluation during vegetative, speech, and singing activities (Carroll et al., 2008; Roehm & Rosen, 2004).

1. The client's nose should be anesthetized. The choice of anesthetic is based on individual examiner's preference. The authors use a combination of 4% plain topical lidocaine and neosynephrine in a 1 to 1 ratio. The side of the nose used is determined by the client anatomy. Select the most patent nasal passage.

2. The flexible fiberoptic endoscope is then passed through the nasal cavity, nasopharynx, and oropharynx, to allow visualization of the larynx and hypopharynx. Any anatomic or functional abnormalities should be documented (Carroll et al., 2008; Roehm & Rosen, 2004).
   a. Note nasal polyposis or other causes of nasal obstruction, as these may affect the client's resonance.
   b. Note any nasopharyngeal masses, including adenoid hypertrophy.

c. With the endoscope at the level of the posterior choanae, have the client say "coca cola" and "ee" to evaluate velar closure.

d. Examine the base of tongue carefully for evidence of mass, tremor, fasciculations, or pooling of secretions.

e. Have the client perform a Valsalva maneuver to look for pooled secretions or a hypopharyngeal mass. This can be done by producing forcible exhalation with the lips closed (thereby closing the glottis).

3. Inspect the valleculae, piriform sinuses, epiglottis, aryepiglottic folds, false vocal folds, and true vocal folds. Particular attention should be paid to masses or lesions, abnormalities of structures, motion abnormalities, and signs of laryngeal irritation (e.g., laryngopharyngeal reflux) (Belafsky, Postma, & Koufman, 2001; Toohill & Kuhn, 1997).

4. Observe the client during quiet respiration for evidence of abnormal adduction if there is suspicion of paradoxical vocal fold motion disorder. A perfume inhalational challenge (asking the client to sniff various odorants, including perfumes) may also be useful to demonstrate this abnormality of motion (Carroll et al., 2008; Roehm & Rosen, 2004).

5. Ask the client to sniff through the nose several times in succession.

6. Alternate "ee" and a sniff. This should be rapidly repeated several times, allowing observation of the range of motion of the vocal folds. Any abnormalities in range of motion, either adduction or abduction, should be noted.

7. Ask the client to produce a low-pitched "ee" and then glide up to a higher pitch in a single breath. This can be done both from low up to high pitch, and from high down to low pitch, to allow assessment of vocal fold lengthening.

8. If there is suspicion of spasmodic dysphonia, ask the client to count from 60 to 70 and from 80 to 90 (Blitzer & Meyer, 2006; Merati, et al., 2005). Other vocal tasks, such as having the client say, "Buy Bob a baseball" or "Pay Paul a penny" may be used specifically to demonstrate abductor spasmodic dysphonia (Roehm & Rosen, 2004).

9. To allow assessment of conversational voice, ask the client an open-ended question, such as, "What did you do yesterday?"

10. Ask the client to perform a simple singing task such as, "Happy Birthday." More complex singing tasks can be utilized, as indicated.

11. Ask the client to hum, sigh, laugh, or whistle.

12. The use of sentences with glottal sounds (such as, "ants are at Erik's apartment") and glides (such as, "we were wearing yellow ones") to assess ventricular hyperfunction, which may be seen in individuals with muscle tension dysphonia.

Instructions:

- *"Say 'coca cola'" (to evaluate the palate).*
- *"Stick your tongue out" (to evaluate base of tongue).*
- *"Puff up your cheeks" (to evaluate hypopharynx).*
- *"Say 'ee'."*
- *"Sniff through your nose 3 times."*
- *"Alternate between a sniff and an 'e'."*
- *"Say 'ee' and slide from a low pitch up to a high pitch."*

- *"Say 'ee' and slide from a high pitch down to a low pitch."*
- *Use additional vocal tasks, as appropriate, as described above.*

Tips

1. The nose should be sufficiently anesthetized, if applicable. Additional anesthetic during the examination usually is not required.
2. The use of topical anesthetic-containing lubricant (e.g., lidocaine jelly) can facilitate comfortable passage of the flexible endoscope through the nasal cavity. However, care must be taken to place the lubricant approximately 5 mm back from the scope lens to avoid diminished visualization.
3. Remain close to the floor of the nose during passage through the nasal cavity. Avoid the nasal septum and turbinates, as pressure in these areas will produce pain.
4. Application of a topical anesthetic (e.g., combination of benzocaine/tetracaine) to the oropharynx may be required in some clients for rigid endoscopy. Most clients can tolerate rigid endoscopy well without this additional step.
5. Proper client positioning is important, to keep the tongue and its base out of the way during rigid endoscopy, and to allow optimal visualization of the larynx.
6. Great care should be exercised to maintain a "centered" view of the vocal folds. This will provide maximal visualization and avoid the inadvertent creation of pseudo-asymmetry and suboptimal evaluation of either vocal fold.

Troubleshooting

1. The client has difficulty tolerating the examination due to gag reflex.
   a. Ensure proper client positioning.
   b. Have the client take short, pant-like breaths.
   c. Keep the client's tongue and jaw adequately protruded to avoid the endoscope touching the base of tongue. It may be helpful to have the client hold his or her own tongue.
   d. If rigid endoscope is used, consider applying topical anesthetic to the oropharynx.
   e. If flexible endoscope is used, retract the endoscope into the nasopharynx.
2. The endoscopic image is out of focus.
   a. Adjust the focus.
   b. Touch the endoscope tip against the client's tongue to defog the lens.
   c. Retract the endoscope, gently wipe, and reapply defogging agent.
3. The vocal folds still cannot be seen, or the entire length of the vocal folds cannot be seen.
   a. Adjust the light.
   b. Adjust the position of the endoscope (may need to be advanced further or withdrawn slightly, or the angle of approach may need to be changed) (Samlan et al., 2010).
   c. Flex the wrist to tilt the tip of the endoscope.
   d. Have the client phonate in a *soft, high* pitch. This lengthens the vocal folds.
   e. Have the client phonate an "oo" (i.e., /u/) sound or hum (/m/)) (Carroll et al., 2008).

DATA ANALYSIS

Videostroboscopic evaluation of the vocal folds requires a detailed knowledge of their proper anatomy and physiology. A thorough review of normal vocal fold physiology is beyond the scope of this chapter. Full and detailed descriptions of normal vocal fold physiology have been well described elsewhere (Duflo & Thibeault, 2007; Samlan et al., 2010; Scherer, 2005; Sulica, 2006). The reader is referred to these sources for additional information.

General Appearance

The general appearance of the vocal folds can provide important information. Some of the features below are better assessed on routine flexible fiberoptic laryngoscopy. However, when possible, they also should be evaluated during videostroboscopy.

- The vocal folds usually are pearly white in color. Changes in color such as erythema can indicate recent phonotrauma or irritation (e.g., laryngopharyngeal reflux) (Hicks, Ours, Abelson, Vaezi, & Richter, 2002; Toohill & Kuhn, 1997).
- A change in vocal fold morphology may reflect pathology. Edema of the vocal folds may be the result of recent illness, phonotrauma, laryngopharyngeal reflux, or chronic inflammation (as occurs in Reinke's edema). Atrophy of the vocal folds results in a bowed and thinned appearance, with accentuation of the ventricle and prominence of the vocal processes (Kashima, Goodwin, Balkany, & Casiano, 2005).
- The presence or absence of mucus as well as its consistency should be noted.

These findings can be an indication of generalized dehydration, postradiation effects, laryngopharyngeal reflux, or postnasal drip (Kashima et al., 2005).

- Structural abnormalities of the vocal folds should be assessed, including vascular ectasias, varices, or webs. A mass or lesion can affect the vibratory characteristics of the vocal folds, due to an increase in mass. The presence of transverse blood vessels is abnormal, as the vessels normally have a longitudinal orientation (Kashima et al., 2005).
- Hyperfunction of the false vocal folds can occur in anterior-to-posterior and/or medial-to-lateral directions and can be evaluated only via flexible laryngoscopy (Samlan et al., 2010) (Figure 8–5). Although this may be an indication of pathology such as muscle tension dysphonia (Belafsky, Postma, Reulbach, Holland, & Koufman, 2002), it is important to realize that it also may be a normal finding in some clients,

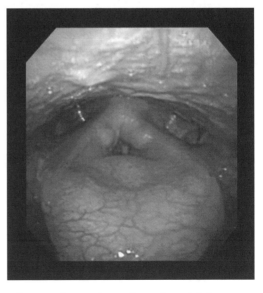

Figure 8–5. Hyperfunctional false vocal fold adduction.

especially with certain speech tasks such as repeated /i/ tasks (Behrman, Dahl, Abramson, & Schutte, 2003; Stager, Neubert, Miller, Regnell, & Bielamowicz, 2003).

Stroboscopy Parameters

Evaluation can be performed during normal, quiet breathing as well as during phonatory tasks. However, the greatest benefit of videostroboscopy is the evaluation of mucosal vibration (see discussion below). Commonly used parameters during a videostroboscopic evaluation include assessment of vocal fold symmetry, amplitude, periodicity, mucosal wave, and closure during vibration.

Symmetry

The free, vibrating edge of the vocal folds should be straight and smooth, and the vocal folds should vibrate as mirror images of one another. Asymmetry of vibration indicates a difference in the mechanical properties or tension of the vocal folds. This could be related to a change in mass of the vocal folds, as occurs in the presence of a cyst or other subepithelial lesion(s). Alternatively, a change in the mucosal wave, as may be seen with epithelial lesions such as papillomas, may also cause vibrational asymmetry. Finally, gross vocal fold motion asymmetry may be present in conditions such as vocal fold paresis.

Amplitude

The amplitude of the vocal folds refers to the horizontal movement away from the midline. This should be symmetric bilaterally. Amplitude is directly influenced by loudness and pitch, varying directly with

loudness and inversely with pitch (Samlan et al., 2010). "Normal" is defined as movement of approximately one-third to one-half of the width of the vocal fold, at modal pitch (Postma et al., 2005; Rosen & Simpson, 2008). Conditions affecting vocal fold mass or stiffness or glottic sufficiency result in decreased amplitude. Examples include vocal fold polyps, cysts, or scarring. Increased amplitude can be seen in conditions of decreased vocal fold tone, such as atrophy, Reinke's edema, or vocal fold edema (Samlan et al., 2010).

Periodicity

The vibration of the vocal folds should be similar from cycle to cycle (given constant pitch and intensity). Periodic vibration of the vocal folds occurs in a regular, rhythmic pattern. Aperiodic vibration of the vocal folds occurs in an irregular pattern (Samlan et al., 2010). As videostroboscopy depends on image sampling of many sequential vibratory cycles, this technique is limited to fairly periodic voices. Voices that are severely aperiodic (often seen in severe dysphonia or aphonia) will be unable to be assessed via videostroboscopy (Connor & Bless, 2007).

Mucosal Wave

In 1974, the cover-body theory was first presented by Hirano. This theory describes the vocal folds as a "body" of muscle (vocalis) enveloped by the pliable, elastic mucosal "cover" (Duflo & Thibeault, 2007; Samlan et al., 2010). The mucosal wave is seen as the movement of the mucosal cover, from the subglottic area up and over the surface of the true vocal folds. Conditions that stiffen the mucosal cover (e.g., mass/lesion, scarring, and sulcus vocalis) will decrease the mucosal wave. An increased mucosal wave will be seen in circumstances where the mucosal cover is more pliable than usual, for example, in Reinke's edema/polypoid degeneration. It also is important at this time to note nonvibrating portions of the vocal folds, known as adynamic segments. These usually are the result of a lesion and/or scarring (Samlan et al., 2010).

Closure

During phonation, the vocal folds should fully or fairly closely approximate one another. Various patterns of closure of vocal folds have been observed in patients with dysphonia (Kaszuba & Garret, 2007; Rosen & Simpson, 2008) (Figure 8-6). A complete closure pattern is seen with full approximation of the vocal folds, at the most comfortable pitch and intensity. In contrast, a gap may be observed in the posterior aspect of the glottis (see Figure 8-6A). These gaps may be a nor-

mal variant, such as in women (especially singers) (Duflo & Thibeault, 2007; Samlan et al., 2010) but also may reflect pathology. An hourglass closure pattern has both anterior and posterior gaps with a point of closure in the mid-membranous vocal fold. This often is seen with mid-vocal fold subepithelial lesion(s) or with vocal fold edema (see Figure 8-6B). An elliptical closure pattern is seen when there is a small area of closure posteriorly, and possibly also anteriorly, but otherwise is open (see Figure 8-6C). A transglottic closure pattern shows incomplete glottic closure during all phases of the vibratory cycle, with the vocal folds never achieving complete or even nearly-complete closure. Finally, irregular closure patterns that do not match any of the above descriptions also may exist.

Duration of the closure also is important. The vocal folds typically are open for approximately two-thirds of one vibratory cycle and are maximally closed for the

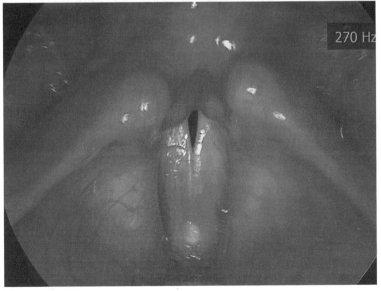

A

Figure 8-6. **A.** Posterior gap in glottal closure. *continues*

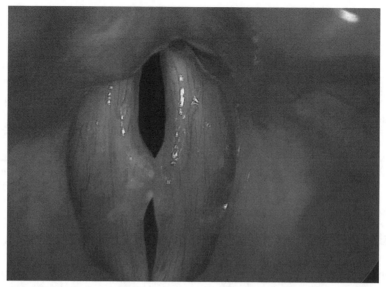

B

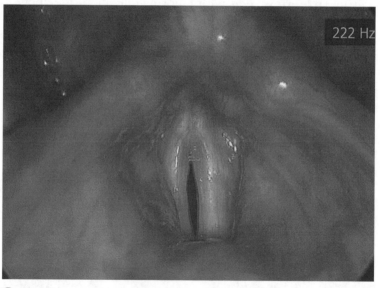

C

Figure 8–6. *continued* **B.** Hourglass closure pattern.
C. Elliptical closure pattern.

remaining third. This finding is both pitch and intensity dependent (Samlan et al., 2010). If the duration of closure is too brief, even though the true vocal folds may completely approximate, the client will have persistent voice complaints, including vocal fatigue. These findings are often seen in clients with vocal fold atrophy, scar, paresis, or thinning of the lamina propria due to aging.

REFERENCES

Behrman, A., Dahl, L. D., Abramson, A. L., & Schutte, H. K. (2003). Anterior-posterior and medial compression of the supraglottis: Signs of nonorganic dysphonia or normal postures? *Journal of Voice, 17,* 403-410.

Belafsky, P. C., Postma, G. N., & Koufman, J. A. (2001). The validity and reliability of the reflux finding score (RFS). *Laryngoscope, 111,* 1313-1317.

Belafsky, P. C., Postma, G. N., Reulbach T. R., Holland, B. W., & Koufman, J. A. (2002). Muscle tension dysphonia as a sign of underlying glottal insufficiency. *Otolaryngology-Head and Neck Surgery, 127,* 448-451.

Blitzer, A., & Meyer, T. (2006). Neurologic disorders of the larynx. In B. J. Bailey, J. T. Johnson et al. (Eds.), *Head and neck surgery-otolaryngology* (4th ed., Vol. 2, pp. 867-894). Philadelphia, PA: Lippincott Williams & Wilkins.

Carroll, T. L., Nunez, R. A., & Rosen, C. A. (2008). Dynamic voice evaluation using flexible endoscopy. E-medicine, updated Feb 19, 2010, *Otolaryngology and Facial Plastic Surgery.* http://www.emedicine.com .

Connor, N. P., & Bless, D. M. (2007). Videostroboscopy. In A. L. Merati & S. A. Bielamowicz (Eds.), *Textbook of laryngology* (pp. 74-83). San Diego, CA: Plural Publishing.

Duflo, S., & Thibeault, S. L. (2007). Anatomy of the larynx and physiology of phonation. In A. L. Merati & S. A. Bielamowicz (Eds.), *Textbook of laryngology* (pp. 31-50). San Diego, CA: Plural Publishing.

Heman-Ackah, Y. D. (2004). Diagnostic tools in laryngology. *Current Opinion in Otolaryngology and Head and Neck Surgery, 12,* 549-552.

Hicks, D. M., Ours, T. M., Abelson T. I., Vaezi, M. F., & Richter, J. E. (2002). The prevalence of hypopharynx findings associated with gastroesophageal reflux in normal volunteers. *Journal of Voice, 16,* 564-579.

Kashima, M. L., Goodwin, Jr., W. J., Balkany, T. J., & Casiano R. R. (2005). Special considerations in managing geriatric patients. In C. W. Cummings et al. (Eds.), *Cummings otolaryngology: Head and neck surgery* (4th ed.). Philadelphia, PA: Elsevier-Mosby.

Kaszuba, S. M., & Garret, C. G. (2007). Strobovideolaryngoscopy and laboratory voice evaluation. *Otolaryngologic Clinics of North America, 40,* 991-1001.

Merati, A. L., Heman-Ackah, Y. D., Abaza, M., Altman, K. W., Sulica, L., & Belamowicz, S. (2005). Common movement disorders affecting the larynx: A report from the neurolaryngology committee of the AAO-HNS. *Otolaryngologic and Head and Neck Surgery, 133*(5), 654-665.

Postma, G. N., Courey, M. S., & Ossoff, R. H. (2005). The professional voice. In C. W. Cummings et al. (Eds.), *Cummings otolaryngology: Head and neck surgery* (4th ed.). Philadelphia, PA: Elsevier-Mosby.

Roehm, P. C., & Rosen, C. A. (2004). Dynamic voice assessment using flexible laryngoscopy—How I do it: A targeted problem and its solution. *American Journal of Otolaryngology, 25*(2), 138-141.

Rosen, C. A., Amin, M. R., Sulica, L., Simpson, C. B., Merati, A. L., Courey, M. S., . . . Postma, G. N. (2009). Advances in office-based diagnosis and treatment in laryngology. *Laryngoscope, 119,* S185-S212.

Rosen, C. A., & Simpson, C. B. (2008). Videostroboscopy and dynamic voice evaluation with flexible laryngoscopy. In C. A. Rosen & C. B. Simpson (Eds.), *Operative techniques in laryngology* (1st ed.). New York, NY: Springer.

Samlan, R. A., Gartner-Schmidt, J., & Kunduk, M. (2010). Visualization of the larynx. In P. W. Flint et al. (Eds.), *Cummings otolaryngology: Head and neck surgery* (5th ed.). Philadelphia, PA: Elsevier-Mosby.

Scherer, R. C. (2005). Laryngeal function during phonation. In R. T. Sataloff, *Professional voice: The science and art of clinical care* (3rd ed.). San Diego, CA: Plural Publishing.

Stager, S. V., Neubert, R., Miller, S., Regnell, J. R., & Bielamowicz, S. A. (2003). Incidence of supraglottic activity in males and females: A preliminary report. *Journal of Voice, 17*(3), 395–402.

Sulica, L. (2006). Voice: Anatomy, physiology, and clinical evaluation. In B. J. Bailey, J. T. Johnson, et al. (Eds.), *Head and neck surgery-Otolaryngology* (4th ed.). Philadelphia, PA: Lippincott Williams & Wilkins.

Toohill, R. J., & Kuhn, J. C. (1997). Role of refluxed acid in pathogenesis of laryngeal disorders. *American Journal of Medicine, 103*(5A), 100S–106S.

Woo, P., & Yanagisawa, E. (2003). The larynx. In K. J. Lee (Ed.), *Essential otolaryngology: Head and neck surgery* (8th ed.) New York, NY: McGraw-Hill.

CHAPTER 9

Stroboscopy in the Voice Clinic: United Kingdom Perspective

JOHN S. RUBIN AND RUTH EPSTEIN

PURPOSES

- To outline the history of development of clinical stroboscopy.
- To provide an overview of the principles of stroboscopy.
- To describe the procedures in conducting strobolaryngoscopy.
- To discuss the scope of need for specialized voice clinic with contemporary imaging techniques with a UK perspective.

DESCRIPTION

This chapter discusses the United Kingdom (UK) perspective on stroboscopy in the voice clinic. The first section of the chapter reviews the history of stroboscopy and the theory behind it. The procedures of carrying out a stroboscopic examination also are described. The second section of the chapter discusses the need for voice clinics in the UK, with an emphasis on the use of specialized imaging techniques like stroboscopy integrated with traditional auditory-perceptual-acoustic voice assessments and quality of life measurements.

INTRODUCTION AND THEORETICAL BACKGROUND

History of Stroboscopy

The concept of stroboscopy is old. The Belgian Joseph Plateau is generally recognized as having intellectual ownership of the concept. In 1832, he developed a device that he called a Phenakistoscope that he turned while viewing images on a separate wheel that rotated. Around that same time, the Austrian Simon von Stampfer also used rotating disks and named the term stroboscope. In 1874, the German physician Max Oertel came up with the idea of, and in 1895 realized, laryngeal stroboscopy, using a wheel with systematic holes or perforations through which light could reflect off a mirror on his head and could pass onto the larynx, thereby creating the illusion of slow motion (Kaszuba & Garrett, 2007). Rotating and/or vibrating mirrors were used relatively early on in stroboscopy. For example, in 1931 Harold Edgerton "invented" the electronic strobe light stroboscope, conceptually using a flashing lamp to study machine parts in movement. This idea was then taken up by General Radio Corporation, who produced a "Strobotach." Edgerton also used this concept with very short blasts of light to develop still photographs of fast moving objects (Wikipedia).

Early problems with illumination, control of flash frequency, and quality of image bedeviled early stroboscopes. In 1960, van den Berg, Timke, Schonharl, and von Leden published a book on laryngeal stroboscopy. This was further popularized in the 1990s by Ford and Bless (1991) and Hirano and Bless (1993).

Physics of Stroboscopy

The human vocal folds have a vibratory range between 60 and over 1200 cycles per second. Stroboscopic light takes advantage of the limitations of the human retina. In accordance with Talbot's law, if a point of the retina is excited by a light stimulus undergoing periodic variations in magnitude at a frequency exceeding the fusion frequency, the visual sensation produced is identical with that produced by a steady stimulus whose magnitude equals the mean magnitude of the variable stimulus taken over one period (Wikipedia).

What this corresponds to physically is that each image remains on the retina for approximately 200 microseconds subsequent to exposure. The light pulse can be advanced with a delta-t generator (Boehme & Gross, 2005) through successive vocal cycles, either at the same point in each cycle or in percentage increments, the stroboscope apparently freezes the vocal folds or allows them to appear to be moving in slow motion, the retina "filling in the missing pieces" by fusing the images it "sees" as motion. This phenomenon of apparent motion is called persistence of vision (Kaszuba & Garrett, 2007). Although knowledge of this phenomenon has been attributed as far back as to Lucretius, the Roman poet, more modern attributions are to the British physician Peter Roget, FRS in 1824 during stroboscopic experiments.

Clinical Applications of Stroboscopy

The stroboscopic examination has become the keystone evaluation of the voice clinic from a diagnostic perspective. In several publications, it has been demonstrated to lead to a modification in diagnosis of 10 to 18% (Cantarella, 1998; Remacle, 1996; Sataloff, Spiegel, & Hawkshaw, 1991; Woo, Colton, Casper, & Brewer, 1991).

Stroboscopy is particularly useful for identifying the effect of pathology on the viscoelastic properties of the vocal folds, both from a standpoint of mass and stiffness. It has been a giant leap forward in this regard, as a flexible nasendoscope may well demonstrate a normal-appearing smooth edge of a vocal fold that is actually severely damaged. Therein comes the change in diagnosis so common in the voice clinic. It has proven particularly helpful in the diagnosis of scarring or tethering, of sulcus vocalis or vergeture, of cysts or other submucosal pathology. Even with relatively obvious pathology such as the spectrum of what is called vocal nodules and polyps, stroboscopy can demonstrate the degree to which the pathology impacts on the biomechanics of the cover and on glottic closure. In cases of cysts, the adynamic segment overlying the cyst may be the only feature that leads one to operate and to explore at surgery the superficial layer of the lamina propria. And in instances of complex pathology or post-surgical/trauma, stroboscopy has proven to be a particularly good guide to surgical intervention whereby one vocal fold may appear edematous but have better vibratory characteristics than its neighbor, and thus not be the side that should be operated on. In cases of early carcinoma or dysplasia, stroboscopy is particularly sensitive to the stiffness inherent to invasion of the superficial layer of the lamina propria, and is a more sensitive tool than any currently available imaging system.

EQUIPMENT FOR STROBOSCOPY

A microphone is used to pick up the frequency of the client's sustained phonation, which in turn triggers the stroboscopic light source. This works well only if the client's vocal cycle is relatively periodic. With very aperiodic vocal production, its advantages are lost or greatly diminished. In theory and often in practice, stroboscopic flashes can be emitted at the same frequency as phonation. This is known as synchronization. They also can be emitted at a variation of frequency (asynchronization) or at any other frequency desired. There are advantages to each. By synchronizing the flashes to the fundamental frequency of the vibrating vocal folds, an apparent stationary, standstill image is produced. By varying the flashes slightly but consistently across different phases of the vocal fold vibratory cycle, it produces apparent slow forward or backward motion, depending on the light flash. The frequency of the light flash is adjusted to be equal to, or an amount above or below the cyclic speed of the object it is lighting. In this manner the object appears stationary, moving forward or backward depending on the flash frequency. By applying it at a fixed setting of frequency with tone generator control, it can be useful in larynges with extreme asynchrony of movement. A further option available on many systems is to move the foot pedal that controls the degree of asynchrony during the examination. This can allow the larynx to be seen in a variety of apparent positions during the examination (Boehme & Gross, 2005).

The stroboscope may be linked to a camera that is embedded into the device used for examining, what is known as a distal chip-tip camera. This typically is found on a digital flexible endoscope. The stroboscope may also be attached to a camera that in turn is attached to the examining device. Such a device may be a flexible nasendoscope, or a rigid 70- or 90-degree endoscope. In turn, this device is connected to some type of recording device. Typically, the recording device (analog or now more commonly digital) will have the capacity for image capture and will be attached to a device for image reproduction.

PROCEDURES FOR STROBOSCOPY

Rigid Strobolaryngoscopy

In our voice clinic, the patient is seated comfortably. Feet should be firmly planted on the floor. The use of local anesthesia is not preferred. The patient's tongue is extended and held by the examiner (or by the patient, particularly the young patient). The patient is instructed to phonate, in the first instance with a "heee" in a comfortable but high frequency. At the same time, he or she is instructed in techniques to elevate the soft palate (surprised look, slight smile, imagining he or she is biting into an apple). The rigid scope is gently advanced toward the posterior two-thirds of the tongue without contacting the uvula, soft palate, fauces, or posterior pharyngeal wall. This works well in most instances. Once the patient is comfortable with this technique, the larynx should be examined during production of high and low pitches, and also during a pitch glide, at low and higher amplitudes.

Flexible Strobolaryngoscopy

The patient is positioned as described in the previous section above. If needed, the nose and postnasal space can be topically anesthetized and decongested with a mixture of 0.25% phenylephrine and 2 to 3% lidocaine using an atomizer. Avoid this if the anatomy of the nose will so allow. After allowing adequate time for decongestion, the flexible scope is inserted through the nose and passed into position above the larynx. There are two schools of thought as to passage of the scope within the nose. One group advocates passage between the inferior and middle turbinate on the basis that the resultant angle makes the remaining examination easier. The other group advocates passage along the floor of the nose medial to the inferior turbinate. They believe that this allows for a more comfortable passage of the scope. Undoubtedly, both techniques have their place, depending on the intranasal anatomy. The advantage of the flexible over rigid scope is that there is much greater latitude of investigations that the examiner can comfortably perform. Subtle movement disorders can be looked for, and the patient can also be asked to sing or read/repeat complex materials.

INTERPRETATION OF STROBOSCOPIC IMAGES

Normal Stroboscopic Vibratory Pattern

Normal vibratory pattern of vocal fold vibration is said to involve three movements (Boehme & Gross, 2005): (1) horizontal, from median to lateral; (2) vertical, from caudad to cephalad; and (3) wavelike, with glottal opening from caudad to cephalad. Normal vocal fold vibration is regular and symmetrical with a complete closed phase like a shutter, and the generation of a "mucosal wave" particularly in the lower frequencies. In the upper frequencies, the amplitude and mucosal waves diminish. With increase in loudness, there is a corresponding increase in amplitude and a more prominent mucosal wave.

Hirano and Bless (1993) identified the following relevant observable characteristics of the vibratory pattern: glottal closure, closure phase, symmetry, amplitude of vibration, periodicity, mucosal wave, and adynamic segments. They developed a Videostroboscopic Rating Scale based on these characteristics at the University of Wisconsin (Hirano & Bless, 1993):

Glottal closure: Boehme and Gross (2005) identified six variations to complete glottal closure: posterior incomplete; incomplete from front to back; hourglass-shaped; arch-shaped; anterior incomplete; and irregular.

Vocal fold symmetry: In the normal larynx, the vocal folds close symmetrically. Should there be a disruption in the vibration, it usually is associated with pathology, either asymmetric mass or stiffness, or unilateral atrophy/diminished mobility.

Amplitude of vibration: Each vocal fold needs to be evaluated separately. When vocal intensity increases so too does the amplitude of vibration. However, amplitude may well decrease with stiffness. The amplitude of vibration is highly dependent on pitch frequency (vocal fold tension) and loudness (subglottal pressure).

Periodicity: Periodicity refers to the regularity of successive vocal vibratory cycles. Normal vibratory activity is regular and periodic.

Mucosal wave: The mucosal wave is a feature of the cover (epithelium and superficial layer of the lamina propria). If it is diminished or is not present, this may be a sign of underlying pathology, often stiffness.

Adynamic segment: This is a useful feature to identify a focal underlying mass or stiffness.

When interpreting the findings, it should be noted that in "normal speakers," males tend to have longer closed phase as well as more complete closure than females. Children have a larger posterior chink and shorter closed phase than adults. The elderly have more asymmetry and larger glottal gaps (Ford & Bless, 1991). Especially when using the rigid scope and holding the tongue in protrusion, a small posterior gap in females is within normal limits.

VOICE CLINICS IN THE UNITED KINGDOM

Historical Development of the United Kingdom Voice Clinics

In the latter part of the 20th century, it became clear that voice disorders were debilitating and that their management required special expertise. As such, in many European countries, a specialism named Phoniatrics, developed. The United Kingdom is one of the few nations in Europe not to have developed the specialty of Phoniatrics. Rather, at the present time, any ear-nose-and-throat surgeon in the United Kingdom with a special interest in laryngology, can forge ties with specialist speech and language therapists, and other individuals interested in the care of the professional voice, and can consider him or herself as a "voice specialist."

That said, in the United Kingdom, it has been evident that the diagnosis of voice disorders requires close collaboration between various professionals who can contribute knowledge and skills concerning the patient's dysphonia. As such, we have seen the development and institution of multidisciplinary voice clinics. These provide the appropriate setting for assessment and treatment of voice disorders using a multidisciplinary team approach. Interest in development of such multidisciplinary clinics began in the late 1970s. Thereafter, voice clinics have been established in an increasing number of centers, consisting in the main of a laryngologist and speech and language therapist with special interest in voice. Other professionals such as scientists, physical therapists, voice coaches, and psychologists also have been incorporated in certain centers.

Scope of Need of Voice Clinics in the United Kingdom

Several estimations (Leske, 1981; Wilson, 1987) have placed the incidence of voice disorders in the United States to be between 3 to 9% of the population. In the United Kingdom, there are no reliable statistics on the incidence of voice disorders as they are not recognized as an occupational disorder by law. Mathieson in 1997 made a determination of 121 cases per 100,000 population in 1997 in relation to individuals being referred to a hospital in London with a voice problem (Greene & Mathieson, 2001). The caveat is that this is likely to be underreported both in terms of incidence and prevalence. This is on the basis that such data only represent individuals who are seen by otolaryngologists, but exclude those who do not have sufficient concerns regarding the state of their voice to warrant a visit to the general practitioners (Greene & Mathieson, 2001).

The Multidisciplinary Voice Clinic in the United Kingdom

It is not surprising, given the scope of the problem, that multidisciplinary voice clinics have become the norm in most major

trusts in the United Kingdom. In 2010, such a clinic represents the current ideal best practice for patients referred to many and perhaps most ENT departments in the United Kingdom. In year 2000, there were 50 recorded voice clinics in the United Kingdom. Subsequently, there has been a significant increase in this type of multidisciplinary voice care; such that, as of November 15, 2009, the British Voice Association Web site identified 108 active voice clinics, a growth of over 100% in a decade. Keystone elements of a specialized voice clinic in the United Kingdom include the following:

1. **Multidisciplinary teamwork:** Multidisciplinary participation of a nucleus of speech and language therapist specialized in voice disorders and ENT surgeon with a special interest in laryngology during the initial history taking and physical examination with the goal of a combined diagnosis and treatment plan.

2. **Equipment:** Specialized equipment permitting detailed and clear visualization of the larynx, with some type of permanent record. At the time of this writing, this usually includes digital stroboscopy with a rigid telescope or flexible fiberoptic device. Many centers are currently purchasing digital chip-tip type of flexible endoscopes, thereby markedly improving visualization. Kymography is available in some centers but, by and large, is still a research tool for the large majority of voice clinics in the United Kingdom as is high-speed photography.

3. **Perceptual and acoustic analysis:** The GRBAS is by far the most commonly used perceptual rating scale in voice clinics in the United Kingdom. Many voice clinics utilize acoustic analysis as an adjunct measurement to voice therapy and treatment.

4. **Quality of life questionnaires:** Questionnaires designed to assess the psychological status of the individual are the norm. The Voice Handicap Index (VHI; Jacobson, Johnson, Grywalski, Silbergleit, Jacobson, & Benninger, 1997) is probably the most common tool utilized in the majority of voice clinics.

5. **Ready access to imaging such as ultrasound, computed tomography (CT) and magnetic resonance imaging (MRI) scanning:** A few clinics have access to dopamine active transporter (DAT) scanners and functional MRI. However, at the time of this writing, these are still research tools and not used regularly in the voice clinic. Clinics have access to barium swallow, but are more likely to request functional endoscopic evaluation of swallow, videofluoroscopy or referral to a gastrointestinal (GI) laboratory for 24-hour pH (or non-pH refluxate) investigation or manometry. (As this document specifically reviews voice clinics, we will not go further into dysphagia investigations although most trusts have swallowing services).

6. **Pathways:** Strict pathways to ensure most efficacious use of time management. This is particularly important as: (1) there is an 18-week limit prescribed nationally in time allowed for complete initial management of a patient including surgery, from the time of the general practitioner referral; and (2) the maximum number of speech therapy sessions allowed is six.

7. **Outcome:** Combined follow-up to review outcome (with as noted above some clinics with specialized speech therapy-led follow-up clinics with expert ENT surgical advice available.)

FUTURE APPLICATIONS OF STROBOSCOPY IN THE VOICE CLINIC

The stroboscope is the backbone of the voice clinic. However, interpretation is skill-dependent on the examiner and it is a subjective form of analysis. Studies have demonstrated only moderate inter-rater correlations for judging specific parameters (kappa = 0.61 to 0.81) (Rosen, 2005). Other limitations include color issues with the computer monitor making color interpretation suspect, and limitation of the technique to relatively periodic vocal fold movements.

More recently, high-speed digital imaging systems have been developed that can observe laryngeal motion capture up to 4000 frames per second, are not dependent on extraction of fundamental frequency for motion extraction, and that initiate recording with the onset of phonation. One recent study in a tertiary center found 63% of data from stroboscopy to be uninterpretable due to the severity of voice disorders tested, whereas 100% of high-speed photography was interpretable (Patel, Dailey, & Bless, 2008).

REFERENCES

Boehme, G., & Gross M. (2005). *Stroboscopy: And other techniques for the analysis of vocal fold vibration*. London, UK: Whurr.

Cantarella, G. (1998). The impact of videostroboscopy on laryngological diagnosis: A retrospective study. *European Archives of Oto-Rhino-Laryngology, 255*(Suppl. 1), 139.

Ford, C. N., & Bless, D. M. (1991). *Phonosurgery: Assessment and surgical management of voice disorders*. New York, NY: Raven Press.

Greene, M. C. L., & Mathieson, L. (2001). *The voice and its disorders* (6th ed.). London, UK: Whurr.

Hirano, M., & Bless, D. M. (1993). *Videostroboscopic examination of the larynx.* San Diego, CA: Singular Publishing Group.

Jacobson, B. J., Johnson, A., Grywalski, C., Silbergleit, A., Jacobson, G., & Benninger, M. S. (1997). The Voice Handicap Index (VHI): Development and validation. *American Journal of Speech-Language Pathology, 6*(3), 66-70.

Kaszuba, S. M., & Garrett, C. G. (2007). Strobovideolaryngoscopy and laboratory voice evaluation. *Otolaryngologic Clinics of North America, 40*, 991-1001.

Leske, M. C. (1981). Prevalence estimates of communicative disorders in the US. Speech disorders, *ASHA, 23*(3), 217-225.

Patel, R., Dailey, S., & Bless, D. (2008). Comparison of high-speed digital imaging with stroboscopy for laryngeal imaging of glottal disorders. *Annals of Otology, Rhinology and Laryngology, 117*(6), 413-424.

Remacle, M. (1996). The contribution of videostroboscopy in daily ENT practice. *Acta Oto-Rhino-Laryngologica (Belgium), 50*, 265-281.

Rosen, C. A. (2005). Stroboscopy as a research instrument: Development of a perceptual evaluation tool. *Laryngoscope, 115*(3), 423-428.

Sataloff, R. T., Spiegel, J. R., & Hawkshaw, M. J. (1991). Strobovideolaryngoscopy: Results and clinical value. *Annals of Otology, Rhinology and Laryngology, 100*, 725-727.

Wilson, D. K. (1987). *Voice problems of children.* Baltimore MD: Williams & Wilkins.

Woo, P., Colton, R., Casper, J., & Brewer, D. (1991). Diagnostic value of stroboscopic examination in hoarse patients. *Journal of Voice, 5*, 231-238.

CHAPTER 10

Laryngoscopic Examination: China Perspective

DEMIN HAN AND WEN XU

PURPOSES

■ To examine vocal fold vibration using stroboscopic light.
■ To examine pharyngeal and laryngeal tissues for identifying abnormal structures.

ASSESSMENT OF VOCAL FOLD STRUCTURE

Visual examination of the larynx is an important investigation in a voice clinic. Prior to any laryngeal examination, the medical history of the patient should be considered carefully. Particular attention should be paid to the condition of the patient. If the patient has any obvious laryngeal obstruction, the examiner must exercise extra precautions during the examination to prevent causing or aggravating any dyspnea. The examination of larynx includes external inspections, indirect laryngoscopy, flexible fiberoptic laryngoscopy, electronic laryngoscopy, strobovideolaryngoscopy, direct laryngos-

copy, and/or other imaging and laboratory examinations.

In Mainland China, indirect laryngoscopy generally is used as a screening procedure in a general laryngology practice. Flexible laryngoscopy is a common tool used to examine patients with nasal, pharyngeal, or laryngeal disorders. Stroboscopy generally is not available except in a few large hospital voice centers. This chapter describes the various laryngoscopic procedures.

Indirect Laryngoscopy

Indirect laryngoscopy (Figure 10–1) is the most common traditional ear, nose, and throat (ENT) examination procedure. This

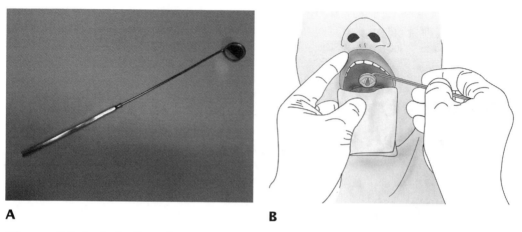

A   **B**

Figure 10–1. **A.** Indirect laryngoscope. **B.** Indirect examination of the larynx.

procedure begins with putting the laryngeal mirror above a naked alcohol flame to prevent fogging of the mirror inside the oral cavity. The patient is asked to protrude his or her tongue and then the examiner grasps the tongue gently with a piece of gauze and gently pulls it forward. The mirror is placed in the oral cavity and the back surface is used to elevate the soft palate. Local anesthetic spray is used to numb any gag reflex. The indirect laryngeal mirror should provide a good view of the laryngeal and hypopharyngeal structures that include the root of tongue, lingual tonsils, epiglottic vallecula, epiglottis, the lateral glossoepiglottic folds, the median glossoepiglottic folds, the aryepiglottic folds, the arytenoids cartilages, hypopharyngeal walls (lateral and posterior), and piriform fossa. Ask the patient to phonate a high-pitched vowel /i/ ("e-e-e-e") sound. This will give a good view of the ventricular folds, the laryngeal ventricle, the vocal folds, and the subglottis. In some patients, a few tracheal rings might also be seen between the vocal folds during respiration. Occasionally, one might find a furled epiglottis, in which case laryngologists refer to an "omega-shaped" epiglottis.

After the larynx has been inspected during quiet respiration, vocal fold movement is inspected during phonation. If the indirect laryngoscopy is not successful due to gag reflex, a small amount of 1% tetracaine hydrochloride topical anesthetic spray may be applied to the surface of the uvula, soft palate, and the posterior wall of the pharynx.

Flexible Laryngoscopy

Indirect laryngoscopy is only a screening procedure of the hypolarynx and larynx. Flexible laryngoscopy (Figure 10–2) may be used as the basic inspection of this area when the result of indirect laryngoscope is not satisfactory. By using a flexible laryngoscope, one can observe not only the laryngeal lesions, but also the changes of the vocal tract in relationship to articulation, swallowing, and respiration in a more natural state. This inspection is conducive to a more complex dynamic voice assessment.

Topical anesthestic spray (1% tetracaine hydrochloride) may be applied to the nostril, the pharynx, and the larynx

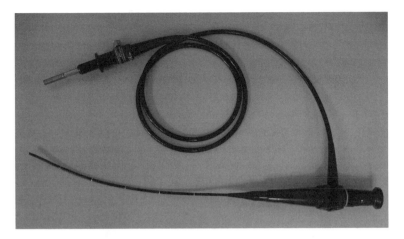

Figure 10–2. Flexible laryngoscope.

if needed. The patient could sit up or lie down supinely. The flexible fibro laryngoscope is inserted into the patient's nostril and passed transnasally under direct visual guide into the oropharynx, hypopharynx and then the larynx. Occasionally, 0.5 to 1% ephedrine also may need to be applied in the nostril to alleviate nasal edema.

Flexible laryngoscopy allows visualization of structures from the anterior nares to the larynx and extending to the upper trachea. This procedure does not interfere with oral articulation and it also is useful in observing velopharyngeal activity. Flexible laryngoscopy also is especially suitable for patients who have a short neck, a hypertrophic tongue, or an "omega-shaped" epiglottis. The optical fiber takes advantage of being flexible, high illumination power so that it can be guided to any direction. The flexible fiberoptic scope usually has an external diameter of 3.2 to 6.0 mm and a length of 300 mm or more. It can be upswept by 90° to 130°, bending down by 60° to 90° with a viewing angle of 50°. The flexible fiberoptic scope can be connected to a video-recording system, camera system, and/or computer system. If needed and properly set up, the flexible laryngoscope also can be used in conjunction with vacuum suction instrument and biopsy forceps for suction and local biopsy.

Electrolaryngoscopy

The electroendoscope (Figure 10–3) was first used in the gastrointestinal tract and bronchoscopic examinations. The electronic nasopharyngolaryngoscopic imaging system was introduced to the market around 1993. It has a higher resolution than the traditional flexible fiberoptic scope. The imaging system uses a charge coupled device (CCD) chip at the tip of the endoscope, which functions as an ultra small camera. The external diameter of the pipe and the tip is around 5 mm. Images are transmitted after being converted into electronic signals. The laryngoscopic system could be connected to a digital image processing system that accepts the electronic signals of the imaging system for real-time processing using image enhancement of intensity, contrast, and image enlargement.

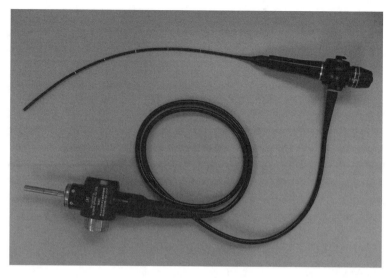

Figure 10–3. Electrolaryngoscope.

Direct Laryngoscope and Microscopic Examination

Direct laryngoscopy and microscopy can be used to observe the laryngeal structures in close details under local or general anesthesia.

ASSESSMENT OF VOCAL FOLD VIBRATION

Vocal folds vibrate approximately 250 times per second while phonating at middle C. According to the law of Talbot, human eyes can only sense five images (video) per second, that is, each image is retained on the retina for 0.2 seconds. Hence, vocal fold vibration is too fast for the eyes to follow. Therefore, conventional indirect laryngoscopy, direct laryngoscopy, or flexible laryngoscopy cannot observe the vibration of vocal folds under continuous light. The vibratory margin of the vocal folds may be assessed using strobo-laryngoscopy, high-speed photography, high-speed video laryngoscopy, videokymography, electroglottography, or photoglottography (Hirano & Bless, 1993; Kendall, 2009; Oertel, 1895; Yangisawa, Owens, Strothers, & Honda, 1983). High-speed laryngoscopy and videokymography are described in separate chapters by Kong and Yiu (Chapter 12), and Švec and Šram (Chapter 11) in this book.

Strobolaryngoscopy

Strobolaryngoscopy allows observation of vocal fold vibration using pseudo-slow-motion of the images.

Basic Principle: Videostrobolaryngoscopy is a special examination technique that uses a strobe light and microphone to synchronize the movements of the vocal folds so they may be viewed in a "slow motion." Stroboscopic light illuminates different points on the continuous movement track of the vocal folds. The different illuminated points combine visually to create an optical illusion of slow motion or static vocal fold vibration. The vocal folds will appear static when the frequency of the strobe light is equal to that of the vocal fold vibration. This static view is useful for observing structures of vocal folds when phonating. The slow-motion effect, which is created by having the stroboscopic light desynchronized with the frequency of vocal fold vibration by approximately 2 Hz, is useful for observing the characteristics of vocal fold vibration. Unlike high-speed photography, stroboscopy does not provide a "true" slow-motion image. This approximation of slow motion, however, provides the necessary clinical information in most instances.

Equipment and Materials: The strobolaryngoscopy system (Figure 10–4) consists of stroboscopic light, rigid endoscope or fiberoptic laryngoscope, microphone, foot switch for triggering the light source, and image recording, video recording system, and display system. A microphone picks up the frequency of the patient's sustained phonation, which triggers the stroboscopic light.

Test Procedures: The patient should sit upright, with his or her shoulders forward and head elevated. Before carrying out the examination, reassure the patient to relax by explaining the procedure and what is expected from him or her. Misty visualization could be prevented by means of heating, airstream blowing, or smearing antifogging agent on the tip of the strobolaryngoscope. The microphone can be fixed on the surface of thyroid cartilage or directly connected to the

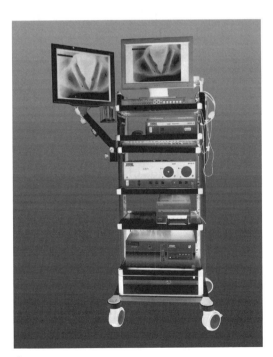

A

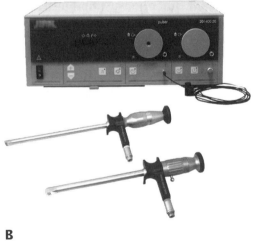

B

Figure 10–4. Strobolaryngoscopy.

laryngoscope. Place the strobolar-yngoscope inside the patient's oral cavity and use the back surface to elevate the soft palate, then rotate the lens to aim at the hypopharynx and the larynx. The patient is asked to phonate vowel /i/ ("e-e-e-e") at his or her comfortable pitch and loudness while the laryngoscope is advancing. The examiner can initiate and control the phase difference between the acoustic impulse and the stroboscopic light (which can be adjusted from 0° to 360°) by using the foot pedal. This allows observation of the static phase or the slow-motion phase during the vibration of the vocal folds.

Analysis of Stroboscopic Images: Stroboscopic interpretation should include the following: the shape and symmetry of the vocal folds, the amplitude of vibration, mucosal wave movements, overall glottal closure, supraglottic involvement, and any other unusual findings. In normal conditions, the vocal folds on both sides are symmetric, mucosal wave is normal, and vibration is in uniform rate. The vibration pattern is affected by the vocal fold tension and the subglottal lung pressure. If lesions are found on the vocal folds, depending on the type and severity, the vibration may appear slow, with small amplitude, weakened or missing mucosa wave and asymmetry of vocal folds. The following is a summary of features to be assessed (Echternach, Arndt, Zander, & Richter, 2009; Hirano & Bless, 1993):

1. **Fundamental frequency of phonation.** Strobolaryngoscopy can display the values of funda-mental frequency. Determine if the fundamental frequency is appro-priate for age and gender of the patient.

2. **Patterns of glottal closure.** The glottal closure is the degree of the greatest closure of the vocal folds in the vibration cycle. Normal vocal folds have complete closure in the closed phase. Incomplete glottal closure will produce breathi-ness. Typical vocal fold vibratory patterns include:

   a. **Complete closure:** the vocal folds come together or fully adducted along their entire length.

   b. **Spindlelike fissure:** vocal fold bowing with incomplete closure in the midmembra-nous portion of the vocal folds, which is often seen in unilateral vocal paralysis or presbylarynges.

   c. **Hourglass-like fissure:** there is contact only in the midmem-branous portion of the vocal folds, which is seen when vocal nodules or vocal polyps are present.

   d. **Anterior gap:** there is a gap anterior to the posterior two-thirds of the vocal folds, which is sometimes seen in the presbylarynges.

   e. **Posterior chink:** there is a small chink between the vocal processes, which commonly is seen in women or is a normal variation in many males and females.

   f. **Irregularity fissure:** there is irregular edge making contact.

g. **Incomplete closure.**

3. **Supraglottic activity.** Supraglottic activity is used to describe excessive or hyperfunctional ventricular fold or supraglottic structure movement during phonation. Such movement would appear as hyperplasia or be described as an "anterior and/or posterior squeeze."

4. **Patterns of vibratory motion**

a. **Amplitude of vibration:** This is the maximum excursion of the vocal folds during phonation. The amplitude decreases with stiffness of the vocal folds at high pitch and increases when the muscle tone reduces (e.g., in patients with presbyphonia or vocal fold paralysis).

b. **Mucosal wave:** The mucosal wave is the traveling wave that crosses from the inferior of the vocal folds to the superior surface during phonation. Pliable cover layer of the vocal folds vibrates around the relative fixed body layer and produces cyclical displacement. One of the great advantages of the stroboscopy is the ability to determine the presence, absence or abnormality of the mucosal wave. The patterns of mucosal wave can be described as:

  ▪ **Lack of mucosal wave:** visible mucosal wave is absent, which is seen mostly in vocal fold scarring or malignant lesions infiltration.

  ▪ **Decreased mucosal wave:** mucosal wave is reduced, and the degree of reduced wave can be classified into mild, moderate, and severe.

  ▪ **Normal mucosal waves:** size and degree of mucosal wave are normal while phonating under a comfortable pitch, loudness, and duration.

  ▪ **Enhanced mucosal waves:** mucosal wave is apparently larger, which is sometimes seen in Reinke's edema.

  To describe mucosal waves, one should also compare the relative displacement of the mucosal wave on both sides. The mucosal waves can give more information of the severity of lesions. The superficial lesion always affects the mucosal wave, and the deep tissue damage may cause abnormal vocal fold vibration. However, the use of high-pitched or unstable phonation often produces a vibratory pattern with no observable mucosal waves.

c. **Nonvibrating portion:** The extent of the portion of vocal folds that does not vibrate during phonation indicates the degree of infiltration of a lesion or scarring on the vocal folds.

d. **Symmetry and periodicity:** With normal phonation, the vocal folds vibrate periodically and both sides are symmetric. Aperiodic cyclic vibration is one of the factors producing noise.

REFERENCES

Echternach, M., Arndt, S., Zander, M. F., & Richter, B. (2009). Voice diagnostics in professional sopranos: Application of the protocol of the European Laryngological Society (ELS). Hals-, Nasen-, Ohren-Heilkunde *HNO, 57*(3), 266–272.

Hirano, M., & Bless, D. M. (1993). *Videostroboscopic examination of the larynx*. San Diego, CA: Singular.

Kendall, K. A. (2009). High-speed laryngeal imaging compared with videostroboscopy in healthy subjects. *Archives of Otolaryngology-Head and Neck Surgery, 135*(3), 274–281.

Oertel, M. J. (1895). Das laryngoskopische untersuchung. *Archives of Laryngology and Rhinology (Berlin), 3*, 1–16.

Yanagisawa, E., Owens, T. W., Strothers, G., & Honda, K. (1983). Videolaryngoscopy. A comparison of fiberscopic and telescopic documentation. *Annals of Otology, Rhinology and Laryngology, 92*, 430–436.

CHAPTER 11

Videokymographic Examination of Voice

JAN G. ŠVEC AND FRANTIŠEK ŠRAM

PURPOSES

- To assess the ability of the vocal folds to vibrate.
- To assess pliability and stiffness of the vocal fold tissues.
- To assess perturbation of the vocal fold vibration.
- To assess the duration of vocal fold closure during vibration.
- To assess left-right asymmetry of the vocal folds during vibration.
- To understand the origin of hoarseness on the vocal fold level.

THEORETICAL BACKGROUND

Vocal fold vibration plays the primary role for producing voice quality. Most voice disorders are caused by disturbed vibrations of the vocal folds. To understand the origins of voice disorders, it therefore is important to understand *how* the vocal folds are disturbed in their vibration.

Traditionally, diagnosis of voice disorders has been based on vocal fold visualization via laryngoscopy. Most commonly, stroboscopic light is used to observe the vibrations of the vocal folds (e.g., Böhme & Gross, 2005; Cornut & Bouchayer, 1998; Faure & Muller, 1992; Hirano & Bless, 1993; Wendler, 1992). However, stroboscopic light allows observing the vibration only when the vocal folds vibrate regularly. The stroboscopic flashes need to be synchronized with the vocal fold vibration, which is technically impossible when the vibrations are irregular. As an alternative, high-speed videolaryngoscopic techniques therefore have been used instead of stroboscopy. These techniques allow capturing the vocal fold vibration with the frame rate exceeding 1000 images per second (e.g., Bless, Patel, & Connor, 2009; Deliyski et al., 2008; Hertegård, Larsson,

& Wittenberg, 2003). The vibration disturbances can then be visualized when the high-speed video recordings are played back at slow speed.

Watching the high-speed videos at slow speed, however, is extremely time consuming. One second of a high-speed video recorded with the frame rate of 4000 images per second takes more than 1 minute to watch at standard video speed and even more when played frame by frame. Techniques therefore have been developed to speed up and facilitate observation of the vocal fold vibration. The most basic method is called "**kymography**." This method selects just a single line from each of the images of the vocal folds and uses these to compose a new image, displaying the vibration of only a selected part of the vocal folds in time (Figure 11–1). Such an image is called a "**kymogram**."

The first kymographic images of the vocal folds were obtained in the 1970s by Volker Gall in Germany who constructed a specially modified photographic camera for this purpose (Gall, 1984; Gall & Freigang, 1974; Gall, Gall, & Hanson, 1971; Gall & Hanson, 1973). The method was called "**photokymography**." Although showing promising results, it remained only in an experimental stage

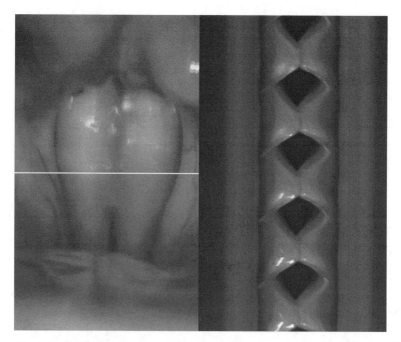

Figure 11–1. The two images provided by the second generation videokymographic camera. The recording was obtained from a 43-year-old male without voice problems. On the left is the standard laryngoscopic image, on the right is the videokymographic (VKG) image showing the normal vibration of the vocal folds at the position indicated by the line on the left. In the VKG image, time runs from top to bottom; the total time displayed is 40 ms.

(Gross, 1985, 1988; Schultz-Coulon, 1990; Schultz-Coulon & Klingholz, 1988). The kymographic method has become more widely known after the invention of "**videokymography**" (VKG) in 1994 (Švec & Schutte, 1996), which is described in this chapter.

Inspired by videokymography, kymographic imaging also has been adopted for extracting the vibration information from the full high-speed video recordings (Deliyski, 2005; Eysholdt, Rosanowski, & Hoppe, 2003; Granqvist & Lindestad, 2001; Larsson, Hertegård, Lindestad, & Hammarberg, 2000; Wittenberg, Tigges, Mergell, & Eysholdt, 2000) and from videostroboscopic recordings (Hertegård et al., 2003; Isogai, 1996; Nawka, 2005; Sung et al., 1999). In these two methods, the kymographic images are called "**digital kymograms**" and "**strobokymograms**," respectively. These two methods differ substantially from videokymography by the fact that the kymograms are extracted from previously recorded videolaryngoscopic recordings by means of **special software**. In contrast to these two methods, **in videokymography, the kymograms are created in the videokymographic camera** and are watched in real time during the laryngoscopic examination. Discussion on the advantages and drawbacks of the three kymographic methods can be found, for example, in Švec and Šram (2002). This chapter focuses on the method of videokymography.

DESCRIPTION

Videokymography is based on a special video camera that can deliver both standard laryngoscopic images as well as the high-speed videokymographic images.

These are captured with a standard video recorder. In the first generation, the camera used a foot switch that allowed switching between the laryngoscopic and videokymographic images (Švec & Schutte, 1996; Švec, Schutte, & Šram, 1997; Švec, Šram, & Schutte, 1999). The current, second generation system, developed in 2006 (Qiu & Schutte, 2006), delivers both these images simultaneously in real time (see Figure 11–1).

The traditional view of the vocal folds (see Figure 11–1, left) is captured by the current videokymographic camera at the frame rate of 25 or 30 images per second (in PAL or NTSC systems, respectively, depending on the corresponding television standard). The kymographic images are delivered at the high-speed rate of 7200 linear images per second. In order to display and save the kymograms simultaneously side by side with the traditional images, the kymographic images are separated into 25 or 30 frames per second, each frame containing 288 (PAL) or 240 (NTSC) VKG image lines (Qiu & Schutte, 2007). The total time displayed in the videokymogram shown on the video monitor is equal to 40 ms (PAL) or 33.3 ms (NTSC).

The schematic display in Figure 11–2 shows the basic vibration characteristics of the vocal folds. In this display, the kymographic features are related to the subsequent phases of the glottal vibratory cycle known from the traditional methods. The vibratory cycle is divided in two basic phases: (1) the **closed phase** and (2) the **open phase**. The open phase is then subdivided into two subphases: (a) the *opening phase*, when the vocal folds are moving laterally (i.e., away from each other), and (b) the *closing phase*, when the vocal folds are moving medially (i.e., closer to each other). Careful observation of the modifications within and across

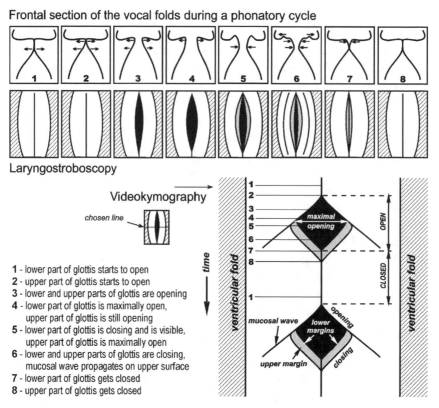

Figure 11–2. Vocal fold vibration, the relationship among the traditional displays and the kymographic display. (From: Švec, J. G., *On vibration properties of human vocal folds: Voice registers, bifurcations, resonance characteristics, development and application of videokymography.* Doctoral Dissertation, University of Groningen, the Netherlands, 2000, Used with permission)

boundaries of these phases, the symmetry between the two vocal folds and the presence of mucosal waves allows differentiating various disturbances of the vocal fold vibrations, which are described in the following sections.

The focus on the vibration disturbances fundamentally differentiates the kymographic methods from the traditional laryngoscopic methods, which describe voice disorders mainly through tissue alterations of the laryngeal structures. Generally, kymography describes voice disorders through vibratory impairments of the vocal folds.

EQUIPMENT AND MATERIALS

The basic equipment for videokymographic examination (Figure 11–3) consists of:

- Videokymographic camera
- Laryngoscope with a standard C-mount objective adapter for the camera
- Continuous light source of high intensity
- Standard video-capturing system with a video monitor
- Microphone for capturing the voice acoustic signal (optional)

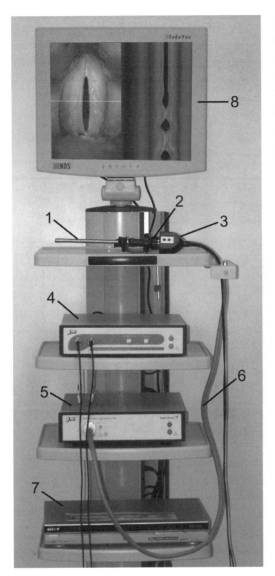

Figure 11–3. The videokymographic equipment: (1) laryngoscope, (2) an objective with a C-mount, (3) VKG camera head, (4) VKG camera unit, (5) endoscopic high-intensity continuous light source, (6) light cable, (7) digital video recorder, and (8) video monitor. (Photo courtesy of Cymo, B.V., Groningen, The Netherlands).

For illumination, a continuous light is used instead of stroboscopic light. As the VKG camera is a high-speed camera, it requires considerably more light than a standard camera for laryngoscopy. The choice of light source is important: insufficient illumination, as well as excessive illumination, causes deterioration of the image quality (Figures 11–4A and 11–4B). A 300-W xenon light source with adjustable intensity and stabilized output has been found to produce images of sufficiently good quality. In some subjects, a 180-W continuous light source (which is present in some stroboscopes as a secondary light source) may be sufficient, but the image quality achieved with such a weaker light source generally is lower (see Figure 11–4A).

Laryngoscope quality is of the same importance as the quality of the light source for obtaining good VKG images. Some laryngoscopes are brighter than others. For instance, older laryngoscopes may not provide as bright images as newer ones, due to deterioration and pollution of the fibers in the light-conducting cables. Before buying a laryngoscope, it is useful to ask the manufacturer of the videokymographic camera for a recommendation on a laryngoscope and a light source well suited for this type of imaging.

For capturing the video signals, videokymography uses a standard video recording system. This usually is a video recorder or a computer. Care should be taken of the video standard. Videokymography can be used in both the PAL as well as the NTSC standards but the camera and the video recording system should always be of the same standard.

Besides the video signals, it is useful to capture the sound during videokymographic examination, which can be recorded together with the video images and stored in the video file. A microphone is needed for this purpose.

The images presented here were obtained with the following equipment:

A. Insufficient light   **B.** Too much light

C. Tilted glottal axis   **D.** Wrong measurement position

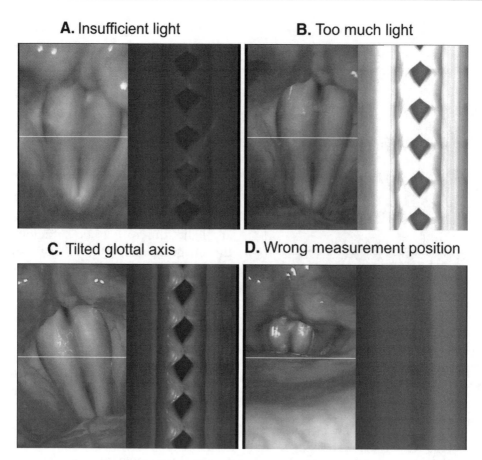

Figure 11–4. Factors negatively affecting videokymographic images: (**A**) insufficient illumination, (**B**) excessive illumination, (**C**) tilted glottal axis, and (**D**) wrong position of the measurement line. Total time displayed in the videokymogram is 40 ms. Notice that there are about 5 vibration cycles in the kymograms in (A), (B), and (C) revealing that the phonation frequency was about 125 Hz (i.e., 5 × 25 Hz).

the second generation videokymographic camera (Cymo, BV), the first generation videokymographic camera (Lambert Instruments, BV), C-mount objective/adapter (optical lens with focal length 32 mm, C1200.32, Cymo, B.V.), laryngoscope (Richard Wolf Lupenlaryngoskop 90°, model 4450.47), the 300-W xenon light source (Richard Wolf Auto LP/FLASH 5135 or Kay Elemetrics 7150), a digital video recording equipment (A/D video converter Canopus ADVC 300 and PC with DiVAS recording software, Xion).

TEST PROCEDURES— GUIDELINES

Inserting the Laryngoscope

Generally, the examination procedure in videokymography is similar to the videolaryngoscopic procedure. The difference between the classic videolaryngoscopic and the videokymographic examination lies especially in the need of more careful positioning of the laryngoscope. Proper positioning of the laryngoscope is important in videokymography, as the clinician should be able to make sure that the measurement line for VKG images is placed at the desirable location on the vocal folds (cf. Figures 11–4C and 11–4D).

As in classical laryngoscopy, the laryngoscope is inserted in the mouth of the client while producing vowel /e/ or /i/ and the laryngoscopic image is followed on a video monitor. Laryngoscopic rules should be followed to prevent or suppress the gag reflex. Care should be taken so that the laryngoscope is not fogged during the examination, which is achieved either by warming the tip of the laryngoscope or applying antifogging solutions on the glass at the tip of the laryngoscope (Cornut & Bouchayer, 1998).

Positioning the Measurement Line for Videokymography

The measurement line is most often aimed at the place of the maximum vibrational amplitude of the vocal folds, perpendicular to glottal axis. To achieve this, the following steps should be done after obtaining the view of the vocal folds on the left side of the screen:

■ In case the glottal axis is in an oblique position on the monitor see (see Figure 11–4C), the camera head should be rotated with respect to the laryngoscope until the vertical position of the glottal axis is achieved (see Figure 11–1). This procedure should be done also when the tilted glottal axis is a typical feature of the investigated larynx (i.e., due to inherent structural asymmetry).

■ The position of the laryngoscope should be adjusted so that the position of the measurement line is approximately in the middle of the vocal folds where their vibration amplitude is maximal (see Figure 11–1). This can be done by slightly tilting the laryngoscope vertically in the mouth.

Focusing the Image

Videokymographic images of high quality require proper focusing of the optical path. The focus can be changed by adjusting the lenses attached to the laryngoscope. A well-focused image can be recognized by sharp contours of the vibrating vocal folds in the VKG image.

Tip—Stabilizing the VKG Image for Better Focus

Have the client phonate a sustained tone at a constant pitch and follow the VKG image on the screen. If the VKG image runs too quickly to be followed, have the client to go up or down in pitch until the VKG image slows down (this phenomenon is analogous to a stroboscopic effect). In the PAL system, a stable VKG image is achieved at the phonational frequencies that are multiples of 25 Hz, that is, 75, 100, 125, 150, 175 Hz, and so forth. At these frequencies, we see 3, 4, 5, 6, 7, and so on vibratory cycles of the vocal folds in the videokymogram on the screen. In the NTSC system, the same effect is observed at multiples of 30 Hz, that is, 90, 120, 150, 180, 210 Hz, and so forth. The pitch-adjustment procedure is particularly useful in singers. It is possible to manipulate the pitch so that the VKG image is practically still on the monitor. The focus of laryngoscope can then be well adjusted by making the VKG images maximally sharp.

Examining Sustained Phonations

As in laryngostroboscopy, examination of sustained phonations is considered to be the most fundamental procedure in videokymography. At the very minimum, the client is asked to phonate at comfortable pitch and loudness (Table 11–1). During the comfortable phonation, the clinician positions the measurement line at the place of maximum vibration amplitude to obtain the most representative videokymogram (see Figure 11–1).

After the representative videokymogram has been obtained, the vocal folds may be scanned from anterior to posterior ("A-P scan") to capture vibration along the whole glottal length (Figure 11–5). This is especially advantageous with organic voice disorders (lesions, polyps, cysts, etc.) in which various parts of the vocal folds may vibrate differently (Schutte, Švec, & Šram, 1998; Švec et al., 2007). The A-P scan

can be done by gently tilting the laryngoscope vertically in the mouth. The scan can be performed in a short time during the sustained phonation—the time of 1 to 2 seconds is sufficient for this purpose. The scanning maneuver often is very helpful when reviewing the examination during playback. The videokymograms from any part of the vocal folds can be visualized in this way. The phonation should be kept approximately constant during the scanning maneuver, however, in order to compare the vibrations from different parts of the vocal folds.

To obtain more information, sustained phonations across different pitches and different intensities can be done following the same procedure as used for the comfortable pitch and loudness.

Additional Phonation Tasks

Useful information also can be obtained from other phonation tasks, depending on

Table 11–1. Phonations and VKG Measurement Positions Used During Videokymographic Examination of Voice

Phonation	VKG Measurement Position
Comfortable pitch and loudness (basic)	• Place of maximum vibration amplitude • A-P scan
Voice onset and offset (hi-hi-hi or he-he-he)	• Place of maximum vibration amplitude
Sustained tones at different pitches (middle, high, low)	• Place of maximum vibration amplitude • A-P scan
Sustained tones at different volumes (soft to loud)	• Place of maximum vibration amplitude • A-P scan
Tones at which the phonations are problematic	• Place of maximum vibration amplitude • A-P scan
Register transitions (in singers)	• Place of maximum vibration amplitude
Cough	• Place of maximum vibration amplitude

the type of voice disorder (see Table 11-1). Voice onset and voice offset provide information on the way the vocal folds start and end their vibration (Figure 11-6). During these events, the vocal folds may exhibit characteristic features, such as asymmetries, abruptness of onset and offset, and so on (Braunschweig, Flaschka, Schelhorn-Neise, & Döllinger, 2008; Dejonckere, 2000; Eysholdt, Tigges, Wittenberg, & Pröschel, 1996; Hertegård, 2005; Mergell, Herzel, Wittenberg, Tigges, & Eysholdt, 1998; Orlikoff, Deliyski, Baken, & Watson, 2009). If the client complains of problems with specific phonations (e.g., high pitch, loud voice, register transitions, etc.), these phonations

A. Start of Anterior-Posterior Scan   **B.** End of Anterior-Posterior Scan

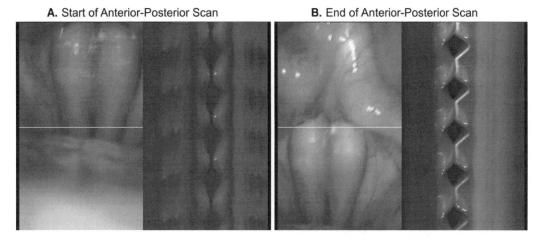

Figure 11-5. Anterior-posterior scan allows examining the vibrations at all parts of the vocal folds. These images were taken (**A**) shortly after the start of the scanning maneuver, capturing the vibrations of the anterior part of the vocal folds, and (**B**) at the end of the scanning maneuver about two seconds later, capturing the vibration of the posterior part of the vocal folds.

A. Voice Onset   **B.** Voice Offset

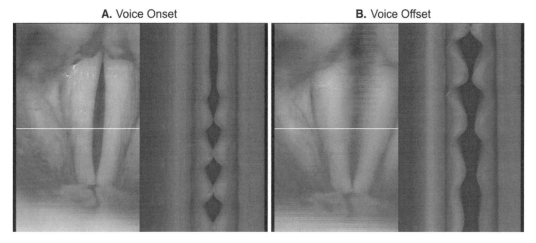

Figure 11-6. (**A**) Voice onset and (**B**) voice offset in videokymography in a male without voice problems. The offset reveals slight left-right asymmetry.

also should be targeted for examination. Furthermore, movement of the vocal folds during coughing can reveal the pliability of the vocal fold tissues, especially in clients who cannot produce voice normally, for example, in psychogenic aphonias.

Factors That Can Affect the Reliability and Validity of the Assessment

For reliable evaluation of videokymographic images, it is important to establish measurement position at the desirable place on the vocal folds (e.g., at maximum vibration amplitude; anterior to, at, and posterior to lesion), make sure that the glottal axis is vertical on the screen (axis tilt up to about 5 to 10 degrees is tolerable), and have sufficient illumination and proper focus of the laryngoscope.

Furthermore, it is important to relate the observed videokymographic vibration pattern to the phonation produced. In soft phonations, the vibration pattern is different from that in loud voice, and the vibration also pattern changes with voice registers (Švec, Schutte, & Šram, 1999).

EVALUATION OF THE VKG IMAGES

After the examination, the recorded videokymographic images should be evaluated. The most basic procedure is based on visual evaluation of the images. Although subjective, visual evaluation is extremely useful as it allows detection of subtle variations in vibration patterns revealing altered functionality of the vocal folds (Bonilha & Deliyski, 2008; Bonilha, Deliyski, & Gerlach, 2008; Fujita, Ferreira, & Sarkovas,

2004; Kim et al., 2003; Mendelsohn, Sung, Berke, & Chhetri, 2007; Schutte et al., 1998; Shaw & Deliyski, 2008; Šram, Schutte, & Švec, 1997; Šram & Švec, 2000; Šram, Švec, & Schutte, 1999; Švec et al., 1999; Tigges, Richter, & Wittenberg, 2005; van Kalkeren, Schutte, Qiu, Švec, & Mahieu, 2006; Verdonck-de Leeuw, Festen, & Mahieu, 2001). Several teams also have been working on automatic quantitative evaluation, but no software is commercially available for this purpose yet (Deliyski et al., 2008; Granqvist & Lindestad, 2001; Larsson et al., 2000; Manfredi, Bocchi, Bianchi, Migali, & Cantarella, 2006; Qiu, Schutte, Gu, & Yu, 2003).

Normal Findings

Sustained phonations at comfortable pitch and intensity normally should present the following properties, which are well visible in the videokymographic images of the vocal folds (Bless, Hirano, & Feder, 1987; Bonilha et al., 2008; Gross, 1988; Hirano, 1981; Hirano, 1992; Shaw & Deliyski, 2008; Švec et al., 2007; Švec et al., 2009):

- Both vocal folds are vibrating
- Ventricular folds are not vibrating
- Vibrational amplitudes of both vocal folds are approximately similar
- Vibrational frequencies of both vocal folds are similar
- The vibrations are regular
- The vibrations are free of aberrations
- The vocal folds touch each other during vibration (PMA*)
- The closed phase takes between 20 and 50% of period duration (PMA*)
- The shape of lateral peaks (i.e., turn from opening to closing) is sharp
- Mucosal waves propagate on the upper vocal fold surface

- No large left-right phase asymmetry is present
- The durations of opening and closing phases are approximately similar

(The features marked with "PMA*" denote that these are valid for the place of maximum vibration amplitude (PMA) of the vocal folds.)

Findings in Voice Disorders

Studies of over 5,000 videokymographic examinations of patients with functional and organic voice disorders have revealed numerous alterations from the normal vibratory patterns, which reveal on different origins of voice disorders. Detailed description and categorization of these for sustained phonations was provided by Švec and his colleagues (Švec et al., 2007; Švec et al., 2009). A summarized list of the altered vibration features and their interpretation is provided in Table 11-2.

The table reveals that alterations of vibration features are related to altered physical and geometrical properties of the vocal folds. These alterations are consequences of pathological processes on the vocal folds, structural asymmetry, malformations, improper neuromuscular functioning, and so forth.

CASE EXAMPLES

Case 1: Patient J.M. (Vocal Fold Cancer)

A 54-year-old male patient, J.M., came for checkup examination to exclude recurrence of carcinoma of the right vocal fold and epiglottal epithelium. The carcinoma was treated 3 years ago by partial frontolateral laryngectomy, epiglottal stripping, and subsequent radiation therapy. Seven months ago, computed tomography (CT) examination of the larynx found no recurrent tumors. His voice was strongly husky, with breathiness but sufficiently sonorous and quite intelligible. There were audible signs of inspiratory stridor. Lymph nodes on the neck were not palpable, the wounds healed well.

Laryngoscopic imaging (Figure 11-7, left) revealed diffusely thickened left vocal fold (lf) of smooth surface and a normal looking left ventricular fold (lv). The right ventricular fold (rv) had reddened smooth surface with two suspicious round bumps with the larger one approximately in the middle of the ventricular fold's length, and the smaller one placed dorsally and a few millimeters caudally. The right vocal fold (rf) was diffusely thickened; the ventral half of the upper surface was unsmooth and of grayish color. The anterior half of the upper vocal fold surface was smooth, with dilated vessels. The most ventral third of the right vocal fold was slightly excaved, causing posterior glottal gap. Gross mobility of the right vocal and ventricular fold was limited and possible only in a restricted range of a few millimeters in the posterior half of the glottis. The gross mobility of the left vocal and ventricular fold was also restricted to few millimeters.

Videokymography (Figure 11-7, right) showed these abnormalities:

- *Complete absence of vibration* on the right vocal fold, indicating very stiff tissues. This was a very serious finding raising a suspicion of cancer invading the body of the vocal fold;
- *Very short closure duration* at the place of maximum vibration amplitude of the left vocal fold, indicating problems with vocal fold adduction;

Table 11–2. Disturbances of the Vocal Fold Vibration and Their Possible Causes

Finding	Possible Cause
Completely absent vibration of the vocal fold	Tumor, scar, excessive mucosal stiffness
Partly absent vibration of the vocal fold	Stiff vocal fold body, dislocated prosthesis
Large vibration of the ventricular fold	Hyperfunction, compensation of glottal insufficiency
Covibration of fluids	Too much fluid or mucus (unclear vocal fold vibration characteristics)
Large cycle-to-cycle variability	Right-left or anterior-posterior asymmetry, or excessively low vocal fold tension
Absence of glottal closure	Serious adduction problem
Short closure duration (1–20%)	Hypoadduction
Long closure duration (>60%)	Hyperadduction
Large amplitude differences	Right-left structural asymmetry of vocal folds
Frequency differences	Unilateral paralysis, serious structural asymmetry
Large phase differences	Right-left asymmetry of tension or mass
Axis shift during closure	Tension asymmetry, niveau difference
Decreased sharpness of lateral peaks	Medial mucosa excessively stiff
Absent or reduced mucosal waves	Mucosa on upper vocal fold surface excessively stiff
Distant mucosal waves	Excessively thick mucosa, Reinke's edema under pliable epithelium
Opening notably shorter than closing	Mucosa more stiff or tensed than optimal
Opening notably longer than closing	Mucosa more pliable than optimal
Sharpened medial peaks	Thinned vocal fold edge
Presence of aberration (any sort)	Various causes
Ripple (aberration)	Localized lesion on vocal fold
Double medial peak (aberration)	Sulcus, furrow on medial vocal fold surface
Medial unsmoothness (aberration)	Defected medial vocal fold shape

Source: Based on Švec, Šram, and Schutte, 2007, 2009.

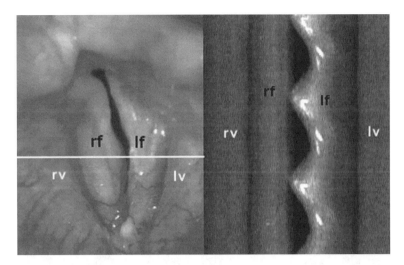

Figure 11–7. Strobolaryngoscopic and VKG images of a male patient with vocal fold cancer on the right. Notice that the right vocal fold (rf) remained completely still during phonation. Total time displayed in the VKG image is 18.4 ms. (Symbols used: rv and lv = right and left ventricular fold, rf and lf = right and left vocal fold.)

- *Decreased sharpness of lateral vibrational peaks* of the left vocal fold; and
- *Absent mucosal waves* on the left, both indicating the mucosa of the left vocal fold is unhealthily stiff.

Based on the videokymographic and videolaryngoscopic findings, the patient was diagnosed with suspected cancerous infiltration of the ventral two-thirds of the right vocal fold as well as with cancerous infiltration on the right ventricular fold. Histologic examination confirmed the malignancy as suspected. Due to the size of the tumor and the patient's medical history, the patient was treated with total laryngectomy.

Case 2: Patient K.B. (Unilateral Vocal Fold Paralysis)

A 64-year-old female patient, K.B., came with the diagnosis of paralysis of the left vocal fold, that developed after virosis 10 years ago causing initial aphonia. She went through voice therapy after which her voice improved. She was reported to speak at raised pitch and complained of vocal fatiguability. The complaints worsened about 7 months ago due to the need of increased vocal effort after sudden worsening of her husband's hearing. Perceptually, her voice was markedly high-pitched, slightly husky, breathy, and strained.

Laryngoscopy (Figure 11–8, left) revealed the left arytenoid cartilage during breathing to be placed almost medially, placed more ventrally than the right one. The left side of the larynx was grossly immobile. On the right side, the gross mobility was normal. The left vocal fold (lf) was thin, slightly concave, in intermedial position, its niveau appeared to be slightly above the right vocal fold. The right vocal fold (rf) showed good gross mobility, crossing the midline at the dorsal

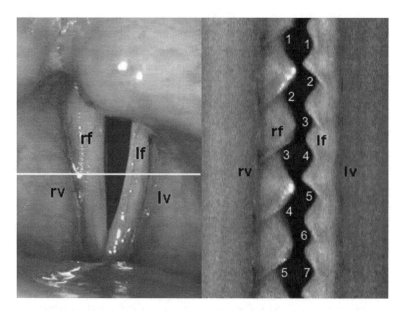

Figure 11–8. Female patient with left vocal fold paralysis. On the left is a laryngoscopic image during breathing; the right image shows the videokymogram during phonation at the position indicated in the left image. Notice the different vibration frequencies of the right (rf) and left (lf) vocal folds (5 versus 7 vibration cycles) and the missing vocal fold contact. Total time displayed in the VKG image is 18.4 ms. The symbols used are the same as those in Figure 11–7.

third of the glottis during phonation. In the anterior two-thirds, there remained a half-moon-shaped glottal gap on the left from the midline.

Videokymography (Figure 11–8, right) showed the following abnormalities:

■ *Absence of glottal closure*, which was indicative of insufficient vocal fold adduction and was typical of vocal fold paralysis (Benninger et al., 1994; Isshiki, Tanabe, & Sawada, 1978; Woodson, 1993). Such an insufficiency is known to cause problems with increasing vocal loudness and with vocal fatiguability.

■ *Left-right frequency differences.* The right vocal fold completed five cycles, whereas the left one completed seven cycles. This was an indication of serious left-right structural asymmetry, also typical of unilateral vocal fold paralysis. The paralyzed vocal fold vibrated at higher pitch than the healthy fold, suggesting the paralyzed fold was stiffer than the healthy one. The two different frequencies of the vocal folds were typical of biphonia (Ouaknine, Garrel, & Giovanni, 2003; Tigges, Mergell, Herzel, Wittenberg, & Eysholdt, 1997).

■ *Large cycle-to-cycle variability* on the nonparalyzed right vocal fold. This could be interpreted as an unsuccessful attempt of the healthy vocal fold to temporarily synchronize with the paralyzed vocal fold. The irregularity is known to cause hoarseness.

■ *Decreased sharpness of lateral peaks* and *shorter mucosal waves* on the paralyzed left vocal fold. This indicated rather stiff medial mucosa of the paralyzed fold. The vibration pattern on this vocal fold reminded that of falsetto register, whereas the sharp lateral peaks on the right were indicative rather of the chest register (Hirano, 1981; Švec, Schutte, & Šram, 1999).

■ *Amplitude was noticeably smaller* on the paralyzed left vocal fold than on the nonparalyzed one. This finding was also indicative of falsetto versus chest register on the left versus the right vocal fold (Hirano, 1981; Švec et al., 1999).

■ *Medial peaks on the paralyzed left vocal fold were sharper* than those of the nonparalyzed vocal fold. This indicated that the medial vocal fold shape of the paralyzed vocal fold was thinner than that of the nonparalyzed vocal fold (Švec et al., 2007; Švec et al., 2009). Such a finding could be explained as a consequence of paralyzed vocalis muscle on the left, causing the vocal fold to be thinner (Hirano, 1975).

Overall, the findings were indicative of typical unilateral vocal fold paralysis. The videokymographic features indicated paralysis of both the vocalis muscle, which caused the altered vocal fold tension and shape, as well as of the posterior cricoarytenoid muscle, which caused the impaired adduction of the vocal process. The patient was recommended for vocal fold medialization procedure (Type I thyroplasty), which improved the voice considerably.

REFERENCES

Benninger, M. S., Crumley, R. L., Ford, C. N., Gould, W. J., Hanson, D. G., Ossoff, R. H., & Sataloff, R. T. (1994). Evaluation and treatment of the unilateral paralyzed vocal fold. *Otolaryngology-Head and Neck Surgery, 111,* 497–508.

Bless, D. M., Hirano, M., & Feder, R. J. (1987). Videostroboscopic evaluation of the larynx. *Ear, Nose and Throat Journal, 66,* 289–296.

Bless, D. M., Patel, R. R., & Connor, N. (2009). Laryngeal imaging: Stroboscopy, high-speed imaging, and kymography. In M. P. Fried & A. Ferlito (Eds.), *The Larynx* (Vol. 1, 3rd ed., pp. 181–210). San Diego, CA: Plural Publishing.

Böhme, G., & Gross, M. (2005). *Stroboscopy and other techniques for the analysis of vocal fold vibration.* London, UK: Whurr.

Bonilha, H. S., & Deliyski, D. D. (2008). Period and glottal width irregularities in vocally normal speakers. *Journal of Voice, 22,* 699–708.

Bonilha, H. S., Deliyski, D. D., & Gerlach, T. T. (2008). Phase asymmetries in normophonic speakers: Visual judgments and objective findings. *American Journal of Speech-Language Pathology, 17,* 367–376.

Braunschweig, T., Flaschka, J., Schelhorn-Neise, P., & Döllinger, M. (2008). High-speed video analysis of the phonation onset, with an application to the diagnosis of functional dysphonias. *Medical Engineering and Physics, 30,* 59–66.

Cornut, G., & Bouchayer, M. (1998). *Assessing dysphonia: The role of video stroboscopy. An interactive video textbook.* Gibraltar, UK: The 3Ears Company.

Dejonckere, P. (2000). Original insights into some vocal fold dynamics by using a single linescan camera. In M. Gross (Ed.), *Aktuelle phoniatrisch-pädaudiologische Aspekte 1999/2000. Band 7* (pp. 53–54). Heidelberg, Germany: Median-Verlag von Killisch-Horn.

Deliyski, D. D. (2005). Endoscope motion compensation for laryngeal high-speed videoendoscopy. *Journal of Voice, 19,* 485–496.

Deliyski, D. D., Petrushev, P. P., Bonilha, H. S., Gerlach, T. T., Martin-Harris, B., & Hillman, R. E. (2008). Clinical implementation of laryngeal high-speed videoendoscopy: Challenges and evolution. *Folia Phoniatrica et Logopaedica*, *60*, 33–44.

Eysholdt, U., Rosanowski, F., & Hoppe, U. (2003). Vocal fold vibration irregularities caused by different types of laryngeal asymmetry. *European Archives of Oto-Rhino-Laryngology*, *260*, 412–417.

Eysholdt, U., Tigges, M., Wittenberg, T., & Pröschel, U. (1996). Direct evaluation of high-speed recordings of vocal fold vibrations. *Folia Phoniatrica et Logopaedica*, *48*, 163–170.

Faure, M. A., & Muller, A. (1992). Stroboscopy. *Journal of Voice*, *6*, 139–148.

Fujita, R., Ferreira, A. E., & Sarkovas, C. (2004). Videokymography assessment of vocal fold vibration before and after hydration. *Revista Brasileira de Otorrinolaringologia*, *70*, 742–746.

Gall, V. (1984). Strip kymography of the glottis. *Archives of Oto-Rhino-Laryngology*, *240*, 287–293.

Gall, V., & Freigang, C. (1974). Zur Larynx-Fotokymografie: Demonstration einiger pathologischer Kehlkopf-Befunde. *Monatsschrift für Ohrenheilkunde und Laryngo-Rhinologie*, *108*, 114–122.

Gall, V., Gall, D., & Hanson, J. (1971). Larynx-Fotokymografie. [In German]. [Larynx-Photokymography]. *Archiv für klinische und experimentelle Ohren- Nasen- und Kehlkopfheilkunde*, *200*, 34–41.

Gall, V., & Hanson, J. (1973). Bestimmung physikalischer Parameter der Stimmlippenschwingungen mit Hilfe der Larynxphotokymographie. [In German]. [Finding physical parameters of vocal cord vibration by use of laryngeal photokymography]. *Folia Phoniatrica*, *25*, 450–459.

Granqvist, S., & Lindestad, P. Å. (2001). A method of applying Fourier analysis to high-speed laryngoscopy. *Journal of the Acoustical Society of America*, *110*, 3193–3197.

Gross, M. (1985). Larynxfotokymographie. *Sprache-Stimme-Gehör*, *9*, 112–113.

Gross, M. (1988). *Endoskopische Larynx-Fotokymografie*. Bingen, Germany: Renate Gross-Verlag.

Hertegård, S. (2005). What have we learned about laryngeal physiology from high-speed digital videoendoscopy? *Current Opinion in Otolaryngology and Head and Neck Surgery*, *13*, 152–156.

Hertegård, S., Larsson, H., & Wittenberg, T. (2003). High-speed imaging: Applications and development. *Logopedics Phoniatrics Vocology*, *28*, 133–139.

Hirano, M. (1975). Phonosurgery: Basic and clinical investigations. *Otologia (Fukuoka)*, *21*(Suppl. 1), 239–440.

Hirano, M. (1981). *Clinical examination of voice*. Vienna, Austria: Springer-Verlag.

Hirano, M. (1992). Stroboscopic examination of the normal larynx. In A. Blitzer, M. F. Brin, C. T. Sasaki, S. Fahn, & K. S. Harris (Eds.), *Neurologic disorders of the larynx* (pp. 135–139). New York, NY: Thieme Medical Publishers.

Hirano, M., & Bless, D. M. (1993). *Videostroboscopic examination of the larynx*. San Diego, CA: Singular Publishing Group.

Isshiki, N., Tanabe, M., & Sawada, M. (1978). Arytenoid adduction for unilateral vocal cord paralysis. *Archives of Otolaryngology*, *104*, 555–558.

Isogai, Y. (1996). Laryngostroboscopy—observation of the travelling wave of the mucous membrane. [In Japanese]. *Larynx Japan*, *8*, 84–91.

Kim, D. Y., Kim, L. S., Kim, K. H., Sung, M. W., Roh, J. L., Kwon, T. K., . . . Sung, M. Y. (2003). Videostrobokymographic analysis of benign vocal fold lesions. *Acta Oto-Laryngologica (Stockholm)*, *123*, 1102–1109.

Larsson, H., Hertegård, S., Lindestad, P. Å., & Hammarberg, B. (2000). Vocal fold vibrations: High-speed imaging, kymography, and acoustic analysis: A preliminary report. *Laryngoscope*, *110*, 2117–2122.

Manfredi, C., Bocchi, L., Bianchi, S., Migali, N., & Cantarella, G. (2006). Objective vocal fold vibration assessment from videokymographic images. *Biomedical Signal Processing and Control*, *1*, 129–136.

Mendelsohn, A. H., Sung, M. W., Berke, G. S., & Chhetri, D. K. (2007). Strobokymographic and videostroboscopic analysis of vocal fold motion in unilateral superior laryngeal nerve paralysis. *Annals of Otology Rhinology and Laryngology, 116*, 85–91.

Mergell, P., Herzel, H., Wittenberg, T., Tigges, M., & Eysholdt, U. (1998). Phonation onset: Vocal fold modeling and high-speed glottography. *Journal of the Acoustical Society of America, 104*, 464–470.

Nawka, T. (2005). *Videostrobokymographie*. Berlin, Germany: Xion Medical.

Orlikoff, R. F., Deliyski, D. D., Baken, R. J., & Watson, B. C. (2009). Validation of a glottographic measure of vocal attack. *Journal of Voice, 23*, 164-168.

Ouaknine, M., Garrel, R., & Giovanni, A. (2003). Separate detection of vocal fold vibration by optoreflectometry: A study of biphonation on excised porcine larynges. *Folia Phoniatrica et Logopaedica, 55*, 28–38.

Qiu, Q., & Schutte, H. K. (2006). A new generation videokymography for routine clinical vocal-fold examination. *Laryngoscope, 116*, 1824-1828.

Qiu, Q., & Schutte, H. K. (2007). Real-time kymographic imaging for visualizing human vocal-fold vibratory function. *Review of Scientific Instruments, 78*, Art. No. 024302.

Qiu, Q., Schutte, H. K., Gu, L., & Yu, Q. (2003). An automatic method to quantify the vibration properties of human vocal folds via videokymography. *Folia Phoniatrica et Logopaedica, 55*, 128–136.

Schultz-Coulon, H.-J. (1990). Mikrofotokymographie des Kehlkopfes. *Sprache-Stimme-Gehör, 14*, 4–10.

Schultz-Coulon, H.-J. & Klingholz, F. (1988). Objektive und semiobjektive Untersuchungsmethoden der Stimme. In G. Kittel & B. Schürenberg (Eds.), *Proceedings of the XVth Congress of the Union of the European Phoniatricians, Erlangen 1988* (pp. 1-87).

Schutte, H. K., Švec, J. G., & Šram, F. (1998). First results of clinical application of videokymography. *Laryngoscope, 108*, 1206–1210.

Shaw, H. S., & Deliyski, D. D. (2008). Mucosal wave: A normophonic study across visualization techniques. *Journal of Voice, 22*, 23-33.

Šram, F., Schutte, H. K., & Švec, J. G. (1997). Clinical applications of videokymography. In G. McCafferty, W. Coman, & R. Carroll (Eds.), *Sydney '97—XVI. World Congress of Otorhinolaryngology-Head and Neck Surgery. Proceedings* (Vol. 2, pp. 1681–1684). Bologna, Italy: Monduzzi Editore.

Šram, F., & Švec, J. G. (2000). Results of videokymographic examinations by functional voice disorders. In M. Gross (Ed.), *Aktuelle phoniatrisch-pädaudiologische Aspekte 1999/2000, Band 7* (pp. 53–56). Heidelberg, Germany: Median-Verlag von Killisch-Horn.

Šram, F., Švec, J. G., & Schutte, H. K. (1999). Possibilities for use of videokymography in laryngologic and phoniatric practice. In P. H. Dejonckere & H. F. M. Peters (Eds.), *Communication and its disorders: A science in progress. Proceedings 24th Congress International Association of Logopedics and Phoniatrics, Amsterdam, the Netherlands, August 23–27, 1998.* (Vol. I, pp. 256–259). International Association of Logopedics and Phoniatrics.

Sung, M. W., Kim, K. H., Koh, T.-Y., Kwon, T.-Y., Mo, J.-H., Choi, S. H., . . . Sung, M. Y. (1999). Videostrobokymography: A new method for the quantitative analysis of vocal fold vibration. *Laryngoscope, 109*, 1859–1863.

Švec, J. G., & Schutte, H. K. (1996). Videokymography: High-speed line scanning of vocal fold vibration. *Journal of Voice, 10*, 201–205.

Švec, J. G., Schutte, H. K., & Šram, F. (1997). *Introduction to videokymography.* [Video tape]. Prague, The Czech Republic: Medical Healthcom.

Švec, J. G., Schutte, H. K., & Šram, F. (1999). Variability of vibration of normal vocal folds as seen in videokymography. In P. H. Dejonckere & H. F. M. Peters (Eds.), *Communication and its disorders: A science in progress. Proceedings 24th Congress International Association of Logopedics and Phoniatrics, Amsterdam, the Netherlands, August 23–27, 1998.* (Vol. I, pp. 122–125). International Association of Logopedics and Phoniatrics.

Švec, J. G., & Šram, F. (2002). Kymographic imaging of the vocal fold oscillations. In J. H. L. Hansen & B. Pellom (Eds.), *ICSLP-2002 Conference Proceedings, Vol. 2. 7th International Conference on Spoken Language Processing, September 16–20 2002, Denver, Colorado, USA* (pp. 957–960). Boulder, CO: Center for Spoken Language Research.

Švec, J. G., Šram, F., & Schutte, H. K. (1999). Videokymografie: nová vysokofrekvenční metoda vyšetřování kmitů hlasivek. [In Czech and in English]. [Videokymography: A new high-speed method for the examination of vocal-fold vibrations]. *Otorinolaryngologie a foniatrie, 48,* 155–162.

Švec, J. G., Šram, F., & Schutte, H. K. (2007). Videokymography in voice disorders: What to look for? *Annals of Otology Rhinology and Laryngology, 116,* 172–180.

Švec, J. G., Šram, F., & Schutte, H. K. (2009). Videokymography. In M. P. Fried & A. Ferlito (Eds.), *The Larynx. Volume I* (3rd ed., pp. 253–274). San Diego, CA: Plural Publishing.

Tigges, M., Richter, B., & Wittenberg, T. (2005). Kymographische Darstellung der Stimmlippenschwingungen. [In German]. [Kymographic imaging of vocal fold vibration]. *Sprache-Stimme-Gehör, 29,* 9–14.

Tigges, M., Mergell, P., Herzel, H., Wittenberg, T., & Eysholdt, U. (1997). Observation and modelling of glottal biphonation. *Acustica-Acta Acustica, 83,* 707–714.

van Kalkeren, T. A., Schutte, H. K., Qiu, Q., Švec, J. G., & Mahieu, H. F. (2006). First clinical experiences of second generation videokymography. In *Proceedings AQL 2006: Advances in Quantitative Laryngology, Voice and Speech Research, October 6–7, 2006, Groningen, the Netherlands.* [CD-ROM] (pp. 1–8). Groningen, The Netherlands: Groningen Voice Research Lab, University of Groningen.

Verdonck-de Leeuw, I. M., Festen, J. M., & Mahieu, H. F. (2001). Deviant vocal fold vibration as observed during videokymography: The effect on voice quality. *Journal of Voice, 15,* 313–322.

Wendler, J. (1992). Stroboscopy. *Journal of Voice, 6,* 149–154.

Wittenberg, T., Tigges, M., Mergell, P., & Eysholdt, U. (2000). Functional imaging of vocal fold vibration: Digital multislice high-speed kymography. *Journal of Voice, 14,* 422–442.

Woodson, G. E. (1993). Configuration of the glottis in laryngeal paralysis. I: Clinical study. *Laryngoscope, 103,* 1227–1234.

CHAPTER 12

Quantitative Analysis of High-Speed Laryngoscopic Images

JIANG PING KONG AND EDWIN M.-L. YIU

PURPOSE

- To analyze vocal fold vibratory pattern and glottal opening using a quantitative analysis program for high-speed laryngoscopic images.

INTRODUCTION AND BACKGROUND

High-speed imaging technology dates back to as early as the 1930s, when Bell Telephone Laboratories first developed its ultra high-speed motion picture filming system and began to study the vibration of vocal folds with a sampling rate of 4000 frames per second (Herriott & Farnsworth, 1938). These images were studied by Farnsworth (1940), and later on by Pressman (1942), Dunker and Schlosshauer (1958), and LeCover and Rubin (1960). Later, Moore and his colleagues (Moore, White, & von Leden, 1962; Moore & von Leden, 1958; Timcke, von Leden, & Moore, 1958, 1959; von Leden, Moore, & Timcke, 1960; von Leden & Moore, 1961) and Flanagan (1958) developed and introduced their system of studying laryngeal physiology using high-speed imaging. However, with the sophisticated operation and data extraction, as well as the extremely high operation cost, high-speed imaging has not gained much popularity in voice research until more recently. The high-speed system involves a large amount of data even for a short duration. The high-speed system can only record images that are a few seconds long. Currently available systems allow recordings between 2 to 8 seconds long depending on the sampling rate.

With the technologic development of digital image processing and high-speed digital imaging systems, the re-emergence of high-speed digital imaging research in voice began in the 1970s with studies carried out at Tokyo University in Japan (Hirose, 2010; Hirose, Kiritani, & Imagawa, 1988, 1991; Imagawa, Kiritani, & Hirose, 1987; Kiritani, Honda, Imagawa, & Hirose, 1986; Kiritani, Imagawa, & Hirose, 1988; Kiritani, Imagawa, Miyazi, Kumada, & Nlimi, 1995; Yoshida, Hirano, Matsushita, & Nakajima, 1972). This system started off with a scan size of 128 (horizontal) × 32 (vertical) pixels with a sampling rate of 2000 frames per second. The system was improved to 256 × 256 pixels later by Kiritani and colleagues in the 1990s (Kiritani, Hirose, & Imagawa, 1993; Kiritani, Imagawa, & Hirose, 1990; Kiritani, Imagawa, Miyazi, Kumada, & Niimi, 1995; Kiritani, Niimi, Imagawa, & Hirose, 1995) with an 8-bit gray scale. The sampling rate subsequently increased to 4000 frames per second. Other signals, such as speech and electroglottographic (EGG) signals, could also be recorded and synchronized with the high-speed images. These synchronized signals are very important when the high-speed images of vocal folds are evaluated in detail.

Basically, there is no major difference between operating high-speed laryngoscopy and traditional videolaryngoscopy. High-speed and traditional video laryngoscopy differ in the sampling rate of video image and the duration of recording that can be made. The traditional videolaryngoscopy captures images with a sampling rate of 25 to 40 frames per second, whereas the high-speed laryngoscopy can capture images with a sampling rate of up to 2000 to 4000 frames per second. Therefore, the images of high-speed laryngoscopy can display much more details of vocal fold vibration. Traditional videolaryngoscopy can record as long as the size of the recording media allows, whereas high-speed laryngoscopy is limited by the sampling rate and is often limited to several seconds.

EQUIPMENT AND MATERIALS

The rapid development of computer and video imaging technologies in recent years has made it possible for high-speed digital imaging systems to be available commercially. Among these are the high-speed laryngoscopy systems from KayPENTAX and Wolf Medical. The high-speed video (HSV) images used in this chapter were obtained using the KayPENTAX system sampled at 2000 frames per second with 128 × 256 pixels gray scale images. Currently, commercial color high-speed systems are also available with 256 × 256 pixels and a sampling of 4000 frames per second.

PROCEDURES FOR CONDUCTING LARYNGOSCOPY

Instructions for conducting a high-speed laryngoscopy are similar to those of the traditional procedure using a rigid endoscope (see Chapters 7, 8, and 9 by Lindestad, Young and Rosen, and Rubin and Epstein in this book).

PROCEDURES IN ANALYZING HIGH-SPEED IMAGES

High-speed digital images are recorded simultaneously with acoustic and electroglottographic (EGG) signals. The images obtained with the high-speed system should be exported to an AVI format.

Before analysis, third party video processing software may be needed to process the AVI file to ensure the images are rotated with the anterior end of the vocal folds facing upward. The software program "High-Speed Video Processing" (HSVP) (Yiu, Kong, Fong, & Chan, 2010) is used for the image analysis. It runs in a MatLab environment and is available at <http://www.hku.hk/speech/voice-handbook>.

Identifying the Glottal Area

The procedures in image processing include: (1) image brightness and contrast adjustment; (2) image rotation and cropping; (3) image motion compensation; and (4) automatic image contrast detection. The aim of these procedures is to identify the glottal area accurately.

Image Brightness and Contrast Adjustment

High-speed image samples generally are low in brightness because of the limitation of the light source when capturing the image. Therefore, prior to image processing, the brightness and contrast of images may need to be adjusted automatically or manually. The range of the gray scale of the image is expanded to cover the full scale of 0 to 255. This is carried out by identifying the range in the gray-scale histogram of digital image. The histogram of an image in Figure 12–1A shows a range between two vertical lines, and the digital data in this range will be extended to cover 0 to 255 in gray scale (there are 256 [0 to 255] shades of grays used in gray scale digital images). The brightness and contrast of this image can be adjusted by changing this range. Figure 12–1B shows the original image, which is relatively dark. Figure 12–1C shows the image adjusted, which is brighter than the original one and can be seen clearly. Figure 12–1D shows the image, which has been adjusted to show a larger contrast.

Image Rotation and Cropping

Endoscopic procedure may not always be able to capture the glottis in vertical

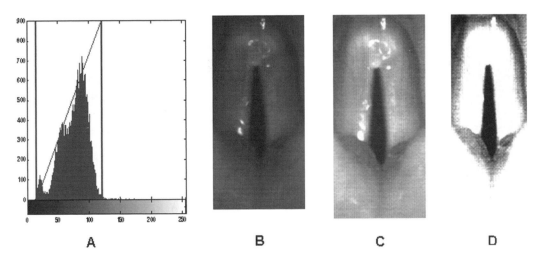

| A | B | C | D |

Figure 12–1. Images for contrast adjustment. **A** shows the histogram of the captured image. **B** is the original image. **C** is the image with brightness adjusted. **D** is the image with contrast adjusted.

alignment with the centre of the image, and therefore the image may need to be rotated before further analysis. Figure 12–2A is the original image, which shows the glottis is not captured in a vertical position. Figure 12–2B is the image being rotated by using the bi-cubic algorithm. Figure 12–2C is the same image shown enlarged and cropped.

Image Motion Compensation

Another factor that would affect the accuracy and validity of digital image processing is the horizontal movement of the endoscope relative to the larynx. This motion complicates the tracking of the dynamic movement of the vocal folds. Figure 12–3 shows the movement

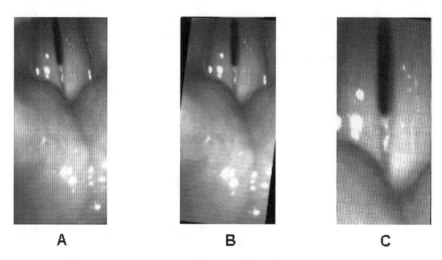

A   B   C

Figure 12–2. Image rotation. **A** is the original image with brightness and contrast adjusted. **B** is the image being rotated by bi-cubic algorithm. **C** shows the image enlarged and cropped.

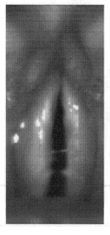
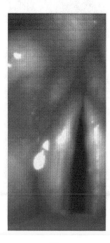

Figure 12–3. Positions of glottis relative to the screen due to motion of the endoscopic camera. (The movement of the endoscope during recording changed the relative position of the glottis captured by the camera.)

A   B

of the endoscope during recording, which changed the relative position of the glottis from the center (Figure 12–3A) to the right side of the screen (Figure 12–3B)

If the dynamic characteristics of the glottis are to be analyzed, the program needs to determine how the glottis has moved. In practice, the analysis system makes use of motion compensation technique to achieve this. Motion compensation refers to the process of detecting and compensating for the camera (endoscope) motion in the image. Details of motion compensation can be found in the paper by Deliyski (2005). In brief, the steps involve computing the displacement vectors (motion trajectories) and then subtracting the motion trajectories from the spatial coordinates

of the original image. Figure 12–4 shows the result after motion compensation. It can be seen that most of the motions have been compensated for after signal processing and the position of the glottis remains relative static in each frame (Figure 12–4).

Automatic Image Contrast Detection

The area of the glottis is calculated based on the pixilated area, which will be affected by how a pixel is determined to be present or not (i.e., 0 or 1). This process is called binarization. The method employed is based on the histogram from the fully opened and fully closed glottis (Figure 12–5A, histograms I and II). After subtraction (Figure

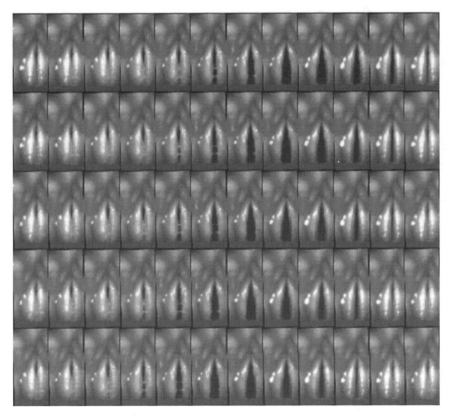

Figure 12–4. Image series after motion compensation. (Note that the glottis remains in a similar location in each frame.)

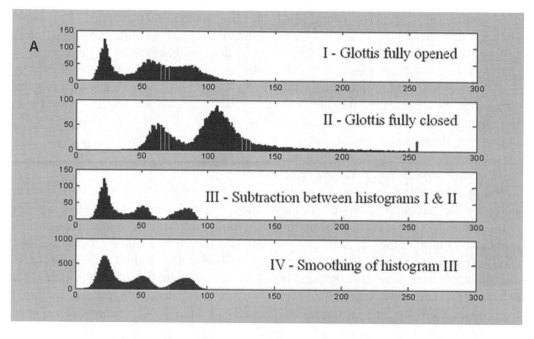

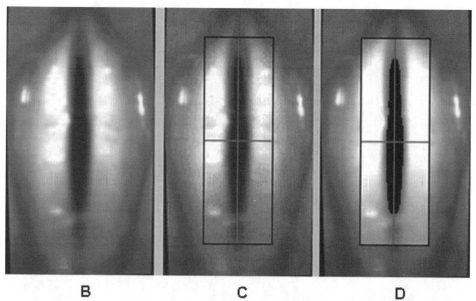

Figure 12-5. Principle of contrast adjustment. **A.** Histograms for contrast adjustment. **B.** Original image. **C.** Manual placement of a window. **D.** Automatic detection of glottis.

12-5A, histogram III) and smoothing (Figure 12-5A, histogram IV), the values at the left and right sides of the first peak were used to determine the automatic contrast adjustment for all images. Each binarized image outlines the shape of the glottis. The outcomes of the images are shown in Figure 12-5 B to D.

Measurement Extraction

After brightness, contrast, rotation, cropping, motion compensation, and binarization have been carried out on the images, the area of the glottis is identified manually by the examiner using a rectangular box. Analysis can then be carried out and the extraction of measurements are outlined in Figure 12–6. Two lines are drawn within the rectangle to divide the glottal area into four regions: A, B, C, and D (see Figure 12–6). A combination of these four regions gives rise to anterior glottis (A+B), posterior glottis (C+D), left glottis (A+C), and right glottis (B+D) (see Figure 12–6). From the center of the glottis (point o in Figure 12–6), the left width (l-o in Figure 12–6), right width (r-o in Figure 12–6),

anterior length (a-o in Figure 12–6), and the posterior length (p-o in Figure 12–6) are defined accordingly. Then fundamental frequency (F0) is defined as reciprocal of period, open quotient (OQ) is defined as a ratio of open phase to period, and speed quotient (SQ) is defined as a ratio of opening phase to closing phase.

The system extracts automatically 13 measurements from the images. They are the: (1) glottal area (GA); (2) left GA; (3) right GA; (4) anterior GA; (5) posterior GA; (6) left glottal width; (7) right glottal width; (8) anterior glottal length; (9) posterior glottal length; (10) ratio of glottal length to glottal width; (11) F0; (12) open quotient (OQ); and (13) speed quotient (SQ).

Operation of the High-Speed Imaging Video Processing System

The interface of the high-speed video processing system is made up of a Display Panel and a Processing Panel. The Display Panel consists of two blocks: Image Display Block and Measurement Display Block. The Processing Panel is made up of four functional blocks: Video and Speech Signal Editing Block, Image Processing Block, Measurement Extraction Block, and Motion Compensation and Automatic Measurement Extracting Block.

Display Panel

Image Display Block. The Image Display Block is made up of three parts (Figure 12–7A). In the middle of this block, there are two sliders, which are used to mark the beginning and the end of the image frames selected. At the top of this block, there are two windows displaying two images. The left window displays the

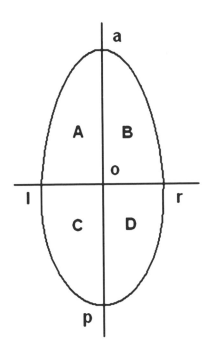

Figure 12–6. Schematic dimensions of glottal measures (o = center; l = left; r = right; a = anterior; p = posterior; A+B = anterior glottis; C+D = posterior glottis; A+C = left glottis; B+D = right glottis)

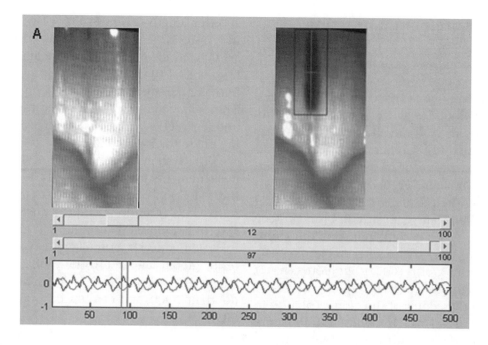

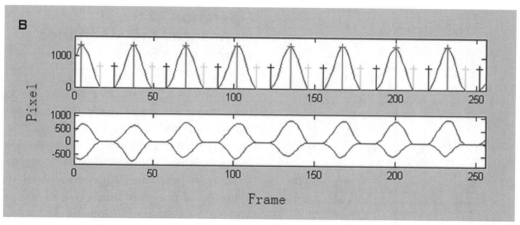

Figure 12–7. Display panel of the high-speed video processing program. **A.** Image display block (The numbers 12 and 97 in the slide indicate the frame number of the two images). **B.** Measurement display block.

frame of the original video file selected by the upper slider, while the right window displays the outcome of processing of the image on the left window. The lower part of this Image Display Block shows the entire segment of two recording channels (speech sound and EGG signals) simultaneously. The two cursors on this plot indicate the relative positions of the selected images.

Measurement Display Block. The Measurement Display Block (Figure 12–7B) is made up of two plots displaying measurements extracted from the processed images. The upper plot displays the dynamic glottal area and points of glottal opening, glottal closure and local maximum glottal area, with which fundamental frequency (F0), open quotient (OQ) and speed quotient (SQ) can be calculated. The lower plot (see Figure 12–7B) shows the left dynamic glottal area (upper tracing) and the right dynamic glottal area (lower tracing) inverted by using a negative value.

Processing Panel

Video and Speech Signal Editing Block. The main function of the Video and Speech Signal Editing Block is for editing the video file, speech sound and EGG signal. There are a total of 16 buttons. The button **Open a video** is used to open a video file and display it in the image windows. The button **Open speech** is used to open a two-channel (speech and EGG signals) acoustical file and display them in the speech sound window just below the image windows. The button **Play video** is used to play a video in the left window of the Image Display Block and the button **Play marked video** is used to play video marked by the two cursors in the Image Display Block. The buttons **Play speech** and **Play EGG signal** are used to play speech sound and EGG signal respectively. The buttons ← **Snd** and ← **Egg** are used to move a speech sound or EGG signal forward respectively, and the buttons **Snd** → and **Egg** → are used to move a speech or EGG signal backward. The buttons **Snd +** and **Egg +** are used to amplify a speech sound or EGG signal and the button **Snd –** and **Egg –** are used to lower the intensity of the signals. These four buttons are used to adjust the synchronization of the speech and video signals if the high-speed

imaging and speech recording systems are not set up to collect synchronized signals simultaneously. The button **Save marked video** is used to save a video marked by the two video cursors, and the button **Save marked speech** is used to save a marked speech and EGG signals.

Image Processing Block. This block has two sliders and 12 buttons for processing the high-speed images. The two sliders are used to adjust the brightness and contrast of the image. The buttons ← **Rotation** and **Rotation** → are used to rotate an image in two different directions with different angles by using the bi-cubic algorithm manually. The button **Transform rotated** is used to transform all the images in the opened file into the images with the rotational angles and direction as selected by the ← **Rotation** or **Rotation** → buttons. The buttons **Zoom in** and **Zoom out** are used to enlarge and restore the image shown in the right image display window in Figure 12–7A. The buttons **Image up**, **Image down**, **Image left**, and **Image right** are used to move an enlarged image in the four directions for selecting a suitable image. The button **Transform enlarged** is used to transform all video images selected in the opened file into the same size as the original image. The button **Transform contrasted** is used to transform all the video images with the adjusted brightness and contrast, and the button **Save transformed** is used to save the processed video images into the opened video file for further use.

Measurement Extraction Block. The Measurement Extraction Block is used for extracting glottal measurements manually. The button **Add window** is used to add an extraction window to select the area of the glottis for measuring. The button **Delete window** is used to delete the extraction window. The buttons **Up, Down, Left,** and **Right** are used to move the extraction window stepwise in four directions to achieve a suitable position. In this system, two parameter extraction windows can be set: one is set for the initial image frame and the second one is set for the final image frame. When the two windows are set, the button **Set window trail** is used to set a trail that tracks the movement of the first window to the second window. This trail is used in the calculation for compensating the movement of the image. The button **Kymography** is used to display the marked video images in the format of kymography. The button **Save montage** is used to save a display of the selected video images in a montage format. The button **Save image** is used to display an image selected by the activated cursor and then save it for further use. The button **Save glottal para** is used to save all the 13 extracted measurements in Microsoft Excel format.

Motion Compensation and Automatic Measurement Detecting Block. This block is designed to carry out motion compensation and extract the measurement automatically. The button **MC all avifile** is used to carry out motion compensation of all image (AVI) files in a folder automatically. The button **Auto ParaExtracting** is used to extract the parameter (measurement) from a video file automatically, after an extraction window is set in the right video display window by the button **Add window**. The 13 measurements will be displayed in another window. The glottal area with the marks (glottal closure and glottal opening and maximum glottal area function), and the left and right areas will be displayed in the parameter plots.

CASE SAMPLES

Three case samples are presented in the following section. These include: (1) a female modal voice, (2) a voice onset and offset, and (3) a quick gliding voice.

Female Modal Voice

Figure 12–8 displays the video images in montage format and the typical glottal measurements of a female modal voice. The average F0, OQ, and SQ are 306 Hz, 70% and 105% respectively. From the contour of glottal area, we can see that the pulse of glottal area appears as a triangle. The left and right glottal areas reach their maximum sizes at different times. The anterior and posterior areas also reach their maximum sizes at different times.

Voice Onset and Offset

High-speed images provide information on voice onset and offset that cannot be obtained simply by acoustic signals, EGG signals, or stroboscopic images. Figure 12–9 displays a series of video montages of a voice onset and the measurements extracted from them. The extracted tracings (see Figure 12–9) show that the vocal folds demonstrated two cycles of pre-vibration, before they reached the normal vibration. Figure 12–10 shows a voice offset and the extracted measurements. It can be seen that the vocal folds vibrated with five further periods from the full vibration before they stopped completely. From the contours of these two samples, it can be seen that the contours of the incomplete vibratory closure look like contours of a sine wave. This means that the speech source has a low power in the high-frequency range.

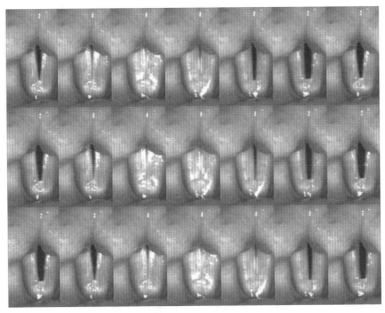

A

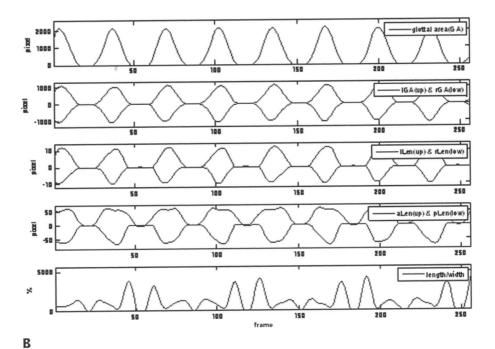

B

Figure 12–8. Video images and extracted glottal measurements of a female modal voice.

157

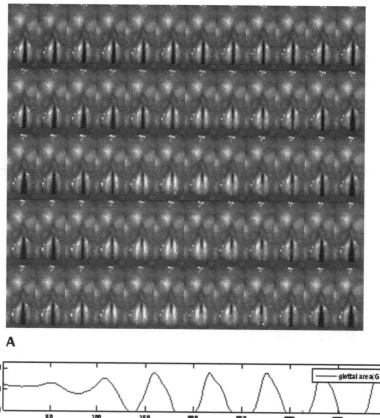

A

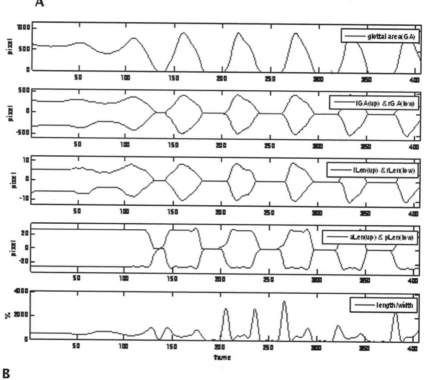

B

Figure 12–9. Video images and extracted glottal measurements of a voice onset.

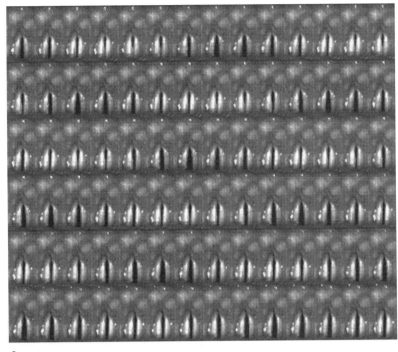

A

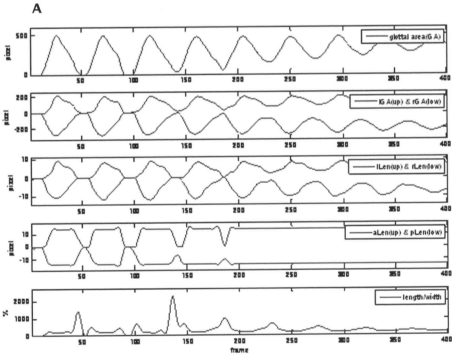

B

Figure 12–10. Video images and extracted glottal measurements of a voice offset.

Quick Gliding Phonation

A gliding pitch requires the vocal folds to change their mass and tension quickly within a short time frame. Figure 12–11 displays a phonation changing quickly from low to high pitch. Figure 12–12 displays the contours of F0, OQ, and SQ from low to high pitch and then back to low pitch again. It can be seen that F0 shows the greatest change. The SQ and OQ do not change much and, indeed, SQ in this phonation context is very small when compared to that in modal phonation. From the contours, it also can be seen that the pitch gliding is not very smooth, and there are irregular periods (see Figure 12–12), hence resulting in higher jitter.

LIMITATIONS AND FURTHER DEVELOPMENT OF HIGH-SPEED IMAGING

High-speed imaging allows the observation of vocal fold vibration directly, and the digital image processing provides quantitative data related to the glottal area. It is important that acoustic signals, and preferably EGG signals, can be captured simultaneously with the high-speed video images. This will allow meaningful analysis of the relationship between the vocal fold vibration and phonation. It also is important that a sufficient sampling rate of high-speed video images can be used. For pitch gliding and falsetto phonation reaching as high as 600 to 800 Hz, a sampling rate of more than 4000 frames or higher per second is necessary. A sampling rate lower than 4000 frames per second would not be fast enough to capture enough frames of data to reconstruct the glottal area images for further signal processing.

Commercially available systems only recommend the use of rigid endoscopes because of the demand for a high-powered light source in high-speed laryngoscopy, although some purpose-built high-speed systems have incorporated flexible endoscopes. The use of a rigid endoscopes limits examinations to only sustained /i/. This makes it difficult for speakers to produce other natural phonation types or running speech, especially voices related to professional performance.

With the improvement in high-speed video imaging technique, better image quality in terms of resolution and color format, a higher sampling rate, faster speed file capturing, and management are made possible. Together with advanced signal processing algorithms for images and acoustic signals, the quality of voice assessment will be improved further in the coming years.

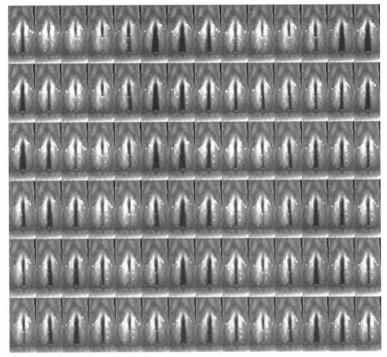

A

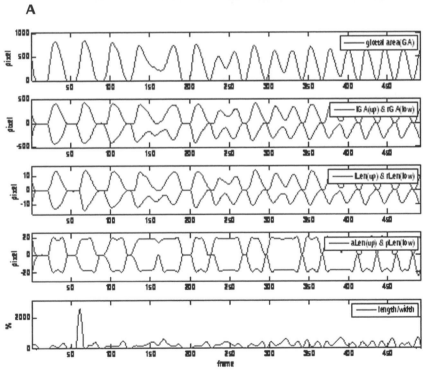

B

Figure 12–11. A quick gliding voice.

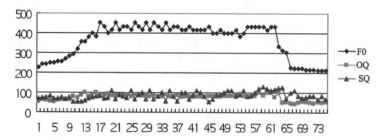

Figure 12–12. Changes of fundamental frequency (F0, Hz), open quotient (OQ, %), and speed quotient (SQ, %) in a gliding pitch phonation.

REFERENCES

Deliyski, D. D. (2005). Endoscope motion compensation for laryngeal high-speed videoendoscopy. *Journal of Voice, 19*(3), 485–496.

Dunker, E., & Schlosshauer, B. (1958). Uber Anspannung und Schwingungsform der Stimmlippen. *Archiv für Ohren-Nasen-Kehlkopfheilkunde, 173,* 497–500.

Farnsworth, D. W. (1940). High-speed motion pictures of the human vocal cords. *Bell Laboratories Record, 18*(1), 203–208.

Flanagan, J. L. (1958). Some properties of the glottal sound source. *Journal of Speech, Language and Hearing Research, 1*(2), 99–116.

Herriott, W., & Farnsworth, D. W. (1938). High speed motion pictures of the vocal cords. *Journal of the Acoustical Society of America, 9,* 274.

Hirose, H. (2010). Investigating the physiology of laryngeal structures. In W. J. Hardcastle, J. Laver, & F. E. Gibbon (Eds.), *Handbook of Phonetic Sciences* (130–152). Oxford, UK: Blackwell Publishing.

Hirose, H., Kiritani, S., & Imagawa, H. (1988). High-speed digital image analysis of laryngeal behavior in running speech. In O. Fujimura (Ed.), *Vocal physiology: Voice production, mechanisms and functions* (pp. 335–345). New York, NY: Raven Press.

Hirose, H., Kiritani, S., & Imagawa, H. (1991). Clinical application of high-speed digital imaging of vocal fold vibration. In J. Gauffin & B. Hammarberg (Eds.), *Vocal fold physiology: Acoustic, perceptual, and physiological aspects of voice mechanisms* (pp. 213–216). San Diego, CA: Singular Publishing Group.

Imagawa, H., Kiritani, S., & Hirose, H. (1987). High-speed digital image recording system for observing vocal fold vibration using an image sensor. *Iyō denshi to seitai kōgaku. Japanese Journal of Medical Electronics and Biological Engineering, 25*(4), 284–290.

Kiritani, S. (1995). *Recent advances in high-speed digital image recording of vocal cord vibration.* Paper presented at the International Congresses of Phonetic Sciences, Stockholm.

Kiritani, S., Hirose, H., & Imagawa, H. (1993). High-speed digital image analysis of vocal cord vibration in diplophonia. *Speech Communication, 13*(1–2), 23–32.

Kiritani, S., Honda, K., Imagawa, H., & Hirose, H. (1986). *Simultaneous high-speed digital recording of vocal fold vibration and speech signal.* Paper presented at the IEEE International Conference on International Conference on Acoustics, Speech, and Signal Processing, 1986. Tokyo, Japan

Kiritani, S., Imagawa, H., & Hirose, H. (1988). High-speed digital image recording for the observation of vocal cord vibration. In O. Fujimura (Ed.), *Vocal physiology: Voice production, mechanisms and functions* (pp. 261–269). New York, NY: Raven Press.

Kiritani, S., Imagawa, H., & Hirose, H. (1990). *High-speed digital image recording for the observation of the vocal cord vibration.* Paper presented at the International Conference on Spoken Language Processing, 1990 (pp. 61–64). Kobe, Japan.

Kiritani, S., Imagawa, H., Miyazi, M., Kumada, M., & Niimi, S. (1995). Quasi-periodic perturbations in pathological vocal fold vibration. *Annual Bulletin Research Institute of Logopedics And Phoniatrics, 29,* 27–33.

Kiritani, S., Niimi, S,. Imagawa, H., Hirose, H. (1995) Vocal fold vibrations associated with involuntary voice changes in certain pathological cases. In: Vocal fold physiology: voice quality control. Vocal Fold Physiology Series, Kurume, Japan, pp 269–281.

Le Cover, M., & Rubin, H. I. (1960). Technique of high speed photography of the larynx. *Journal of the Biological Photographic Association, 28,* 133.

Moore, G. P., White, F. D., & von Leden, H. (1962). Ultra high speed photography in laryngeal physiology. *Journal of Speech and Hearing Disorders, 27*(2), 165–171.

Moore, P., & von Leden, H. (1958). Dynamic variations of the vibratory pattern in the normal larynx. *Folia Phoniatrica et Logopaedica, 10*(4), 205–238.

Pressman, J. J. (1942). Physiology of the vocal cords in phonation and respiration. *Archives of Otolaryngology-Head and Neck Surgery, 35*(3), 355–398.

Timcke, R., von Leden, H., & Moore, G. (1958). Laryngeal vibrations: Measurements of the glottic wave; Part I. The normal vibratory cycle. *Archives of Otolaryngology-Head and Neck Surgery, 68,* 1–19.

Timcke, R., von Leden, H., & Moore, G. (1959). Laryngeal vibrations: Measurements of the glottic wave: Part II. Physiologic variations. *Archives of Otolaryngology-Head and Neck Surgery, 69*(4), 438–444.

von Leden, H., & Moore, P. (1961). Vibratory pattern of the vocal cords in unilateral laryngeal paralysis. *Acta Oto-Laryngologica, 53*(2–3), 493–506.

von Leden, H., Moore, P., & Timcke, R. (1960). Laryngeal vibrations: Measurements of the glottic wave: Part III. The pathologic larynx. *Archives of Otolaryngology-Head and Neck Surgery, 71*(1), 16–35.

Yiu, E.M.-L., Kong, J., Fong, R., & Chan, K.M.K. (2010). A preliminary study of a quantitative analysis method for high-speed laryngoscopic images. *International Journal of Speech Language Pathology, 12*(6), 520–528.

Yoshida, Y., Hirano, M., Matsushita, H., & Nakajima, T. (1972). A new apparatus for ultra high-speed cinematography of the vibratory vocal cords. *Journal of Otolaryngology of Japan, 75,* 1256–1261.

CHAPTER 13

Electroglottography: Speech Studio Laryngograph

RUTH EPSTEIN

PURPOSE

- To obtain information about vocal fold contact across time using noninvasive procedures.

THEORETICAL BACKGROUND

Electroglottography (EGG), also called electrolaryngography (Abberton, Howard, & Fourcin, 1989; Baken, 1992), is a noninvasive method commonly used to evaluate vocal fold contact during phonation across time. It is based on the principle that human tissue is a good conductor of electricity. A low electrical current is passed between the vocal folds via a pair of surface electrodes placed on either side of the thyroid laminae. As the vocal folds open and close, changes occur in electrical impedance. The impedance rises when the glottis opens and drops as the vocal folds approximate. These changes in electrical impedance are depicted in a waveform of the glottal cycle as a function of

time. In addition to the waveform captured by the surface electrodes, a microphone can be used to capture the speech signal simultaneously to the laryngeal signal. Many studies conclude that EGG output is strongly related to kinematic events of vocal fold vibration on the basis of the assumption that the output of the EGG is related to the dynamic area of the medial contact of the two vocal folds during phonation (Berke, Hantke, Hanson, & Gerratt, 1986; Fant, Ondrackova, Lindqvist, & Sonesson, 1966; Fourcin, 1974; Scherer, Druker, & Titze 1988).

The electroglottograph monitors vocal fold closure and provides a basis for measuring vocal fold vibration during phonation (Abberton et al., 1989). The output is an EGG waveform, also known as an Lx (larynx excitation) waveform, which shows duration, coordination, and relative vocal fold contact patterns within a glottal cycle. The signal basically is unaffected by other activities in the vocal resonance tract or environmental acoustic noise. The apex of the waveform indicates the closed phase of the vibratory cycle, where there is maximum contact of the vocal folds and hence maximum conduction of the current. The trough in the waveform shows the open phase of the cycle and minimum conduction of the current. Nevertheless, the orientation of the Lx waveform is somewhat arbitrary. Some manufacturers have used an inverted, mirrored, Lx waveform.

Details of vocal fold vibration can be related to the Lx cycle. The Lx waveform has four main features (Abberton et al., 1989) (Figure 13–1):

1. A steep rising edge, which corresponds to the vocal fold closing.
2. A maximum peak, which corresponds to maximum vocal fold closure.
3. A falling edge, which corresponds to vocal fold opening.
4. A trough, which corresponds to vocal fold open phase.

The shape and length of these phases can change with voice quality.

The technique has its limitations. For example, variations in adipose neck tissue thickness, extrinsic muscle contraction,

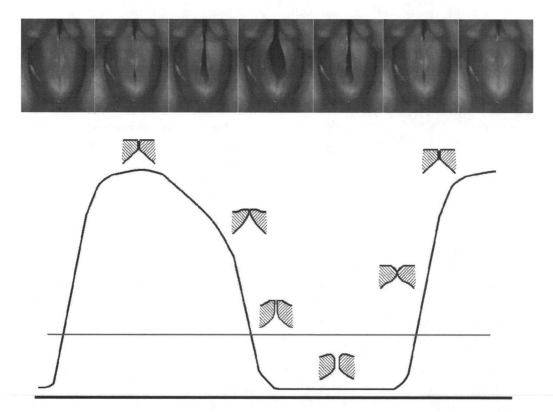

Figure 13–1. The EGG waveform and its relationship to soft tissue contact with simultaneous stroboscopic images of the vocal folds. (Courtesy of Pedro Amarante)

blood vessel constriction and dilation, and electrode placement can produce errors in the measurement. Using high-pass filtering of the raw EGG signal or dual-channel EGG can reduce some of the errors in measurement (Rothenberg, 1992). EGG is increasingly used for the assessment of vocal pathology. It also is used by clinicians as a tool in voice therapy (Baken & Orlikoff, 2000; Fourcin & Abberton, 1971).

nized to the edge of the displayed EGG waveform.

■ EG-2 standard and PCX series electroglottograph (EGG) (Glottal Enterprises). These two models offer dual channel electrodes that provide a quantitative indication of vertical laryngeal movement, in addition to standard features available on the Laryngograph and KayPENTAX models.

DESCRIPTION

Several EGG systems are available commercially:

■ Laryngograph microProcessor using Speech Studio software (Laryngograph Ltd). The Laryngograph microProcessor provides the EGG and acoustic waveforms. These input to a host personal computer via a specified USB interface and produce accurate analyses of vocal fold contact behaviors in both sustained vowels and connected speech. It can be used in conjunction with the Laryngograph Ltd. stroboscopy system.

■ The Electroglottograph (EGG) (KayPENTAX Model 6103). The Electroglottograph can be used in conjunction with the KayPENTAX Computerized Speech Lab (CSL) or with KayPENTAX computer-integrated stroboscopy system (e.g., the Digital Strobe). A software option for CSL (Real-Time EGG Analysis) provides a real-time EGG display. In the KayPENTAX Digital Strobe system, the EGG waveform can be displayed concurrently with the vibrating vocal folds. The observed video frame of stroboscopic data is time-synchro-

EQUIPMENT AND MATERIALS

This chapter describes the use of Laryngograph microProcessor with Speech Studio software (Figure 13–2).

■ Recording software: Laryngograph Speech Studio software.

■ Standard passage such as North Wind and the Sun (International Phonetic Association, 1999) or The Rainbow Passage (Fairbanks, 1960).

■ Alcohol swab for cleaning the skin surface.

TEST PROCEDURES

1. Before placing the electrodes, clean the client's neck skin surface with alcohol swab. Then, place the surface electrodes on either side of the thyroid laminae. The placement of the electrodes should be secured with a neck band (Figure 13–3).

2. Explain the procedure to the client before obtaining the EGG waveform.

   Instruction: *"We are going to analyze your voice today. I will*

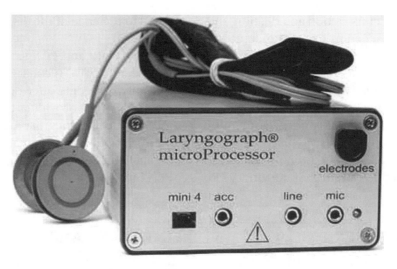

Figure 13–2. The Laryngograph® microProcessor.

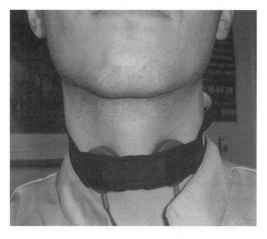

Figure 13–3. Placement of the EGG electrodes (Courtesy of Pedro Amarante)

place these two electrodes on your neck and will ask you to say "ah" using your comfortable voice for three seconds." The vowel /a/ is commonly used due to neutral vocal tract configuration. Other vowels can be used if deemed appropriate.

■ Get the client to say "ah" and watch the waveforms generated while moving the electrodes vertically until a good signal with maximum amplitude is obtained. Click the **microphone** icon on the screen. This will open the speech screen that will display the data.

■ Click the **Record** button. Enter the client's details and click **OK**. This will automatically start the recording. Once the signal is obtained, click the **Stop** button. This will result in display of all the data recorded.

■ To better visualize the data, do a right click on the mouse and select **scale-to-fit**. This will provide a display of the signal of the entire duration.

■ Left click on the mouse and drag to highlight the section to be analyzed. This will result in automatic display of fundamental frequency (Fx), closed quotient (Qx), the time in seconds from the start of the recording, and loudness in dBs (Rms).

■ Click the **MDVP** icon on the screen for a multidimensional voice profile report of the selected section. Note that sustained vowel analyses must not be applied to connected speech.

3. The connected speech profile is then recorded. Ask the client to read aloud a standard passage using his or her habitual voice. Follow the steps above to record the signal.

Instruction: *"Would you please read aloud this passage in your comfortable conversational voice. Take time to familiarize yourself with the passage."* The passage should be read once only.

■ Left click on the mouse and drag to highlight the section to be analyzed. Click the **QA** (Quantitative Analysis) icon for analysis. The Speech Studio software offers various options of predefined graph groups for display. Predefined graph groups can be selected under **Analysis** from the menu, then **QA Settings**. Note that connected speech analyses must not be applied to sustained vowels.

DATA ANALYSIS

EGG may be interpreted with calculations reflecting the contact phase of the vibratory cycle, such as the contact quotient (CQ), or by evaluating the geometry of the Lx waveform itself. The waveform is analyzed by means of temporal representations. Quantitative measurements of parameters such as glottal cycle duration (related to the waveform period from which the frequency can be extracted), opened and closed phases of the vocal folds, and closure quotient (ratio between open and closed phase) are calculated using digital signal processing techniques. These data provide the clinician with information on the degree of hoarseness and quality of the vocal register (Godino-Llorente et al., 2006). In addition to the Lx waveform, the speech (Sp) waveform is also displayed during the EGG analysis, from which a number of additional parameters can be obtained. For example, amplitude, spectrogram, long-term average spectrum, formants and harmonics, speech tracing, and frequency and amplitude tracing.

Closed quotient (Qx), also described as contact quotient (CQ), is derived from the Lx waveform and is the fraction of time the glottis is considered closed. As standardized by the Laryngograph Speech Studio software, the time width of the closed phase at the 70% down from each positive peak of the Lx waveform is divided by the total time of each cycle, to provide the percentage of the contact phase. The 70% criteria is a standardized default for Laryngograph Speech Studio software.

Characteristic Features of Lx Waveform

The shape and the length of different phases can change with vocal quality. The evaluation of the EGG waveform is subjective and is based on the expertise of the clinician. Characteristics of a normal waveform in modal register at a comfortable pitch and intensity include a well- defined point of contact onset, a steep slope for increasing contact, a "knee" in the open phase (particularly in males), and an open phase (Mayes et al., 2008) (Figure 13–4).

Deviant waveform as seen in breathy voice quality is characterized by small closure peaks, which are more symmetrical than those of normal voice. The open phase in each cycle is relatively longer, marked by a long plateau between the end of separation and the beginning of contact (Fourcin, 1981) (Figure 13–5).

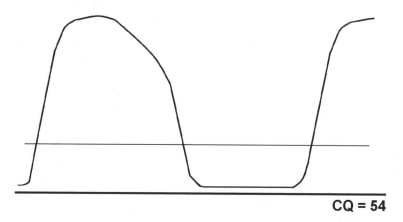

CQ = 54

Figure 13–4. Lx of a normal voice. Well-defined closure depicted in the vertical rise of the waveform from the baseline. The contact quotient (CQ) is around 50%. Additionally, the knee point is usually noticeable indicating the "pealing" of the vocal folds as they come apart. (Courtesy of Pedro Amarante)

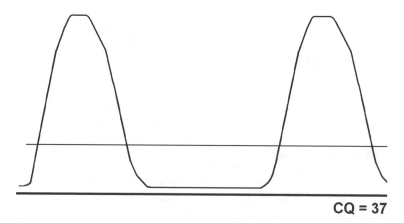

CQ = 37

Figure 13–5. Lx of a breathy voice. The contact quotient (CQ) is usually reduced (e.g., 37%). This reduction of CQ indicates that the vocal folds are spending more time being opened than closed for each vocal cycle. It typically is accompanied by an increased noise on the spectrogram signal due to the turbulence caused by the air escaping through the vocal folds. (Courtesy of Pedro Amarante)

Pressed voice quality is characterized by an extended closed phase and the vocal folds only open for a small amount of time (Figure 13-6).

NORMATIVE DATA

Quantification of phases of the vocal fold cycle on the basis of Lx is of questionable validity (Baken, & Orlikoff, 2000). This is because the criterion level set at 70% is adjustable. Furthermore, the application is limited to certain individuals due to anatomical variation such as excessive adipose tissue. Quantitative measures of Lx are relevant to the evaluation of voice disorders and provide qualitative descriptions of laryngeal actions, particularly when used in conjunction with other types of measures such as stroboscopy (Karnell, 1989; Vieira & NcInnes, 1997).

The EGG signal has been characterized in terms of a contact phase, represented by increasing or decreasing vocal fold contact, as well as a minimal contact phase, marked by an apparent lack of vocal fold contact (Orlikoff, 1998). A number of quantitative parameters, which describe the EGG signal, have been developed on the basis of this assertion. The contact quotient is a ratio of the contact phase duration to the fundamental period (Orlikoff, 1991; Scherer et al., 1995). The normative range of the contact quotient is 0.4 to 0.6 for both males and females, indirectly reflecting vocal fold adduction energy (Table 13-1). The contact index, defined as the difference between the durations of increasing and decreasing vocal fold contact divided by total contact phase duration, reflects contact symmetry. This measure ranges between 0.4 and 0.6 for both males and females in modal register (Orlikoff, 1991). Falsetto register phonation is associated with a contact index close to 0, whereas pulse register phonation is associated with a contact index close to −0.8 (Aronson & Bless, 2009; Baken & Orlikoff, 2000).

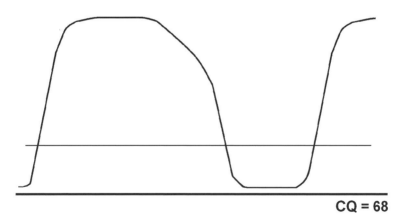

CQ = 68

Figure 13-6. Lx of a pressed voice. The contact quotient (CQ) is usually increased due to excessive tension on the vocal folds contact area/surface (e.g., 68%). The graph presents an extended closed phase and the vocal folds only open for a small amount of time. The voice usually sounds strangled and strained. (Courtesy of Pedro Amarante)

Table 13–1. Normative Data with Traditional Display of Values in Percentage of Closed by Open Time

Type of Phonation	Contact Quotient (CQ)	Percentage (%)
Normal	0.4–0.6	47%
Pressed	0.7–1.0	67%
Breathy	0.1–0.3	32%

CASE STUDY

M.H., a 42-year-old male banker, was referred by a laryngologist. Videolaryngostroboscopy demonstrated diminished movement of the left vocal fold, which gave the diagnosis of left vocal fold palsy. M.H. reported a 3-week history of vocal weakness following an upper respiratory tract infection and long-haul air travel. His voice was hoarse when he boarded the plane in New York and became very weak and breathy on arrival in London. Perceptually, his voice was characterized as high-pitched, moderately breathy, rough, and effortful. Pitch and loudness range were reduced markedly. EGG evaluation was carried out, which provided information on the closure phase. The preintervention EGG waveform was classified as abnormal. The following features were observed (Figure 13–7):

■ The waveform was characterized by a "sinus wave" pattern, with an irregular onset and short contact phase.
■ Reduced closed quotient (Qx).
■ There was a relatively long open phase in each cycle, marked by a long plateau between the end of separation and the beginning of contact.
■ The speech signal demonstrated small positive peaks.

The Titze semiocclusion exercises (Titze, 2006) were demonstrated to M.H., with the aim of improving vocal fold apposition and vocal clarity. He was advised to practice the exercises frequently. He was seen for four sessions of voice therapy over a period of 3 weeks. Postintervention evaluation suggested an improvement in voice quality that was reflected in the EGG waveform. Review by the laryngologist demonstrated good compensatory closure of the right vocal fold and improved closure pattern. M.H.'s voice sounded clearer with reduced strain. EGG assessment showed (Figure 13–8):

■ Improved symmetry of the waveform.
■ Increased closed quotient (Qx).
■ The closure phase and the 'knee' in the Lx separation phase are better defined and regular.
■ The open phase is shorter than pretreatment.
■ The speech signal demonstrates rapid vocal fold closures, with steep vertical variations.

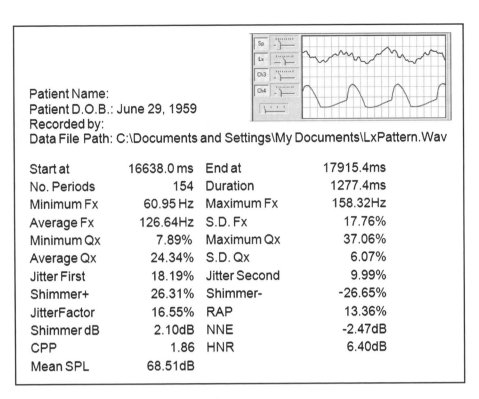

Patient Name:
Patient D.O.B.: June 29, 1959
Recorded by:
Data File Path: C:\Documents and Settings\My Documents\LxPattern.Wav

Start at	16638.0 ms	End at	17915.4ms
No. Periods	154	Duration	1277.4ms
Minimum Fx	60.95 Hz	Maximum Fx	158.32Hz
Average Fx	126.64Hz	S.D. Fx	17.76%
Minimum Qx	7.89%	Maximum Qx	37.06%
Average Qx	24.34%	S.D. Qx	6.07%
Jitter First	18.19%	Jitter Second	9.99%
Shimmer+	26.31%	Shimmer-	-26.65%
JitterFactor	16.55%	RAP	13.36%
Shimmer dB	2.10dB	NNE	-2.47dB
CPP	1.86	HNR	6.40dB
Mean SPL	68.51dB		

Figure 13–7. Case study: Initial assessment.

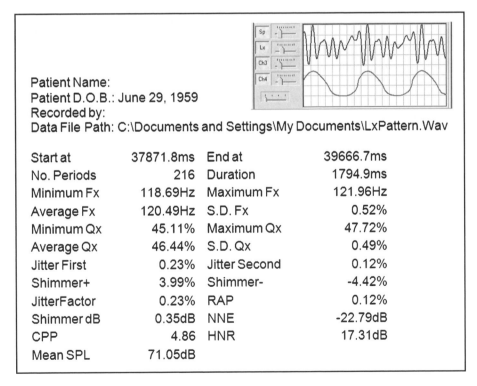

Patient Name:
Patient D.O.B.: June 29, 1959
Recorded by:
Data File Path: C:\Documents and Settings\My Documents\LxPattern.Wav

Start at	37871.8ms	End at	39666.7ms
No. Periods	216	Duration	1794.9ms
Minimum Fx	118.69Hz	Maximum Fx	121.96Hz
Average Fx	120.49Hz	S.D. Fx	0.52%
Minimum Qx	45.11%	Maximum Qx	47.72%
Average Qx	46.44%	S.D. Qx	0.49%
Jitter First	0.23%	Jitter Second	0.12%
Shimmer+	3.99%	Shimmer-	-4.42%
JitterFactor	0.23%	RAP	0.12%
Shimmer dB	0.35dB	NNE	-22.79dB
CPP	4.86	HNR	17.31dB
Mean SPL	71.05dB		

Figure 13–8. Case study: Postintervention.

REFERENCES

Abberton, E. R., Howard, D. M., & Fourcin, A. T. (1989) Laryngographic assessment of normal voice: a tutorial. *Clinical Linguistics and Phonetics, 3*(3), 281–296.

Aronson, A., & Bless, D. (2009). *Clinical voice disorders*. New York, NY: Thieme.

Baken, R. J. (1992). Electroglottography. *Journal of Voice, 6*, 98–110..

Baken, R. J., & Orlikoff, R. F. (2000). *Clinical measurement of speech and voice* (2nd ed.). San Diego, CA: Singular.

Berke, G. S., Hantke, D. R., Hanson, D. G., & Gerratt, B. (1986). An experimental model to test the effect of change in tension and mass on laryngeal vibration in vivo. *Proceedings International Conference Voice*, 2;ii-1–ii-8.

Fairbanks, G. (1960). *Voice and articulation drillbook*. New York, NY: Harper and Row.

Fant, G., Ondrackova, J., Lindqvist, J., & Sonesson, B. (1966). Electrical glottography. *Quarterly Progress and Statue Report, 4*, 15–21

Fourcin, A. J. (1974). Laryngographic examination of vocal fold vibration. In B. Wyke (Ed.), *Ventilatory and phonatory control systems: An international symposium*. London, UK: Oxford University Press.

Fourcin, A. J. (1981). *Laryngographic assessment of phonatory function*. ASHA Reports, *11*, 116–128.

Fourcin, A. J., & Abberton, E. (1971). First applications of a new laryngograph. *Medical and Biological Illustration, 21*, 172–182.

Godino-Llorente, J., Saenz-Lechon, N., Osma-Ruiz, V., Aguilera-Navarro, S., & Gomez-Vilda, P. (2006). An integrated tool for the diagnosis of voice disorders. *Medical Engineering and Physics, 28*(3), 276–289.

International Phonetic Association. (1999). *Handbook of International Phonetic Association: A guide to the use of International Phonetic Alphabet*. Cambridge, UK: Cambridge University Press.

Karnell, M. P. (1989). Synchronized videostroboscopy and electroglottography. *Journal of Voice, 3*, 68–75.

Mayes, R. W., Jackson-Menaldi, C., DeJonckere, P. H., Moyer, C., & Rubin, A. D. (2008). Laryngeal electroglottography as a predictor of laryngeal electromyography. *Journal of Voice*, 756–759.

Orlikoff, R. F. (1991). Assessment of the dynamics of vocal fold contact from the electroglottogram: Data from normal male subjects. *Journal of Speech and Hearing Research, 34*, 1066–1072.

Orlikoff, R. F. (1998). Scrambled EGG: The uses and abuses of electroglottography. *Phonoscope, 1*, 37–53.

Rothenberg, M. (1992). A multichannel electroglottograph. *Journal of Voice, 6*, 36–43.

Scherer, R., C., Druker, D. C., & Titze, I. ??(1988). Electroglottography and direct measurement of vocal fold contact area. In O. Fujimura (Ed.), *Vocal physiology: Voice production, mechanisms and functions*. New York, NY: Raven Press.

Scherer, R. C., Vail, V. J., & Guo, C. G. (1995). Required number of tokens to determine representative voice perturbation values. *Journal of Speech and Hearing Research, 38*, 1260–1269.

Titze, I. R. (2006). Voice training and therapy with a semi-occluded vocal tract: Rationale and scientific underpinnings. *Journal of Speech, Language and Hearing Research, 49*, 448–459.

Vieira, M. N., McInnes, F. F., & Jack, M. A. (1997). Comparative assessment of electroglottographic and acoustic measures of jitter in pathological voices. *Journal of Speech, Language and Hearing Research, 40*, 170–182.

SECTION III

Laryngeal Muscle Activities

CHAPTER 14

Assessing Vocal Hyperfunction Using Surface Electromyography

AMY Y.-H. WONG AND ESTELLA P.-M. MA

PURPOSES

- To capture and analyze electrical activities of an individual's muscles when the corresponding target muscles contract.
- To serve as biofeedback in the treatment and rehabilitation of a wide range of hyperfunctional voice disorders, neuromuscular disorders, and swallowing disorders.

INTRODUCTION

Vocal hyperfunction can be characterized by an excessive and/or imbalanced muscle tension around the laryngeal and perilaryngeal regions during phonation (Freeman & Fawcus, 2000; Hillman, Holmberg, Perkell, Walsh, & Vaughan, 1989; Redenbaugh & Reich, 1989). Surface electromyography (SEMG) provides a noninvasive and objective measure of muscle activities and strength during muscle contraction.

The literature has reported clinical usefulness of SEMG to differentiate between hyperfunctional and normal voices. Stemple, Weiler, Whitehead, and Komray (1980) measured the activities of perilaryngeal muscles in individuals with vocal nodules using SEMG. They found that individuals with vocal nodules exhibited significantly greater SEMG levels over perilaryngeal area than vocally healthy controls both at rest and during phonation. Hocevar-Boltezar, Janko, and Zargi (1998) studied the SEMG characteristics of different muscle sites in the lower face and anterior neck during silence and vowel production in vocally healthy individuals and patients with muscle tension dysphonia (MTD). Their results revealed that the majority of the patients with MTD demonstrated significantly greater SEMG activities in supralaryngeal and perioral muscles than controls with normal voice. Redenbaugh and Reich (1989) compared vocally hyperfunctional speakers and vocally normal speakers using SEMG. In their study, each participant's absolute SEMG levels during sustained vowel prolongation and passage reading aloud tasks were also used to derive proportions relative to his or her own rests EMG, maximal SEMG, and 50% maximal SEMG. The authors found that individuals with hyperfunctional dysphonia demonstrated significantly higher absolute SEMG levels than vocally healthy controls during rest, sustained vowel prolongation, and passage reading. Significant group differences also were found after normalization relative to the maximal and 50% maximal SEMG levels. The authors concluded that normalizing SEMG signals is a valid procedure to differentiate between hyperfunctional and healthy normal voices.

SEMG also has been used as a voice training tool for providing augmented feedback for dysphonic individuals to reduce their laryngeal muscle tensions (Allen, Bernstein, & Chaitr, 1991; Andrews, Warner, & Stewart, 1986; Stemple et al., 1980). Another study found that the use of SEMG biofeedback was successful in helping to eliminate vocal nodules as well as releasing excessive tensions in laryngeal area after undertaking eight sessions of SEMG biofeedback training (Stemple et al., 1980). Another study found SEMG to be effective in a group of individuals with hyperfunc-

tional dysphonia (Andrews et al., 1986). A case study by Allen and colleagues (1991) showed that SEMG biofeedback helped a young boy with hyperfunctional dysphonia and vocal nodules to reduce laryngeal muscle tension. These positive results from the literature show promising results with the use of SEMG in voice therapy.

DESCRIPTION

Several systems are commercially available for recording SEMG signals, namely, the PowerLab of ADInstrument (Colorado Springs, CO), the Bortec system (Bortec Biomedical, Canada), and the Delsys Bagnoli system (Delsys Inc, Boston, MA). This chapter uses the PowerLab system to illustrate the procedures and precautions of recording electromyographic voltages.

EQUIPMENT AND MATERIALS

- Recording software and hardware: Scope program of the PowerLab system (http://www.adinstruments.com/solutions/research/EMG/) by ADInstruments (Colorado Springs, CO) with Dual Bio Amp (ML 135).
- Electrodes: silver/silver chloride electrodes (10 mm in diameter) with connecting wires, and dry earth strap.
- Accessories for recording: skin prepping abrasive gel (Nuprep), alcohol swab, conduction cream (TEN 20, 228 g), adhesive tape, gauze pad, and standard passage such as "North Wind and the Sun" (International Phonetic Association, 1999).

TEST PROCEDURES

Setting Up Before Recording

1. Start the Scope program (Figure 14–1).
2. Adjust the **amplifier** and **filter** settings on the right column:
   a. Amplifier: Select a range of **500 µV** for capturing the muscle activities around perilaryngeal regions, namely, the orofacial area (buccinator, risorius) and the thyrohyoid area (thyrohyoid, omohyoid, sternohyoid, and platysma muscles).
   b. Filter setting: Select the band-pass filter from **10 to 500 Hz** for both Input A and Input B.
   c. Change the sampling speed to **1280/s** and time to **5 seconds**.

Attaching the Surface Electrodes

1. The electrodes need to be prepared before the recording procedures proceed. Fill the concave side of each electrode with conduction cream (Figure 14–2).
2. Explain to the client the test procedures.

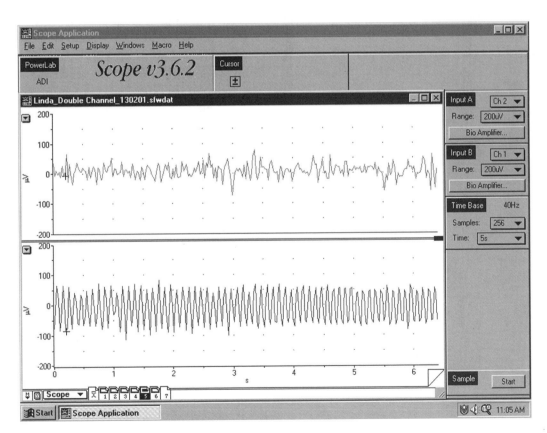

Figure 14–1. Main display screen of the Scope program.

Instructions: *"Today, we are going to assess the muscle activities of your face and neck muscles. You will be asked to read aloud a set of phrases. Your performance will be captured and recorded by the surface electromyography (SEMG). Two pairs of electrodes connected to the SEMG will be attached* to your face and neck for the measurement of muscle activities during speaking."

3. Two steps are carried out for skin preparation before securing the surface electrodes on the muscle sites:
   a. Rub skin prepping electrolyte gel onto the client's orofacial and thyrohyoid areas with a gauze pad. This reduces the impedance at the sites of contact (Day, 2002).
   b. Use an alcohol swab to cleanse the muscle sites.

4. After the skin preparation procedure, firmly attach the electrodes onto the client's orofacial and thyrohoyid areas using adhesive tape. Attach a pair of electrodes over the orofacial area (Channel One), with the electrodes being 1 cm away from either lip corner. Attach the other pair of electrodes over the thyrohyoid area (Channel Two), with the electrodes being 0.5 cm away from either side of the midline of the thyrohyoid membrane (Figure 14–3A).

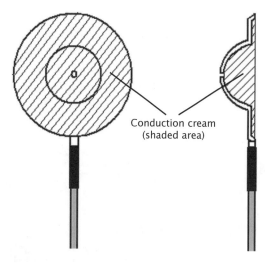

Conduction cream
(shaded area)

Figure 14–2. Surface EMG electrode.

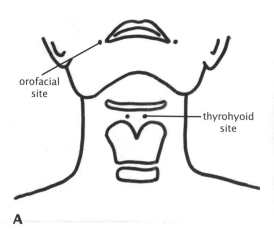

orofacial
site

thyrohyoid
site

A

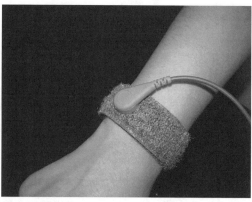

B

Figure 14–3. A. Sites for surface electrodes placement and **B.** earth strap placement

5. Attach a dry earth strap firmly around the client's wrist to ensure the electrical signals will be grounded (Figure 14–3B).

6. After the electrodes and the dry earth strap are secured in place, ask the client to rotate his or her head to ensure no movement artifact is shown in the SEMG recording. He or she should sit straight against the back of the chair in a relaxed posture and relax the hands, and the legs. Keep the mouth closed lightly before speaking.

Instructions: *"Now, I would like you to rotate your head to see if the electrodes are securely attached. Rest your hands on your lap in your most comfortable or relaxed manner. Relax your hands so that your fingers form a bowl shape and sit straight against the chair. Keep your mouth closed naturally and relax before recording."*

(**Note:** The connecting wires, which are connected with the silver/silver chloride electrodes, should be wrapped with insulator and separated at a constant distance and rested on the client's lap to prevent crosstalk between the two wires [De Luca, 1997].)

Capturing SEMG Signals

1. Before making a recording, ask the client to sustain the vowel /i/ to ensure the PowerLab can detect the contractions of the orofacial muscles and thyrohyoid muscles.

Instructions: *"I want you to say "ee" for 5 seconds when I signal the*

'okay' sign. We will repeat this task three times. Remember to take a short pause after each trial."

2. After the system is checked, record the muscle activities while the client is at rest. Ask the client to close his or her eyes and relax for one minute.

Instructions: *"I want you to close your eyes and take a rest for one minute."*

3. Ask the client to read aloud some connected speech (e.g., phrases). Remind the client not to swallow before and after reading each stimulus.

Instructions: *"Now, I want you to read aloud some sentences to assess your facial and neck muscle activities during speaking. Please use your most comfortable pitch and loudness while reading aloud."*

4. Apart from recording the production of sentences, ask the client to read aloud the standard passage "North Wind and the Sun" (International Phonetic Association, 1999) using his or her habitual voice. Allow time for the client to familiarize him or herself with the passage before recording.

Instructions: *"Please read aloud the standard passage with your most comfortable pitch and loudness."*

5. After the recordings are done, remove the electrodes. Provide a wet paper towel to the client to clean his or her face and neck areas.

Instructions: *"Now, I will help you to remove the electrodes from your* *face and neck. Here is a wet paper towel for you to wipe away the gel from your face and neck areas."*

Recording the Maximal and Submaximal Voluntary Contraction

1. Two nonspeech maximal voluntary contraction tasks are then carried out for the normalization process. To achieve the maximal voluntary contraction (MVC) for orofacial site, ask the client to retract his or her own lips at his or her maximum extent for 6 seconds. Allow a one-minute rest between trials to avoid muscle fatigue.

   Instructions: *"I want you to retract your lips as hard as you can. Hold it for about 6 seconds. We will repeat the task five times."*

2. To achieve the MVC for thyrohyoid site, ask the client to place the chin on a stationary platform and flex the neck by exerting a maximal downward force on the platform for six seconds. Allow a one-minute rest between trials to avoid muscle fatigue.

   Instructions: *"I want you to place your chin on this platform. Flex your neck and exert as hard as you can. Hold it for about 6 seconds. We will repeat the task five times."*

3. To achieve 50% of the maximal voluntary contraction (50% MVC), repeat the steps above for achieving MVC but subjectively embody half the effort expended during the MVC for 6 seconds. The clinician can introduce to the client a self-rating scale:

the force exerted for MVC is given an arbitrary value of 10 units and he or she is required to exert a force of 5 units for the 50% MVC.

Instructions: *"We will do these tasks again. Please use half the effort that you have just used during the maximum trials. We will repeat each task five times."*

DATA ANALYSIS

1. Load the file that is to be analyzed.
2. Select **Selection** from the **Windows** drop-down menu. The **Set Selection** box will then appear on the screen. Input the time period to be analyzed and the range of voltage for Channel A and B (the authors recommend −400 to +400 μV). Click **OK** and the chosen time period will be highlighted automatically by the software.
3. Select **Computer Functions** from the **Display** drop-down menu. The Computed Functions box will then appear. Select **Square** under **Function** for Channel A and B. Press **OK**.
4. Select **Data pad** from the **Windows** drop-down menu. The root-mean-square (RMS) voltages of the selected waveform will be displayed in the data pad.

NORMATIVE DATA

Limited normative SEMG data have been reported in the literature. Readers can refer to the results reported in the study by Redenbaugh and Reich (1989) for reference (Table 14–1).

Table 14–1. Means and Standard Deviations of SEMG Measures Reported in Redenbaugh and Reich (1989)

Measures	Hyperfunctional		Control	
	Mean	SD	Mean	SD
At rest (in microvolts, μV)	3.37	1.33	1.10	0.37
Resisted-force maneuver				
MVC (in μV)	70.32	11.79	67.11	10.14
50% MVC (in μV)	29.32	9.24	32.06	17.80
Vowel				
Absolute level (in μV)	14.55	6.26	2.49	0.89
Normalized value: AL/rest	4.81	1.84	2.42	0.93
AL/MVC	0.22	0.12	0.04	0.01
AL/50% MVC	0.61	0.49	0.09	0.03
Passage				
Absolute level (in μV)	21.49	6.70	6.36	1.78
Normalized value: AL/rest	7.68	4.17	6.13	1.57
AL/MVC	0.32	0.13	0.09	0.02
AL/50% MVC	0.86	0.54	0.23	0.09

AL = absolute level; MVC = maximal voluntary contraction.

SEMG signals were recorded by two electrodes attached to the anterior neck area over the thyrohyoid membrane.

CASE STUDY: CLIENT M.P. (BILATERAL VOCAL NODULES)

M.P., a high school teacher, was diagnosed with bilateral vocal nodules by an otolaryngologist. She complained of difficulties in projecting her voice when teaching in class. She frequently had sore throat and even lost her voice after a day of teaching. Perceptually, M.P.'s vocal quality was described as mildly breathy, moderately rough, and moderately strained. Hard glottal attacks were noted during conversations. Relaxed phonation training was recommended.

The relaxed phonation training consisted of eight sessions. Each training session lasted for 30 minutes and was held twice a week for 4 consecutive weeks. During each session, M.P. was required to read aloud some sentences with the surface electrodes attached to her orofacial and thyrohyoid areas. The pretraining results indicated that M.P. showed excessive muscle tensions around her neck when reading aloud the training stimuli. After each practice trial, the root-mean-square values of SEMG signals recorded at her thyrohyoid site were calculated and presented to her as biofeedback. She was told that the values represented the strained quality of her voice with the larger the number the more strained her voice. Therefore, M.P.'s attention was directed to external aspects of her voice production. Attempts were made to avoid directing M.P.'s attention to biomechanics (internal) aspects of voice production (e.g., the values represented muscle tension at the thyrohyoid site with the larger the number the more tension in the neck muscles). M.P. was told to try to bring a smaller value.

The posttraining assessment indicated a great drop of EMG voltages from 20.46 µV (pretraining) to 12.26 µV (post-training). The EMG voltages recorded from the orofacial area also indicated a decrease from 23.24 µV (pretraining) to 15.89 µV (post-training). Visual examination of the larynx revealed a reduction in size of the nodules. This suggested that M.P. has shown improvement after the eight-session relaxation training.

Acknowledgment. This chapter was supported in part by grant from the Faculty of Education Research Fund at the University of Hong Kong awarded to the second author.

REFERENCES

Allen, K. D., Bernstein, B., & Chait, D. H. (1991). EMG biofeedback treatment of pediatric hyperfunctional dysphonia. *Journal of Behavioral Therapy and Experimental Psychiatry, 22,* 97–101.

Andrews, S., Warner, J., & Stewart, R. (1986). EMG biofeedback and relaxation in the treatment of hyperfunctional dysphonia. *British Journal of Disorders of Communication, 21,* 353–369.

Day, S. (2002). *Important factors in surface EMG measurement.* Calgary, Alberta, Canada: Bortec Biomedical Ltd. Retrieved from http://www.bortec.ca/pages.

De Luca, C. J. (1997). The use of surface electromyography in biomechanics. *Journal of Applied Biomechanics, 13*(2), 135–163.

Freeman, M., & Fawcus, M. (2001). *Voice disorders and their management* (3rd ed.). London, UK: Whurr Publishers..

Hillman, R. E., Holmberg, E. B., Perkell, J. S., Walsh, M., & Vaughan, C. (1989). Objective assessment of vocal hyperfunction: An experimental framework and initial results. *Journal of Speech and Hearing Research, 32,* 373–392.

Hocevar-Boltezar, I., Janko, M., & Zargi, M. (1998). Role of surface EMG in diagnostics and treatment of muscle tension dysphonia. *Acta Otolaryngologica, 118*(5), 739–743.

International Phonetic Association. (1999). *Handbook of the International Phonetic Association: A guide to the use of the International Phonetic Alphabet.* Cambridge, UK: Cambridge University Press.

Redenbaugh, M. A., & Reich, A. R. (1989). Surface EMG and related measures in normal and vocally hyperfunctional speakers. *Journal of Speech and Hearing Disorders, 54,* 68–73.

Stemple, J. C., Weiler, E., Whitehead, W., & Komray, R. (1980). Electromyographic biofeedback training with patients exhibiting a hyperfunctional voice disorder. *Laryngoscope, 90*(3), 471–476.

CHAPTER 15

The Applications of Surface Electromyography to Assess Stressor-Evoked Changes in Extralaryngeal Functioning

MARIA DIETRICH AND RICHARD D. ANDREATTA

PURPOSES

- To assess extralaryngeal functioning during exposure to an acute psychological stressor.
- To assess extralaryngeal behaviors within and between clients in a seminaturalistic setting.

THEORETICAL BACKGROUND

Muscle tension dysphonia (MTD) is common among individuals with voice disorders and can be observed as primary MTD (MTD I) or secondary MTD (MTD II). According to the *Classification Manual for Voice Disorders* (CMVD-1) (Verdolini, Rosen, & Branski, 2005), MTD I occurs in the absence of a structural, neurologic, or psychogenic disorder and based on current knowledge lacks a specific etiology. In contrast, MTD II is a compensatory behavior in response to a known underlying condition such as vocal fold lesions or glottal insufficiency. The CMVD-1 states that both MTD I and II present with excessive or atypical laryngeal movements during phonation, which are considered the proximal cause for MTD (Angsuwarangsee & Morrison, 2002; Aronson, 1990; Koufman & Blalock, 1982; Morrison, Nichol, & Rammage, 1986; Morrison & Rammage, 1993; Roy, 2003; Roy, Bless, Heisey, & Ford, 1997; Roy & Leeper, 1993). In other words, there may be variability in the magnitude and pattern of patients' laryngeal behavior associated with MTD. Common complaints of patients with MTD include increased vocal effort during phonation and vocal fatigue (Solomon, 2008).

Unfortunately, systematic assessment of laryngeal muscle "tension" in muscle *tension* dysphonia is rare. Surface electromyography (SEMG) is a practical and noninvasive tool that is useful for measuring such tension. A number of studies have used SEMG to measure extralaryngeal muscle activity in patients with hyperfunctional voice disorders with and without vocal fold lesions (Andrews, Warner, & Stewart, 1986; Hočevar-Boltežar, Janko, & Žargi, 1998; Redenbaugh & Reich, 1989; Stemple, Weiler, Whitehead, & Komray, 1980). These studies, however, varied widely on participant selection criteria, instrumentation, muscle sites sampled, electrode placement, and procedures. Only limited data are available that assess extralaryngeal muscle activity across phonatory, speech, and nonspeech tasks. Although it is difficult to compare the results across studies, data have emerged to show that at least some patients with MTD exhibit increased extralaryngeal muscle activity in anticipation of and during vocalization as compared to vocally healthy controls.

The applications of SEMG are manifold. These include the frequent use in psychophysiology and emotion research (Fridlund & Cacioppo, 1986). MTD I is the condition affecting voice that most often has been linked to psychological factors such as introverted personality, stress reactivity, and increased life stress (Aronson, 1990; Roy, 2003; Roy & Bless, 2000; Seifert & Kollbrunner, 2005). These issues were formalized as "trait theory of voice disorders" (Roy & Bless, 2000; Roy, Bless, & Heisey, 2000a). According to this theory, individuals who are introverted (versus

extroverted) have a tendency to react with anxiety and behavioral inhibition to novelty and threat. In turn, this disposition produces maladaptive laryngeal behavior such as MTD. Elevated trait stress reactivity may potentiate and maintain any increased or dyscoordinated laryngeal activity. However, the precise neurobiological and pathophysiologic processes directly linking stress and behavioral inhibition with MTD I are largely unknown.

Psychophysiology is the study of physiology as it relates to various aspects of psychological or behavioral function. Therefore, psychophysiologic experiments can serve as a window into processes characteristic of MTD I. The psychophysiologic processes under investigation can be varied based on theories or clinical findings in voice science. For example, personality and stress on the one hand, and extrinsic and intrinsic laryngeal muscle activity on the other hand are psychological and physiologic processes of interest in MTD I. Ideally, experiments will yield valid and reliable clinical markers of MTD I (e.g., a quantifiable personality, muscular, or biomechanical profile). Furthermore, those markers should be tested for their sensitivity and specificity to differentiate individuals with MTD I from individuals with other voice disorders such as vocal nodules (cf. Roy, Bless, & Heisey, 2000a, 2000b, for sensitivity and specificity based on personality). Psychophysiologic profiles may be particularly useful as a screening tool in the early stages of voice disorders. For example, a teacher may present with initial vocal effort and vocal fatigue consistent with MTD but may develop MTD I or vocal fold lesions with MTD II depending on this individual's psychophysiologic profile. Based on this information, the clinician can make an informed decision about the most appropriate course of treatment.

In this context, SEMG is a useful tool to provide the clinician with a means to objectify extralaryngeal muscle activity and muscle activity *patterns* (e.g., laryngeal elevation versus depression, cocontraction) within and between clients and across a range of tasks. Objective observations are an informative counterpart to subjective correlates of muscle tension such as perceived vocal effort.

Two psychophysiologic experiments described in the literature aimed to test the trait theory of voice disorders; van Mersbergen, Patrick, and Glaze (2008) and Dietrich (2008) used SEMG of the extralaryngeal muscles to investigate emotion- and stressor-evoked changes in extralaryngeal functioning, respectively, in individuals with and without MTD I (van Mersbergen et al., 2008) and in high and low extroverted vocally healthy individuals (Dietrich, 2008). Although various emotion and stress induction tasks have been described in the literature, the most effective ones are social-evaluative stressors (Dickerson & Kemeny, 2004). For example, public speaking performed while being observed and under time pressure is a well-established laboratory protocol that induces moderate psychosocial stress with significant increases in autonomic cardiovascular activity (e.g., blood pressure) and subjective stress ratings (cf. *Trier Social Stress Test* [TSST; Kirschbaum, Pirke, & Hellhammer, 1993]). Using public speaking as stressor would be akin to a challenge or perturbation to phonatory control. Perturbation paradigms typically are underused in voice and speech areas, but, nonetheless, are powerful designs to test the function of a mechanism and to locate operational factors and weaknesses. Understanding a client's extralaryngeal behavior during stressor exposure will enrich clinical assessment and the therapy process. This additional component for individuals with MTD will provide information about baseline extralaryngeal behavior and treatment progress under more realistic environmental conditions.

DESCRIPTION

Surface electromyography (SEMG) is a widely used and noninvasive means of assessing the functional health and integrity of the neuromotor systems underlying voluntary behaviors in humans. In general, EMG represents a range of methods designed to record the small electrical currents that are generated by muscle cells during the process of excitation-coupling and motor unit activity (Cram & Kasman, 1998). Although EMG has its historical roots in motor control research, today EMG is a commonly used clinical-grade procedure for diagnosing neuromotor dysfunction and for profiling the effects of emotional display and stress. Stressor-evoked changes and muscle activity in part may be linked to autonomic nervous system activity (Goldstein, 2001). These autonomic influences are suggested to produce a general change in the resting tone of muscle fibers and increase the muscle's responsiveness to stressors (McNulty, Gevirtz, Berkoff, & Hubbard, 1994). Such interpretations are possible because of the strong relationship between quantitative measures of EMG activity and observable behavior (Luschei & Finnegan, 2008).

It should be noted that the anterior neck, in and around the area of the thyroid cartilage, has a number of strap muscle groups that can elevate and depress the laryngeal complex. These muscle groups are arranged in a manner whereby significant overlapping occurs (Zemlin, 1998).

This anatomic feature makes it difficult to isolate the SEMG activity of one muscle group from another, because SEMG is a volume conducted signal that reflects the summed activity of motor unit potentials directly under the active electrode elements. However, as the intent of the SEMG signal in the context of this chapter is for the general evaluation of reactivity to situational stressors, SEMG functions as a satisfactory, although gross, indicator of stress and laryngeal behavior.

EQUIPMENT AND MATERIALS

The summation of electrical currents generated by a population of muscle cells can be easily recorded using any of a number of available systems and self-adhesive or re-usable EMG electrodes. Commercially available systems for recording EMG run the gamut from research to clinical grade, with each possessing different recording capacities and instrumentation features. The specific choice of an EMG system can be personal and driven by factors such as the experience of the user, the quality of recordings needed, and cost. Regardless of the specific brand of system used, all systems should be rated for use with humans and have the following basic components: silver/silver-chloride (Ag/AgCl) recording electrodes (e.g., 4 mm diameter); interface cables that allow the electrode leads to connect to other signal processing hardware; band-pass filters; an adjustable differential amplifier; a notch filter (60 Hz) for attenuating power line noise; an analog to digital converter (A/D—16-bit minimum); a visual display (monitor or oscilloscope); and a computer. Also necessary among the desired features is a suite of control software that will allow recording parameter

tuning and adjustments, data acquisition, digitization, and, if possible, post hoc analysis. From the authors' experience, two commercially available systems, the Power-Lab EMG system (http://www.adinstruments.com/solutions/research/EMG/) by ADInstruments (Colorado Springs, CO), and the Neurodata Amplifier system (http://www.grasstechnologies.com/products/ampsystems/15.html) by Grass—AstroMed (West Warwick, RI), meet most of these basic requirements. They are suitable for clinical EMG applications because of their relative ease to set up and operate. The following parameter settings for hardware components are suggested as a starting point and can be applied to most EMG systems:

1. band-pass filter setting of 30 to 2500 Hz;
2. A/D sampling rate of 5000 Hz to ensure capture of the full range of spectral energy in the EMG signal;
3. notch filter set to 60 Hz;
4. amplifier gain set at 10,000 times.

Once the particular system is set up and configured, another important consideration is the placement arrangement of the surface electrodes over the muscle of interest. For the vast majority of clinical applications, a bipolar configuration with differential amplification (DA) and common mode rejection (CMR) will provide the best signal fidelity in most environments. A bipolar configuration uses two electrodes separated from each other by some predetermined distance (based on the length of the muscle of interest) as the active recording elements, with a third electrode placed anywhere on the body to act as a reference source (e.g., bony prominence of the elbow) (De Luca, 1997, 2002). In this arrangement, the DA and CMR processes allow for the elimination of common nuisance effects (such as 60-Hz line noise) in the signal, with isolation and amplification of the biopotential that one is actually interested in.

Prerecording Procedures

1. Preparation for Electrode Placement

Procedurally, surface electrode placement requires abrasion of the skin and cleaning (vigorous wiping with an alcohol prep pad will suffice for both) of the area overlying the muscle of interest. In addition, the use of an electrolyte medium is needed to interface the recording head of the surface electrode with the skin surface. One can purchase electrode types that are preloaded with an electrolytic gel covering the electrode head or that require user to apply the media. Typically, the preloaded varieties are disposable and come with a peel away adhesive for easy application. Although they are simple to use, we have found that it is more cost effective to purchase reusable electrodes with add-on adhesive collars, but the choice is ultimately up to the user's needs.

2. Electrode Placement

Two paramedial locations are suggested for biopotential monitoring to obtain gross information regarding laryngeal elevation and depression: a submental and sternohyoid region placement. With a bipolar configuration, the electrodes should be placed in parallel to the fiber orientation of the muscles to maximize recording sensitivity and selectivity (De Luca, 2002). Given that the muscles in the submental and anterior neck are rather short, an interelectrode distance of approximately 1 cm is adequate to obtain a high-fidelity differential signal. For the submental area, electrodes should be placed along a paramedial and longitudinal orientation from just below the inferior ridge of the mandible directly lateral the mental tubercle. For the sternohyoid region placement, palpate the thyroid prominence along the midline until locating the cricothyroid space and then shift laterally approximately 2 centimeters to place the electrodes over the sternohyoid area. Clinicians should note that the variations in individuals' laryngeal anatomy have to be taken into account when placing the electrodes.

3. Validity and Reliability of Recordings

Confirmation of Electrode Placement. Once the skin is prepared, placements identified, and the electrodes placed, confirmation tasks should be performed and evaluated to ensure correct electrode placement. To confirm sternohyoid placements, have the clients try to open their mouths against a resistance (e.g., the clinician can place his or her thumb under the client's jaw to provide resistance while the client attempts to open the mouth) (Zemlin, 1998). Swallowing a bolus of water or a dry swallow can effectively confirm both submental and sternohyoid placement; and posturing the tip of the tongue against the hard and soft palate will engage the submental muscles. In addition, a sustained /i/ with high pitch will engage the submental complex whereas a sustained /u/ will engage the infrahyoid musculature (Borden, Harris, &

Raphael, 2003). The electrodes may have to be repositioned as needed to ensure valid electrode placements, as indicated by maximal biopotential activity synchronized in time with the behavioral conformation tests.

Movement Artifact. Movement artifacts are problematic and should be preemptively addressed. Check the absence of movement artifact by having the client rotate the head. Long electrode cables also can be taped to a client's shirt. Most importantly, the client should be seated comfortably and keep as still as possible during the recordings. Any chair with a headrest would be ideal to minimize head movements during vocalizations and speech (e.g., examination chair, dental chair). Additional molds to stabilize a client's head are advisable (Figure 15–1). Alternatively, an elastic headband around the headrest and the forehead will cue the client to hold still and thus will reduce extraneous movements.

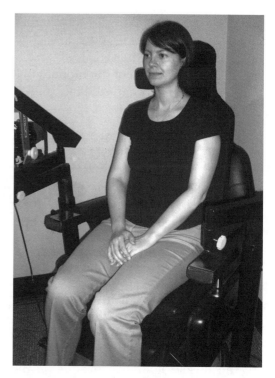

Figure 15–1. Example of an optimal posture for surface EMG recordings during speech.

4. Reference Voluntary Contraction Tasks

It is important to mention that interpretation and comparison of the EMG signal, both within and between clients, is not an entirely straightforward process. Many investigators look into normalization procedures to help solve problems that arise from these factors. The most frequently used strategy is to reference SEMG activity to a predetermined level of muscle activity. Two example methods are maximum voluntary contraction (MVC) and the reference voluntary contraction (RVC). MVC is the maximal contraction effort and RVC is a target level of effort, typically 50% of the MVC, and all subsequent recordings are referenced back as a percentage of this known value. Both MVC and RVC are known to have adequate test-retest reliability (Cram & Kasman, 1998). However, it should also be noted that MVC typically achieves lower reliability than submaximal contraction, for example, up to 50% RVC (De Luca, 1997; Soderberg, 1992). In fact, the orofacial muscles usually operate below 20% MVC during speech (Netsell, 1982).

Therefore, we recommend 50% RVC for the normalization procedure. The procedures should include practice trials (100% and 50%), visual feedback, and motivation of the clients to perform their best. An isometric resistive mandible depression task will serve the purpose of engaging infrahyoid musculature (Juul-Kristensen, Laursen, Pilegaard, & Jensen, 2004; Zemlin, 1998) and also suprahyoid musculature if the tongue is pressed against the palate at the same time (lips and teeth lightly closed during mandible depression). Alternatively, an effortful swallow or Mendelsohn maneuver will be suitable to engage the submental musculature. For 50% RVC, instruct the clients to subjectively embody half the effort of force during mandible depression expended as compared to 100% (MVC). Each RVC for the mandible depression task should be held for 5 seconds and repeated three times with intermittent one-minute recovery periods to avoid muscle fatigue (De Luca, 1997; LeVeau & Andersson, 1992; Soderberg, 1992). At the end, the client should receive 2 minutes of rest before proceeding with voice and speech tasks.

Instructions: *"Please put your thumbs next to each other under your jaw. Now, try to open your mouth while your thumbs are providing resistance at the same time.* (For 100% MVC:) *Please try as hard as possible, ok? Please hold the position for 5 seconds and pay attention to the height of the signal for later comparison.* (For 50% RVC:) *Please use half of the effort that you used during the maximum trial, ok? Please hold the position for 5 seconds and let the signal only rise halfway compared to the maximum trial.* (assist the client with timing)

Recording Procedures

Refer to the specific instrumentation manuals for details regarding triggering and digitization of events in marking the beginning and end of tasks. The suggested recording procedures include several phases as summarized in Table 15–1:

Table 15–1. Overview of Procedures

Phase	Protocol	Duration
Preparations	Set up SEMG RVC (add 2 min. recovery)	variable
Baseline speech	CAPE-V "Rainbow Passage"	5 min.
Rest	Silent	10 min.
Stress anticipation	Silent	2 min.
Stress	(a) Sustained "ah" and "We were away a year ago" (b) Public speaking	5 min.
Recovery	Silent	7 min.
Repeated baseline speech	CAPE-V "Rainbow Passage"	5 min.

SEMG, surface electromyography; RVC, reference voluntary contraction; CAPE-V, Consensus Auditory Perceptual Evaluation of Voice.

1. rest (silent baseline),
2. voice and speech baseline 1,
3. anticipation of stress (silent), voice and speech during stress (public speaking),
4. recovery (silent), and
5. repeated voice and speech baseline 2.

Both tonic (background or constant activity) and phasic (intermittent activity) extralaryngeal muscle activity is captured throughout the protocol while exposure to stress is manipulated. The duration of the rest and recovery phases has been determined based on concurrent cardiovascular recordings such as blood pressure and heart rate. The rest phase should provide sufficient time for the client to recover from baseline speech tasks and to achieve a general physiologic resting state before the onset of the stressor. The length of the recovery phase has been chosen to capture a physiologic recovery slope and a return to baseline.

1. Baseline Speech

The stimuli for voice and speech production are based on the Consensus Auditory-Perceptual Evaluation of Voice (CAPE-V; Kempster, Gerratt, Verdolini Abbott, Barkmeier-Kraemer, & Hillman, 2009) and the phonetically balanced Rainbow Passage (Fairbanks, 1960). Consensus suggestions for adequate acoustic stimuli and appropriate recording parameters also can be found in Titze (1995). The combination of the CAPE-V sentences and the Rainbow Passage creates a speech sample that is roughly of similar length as the public speaking task (5 minutes). It is helpful if the stimuli are displayed on a computer monitor.

Instructions: *"We will now start with speech recordings. We will record*

your muscle movements and speech. Please use your comfortable pitch and loudness. Please keep looking straight ahead."

"Please sustain /a/ (/i/) for 3 to 5 seconds." (monitor length of vowels)

"Please read the following sentences: (1) The blue spot is on the key again. (2) How hard did he hit him? (3) We were away a year ago. (4) We eat eggs every Easter. (5) My mama makes lemon jam. (6) Peter will keep at the peak." (monitor continuous voicing for all-voiced sentence, "We were away a year ago")

"Please read the Rainbow Passage (Appendix 15-A)."

2. Rest

The rest phase will be 10 minutes before the onset of the stressor. However, muscle activity does not have to be recorded for the entire duration. Rather, at minimum, the last minute should be captured as resting baseline.

Instructions: *"We will now continue with a 10-minute, undisturbed, resting period. We will record your muscle activity. Please keep looking straight ahead. Try to move as little as possible and please do not fall asleep."*

3. Public Speaking Stressor

The stressor portion will consist of three parts: anticipation period, standard voice and speech sample, and public speaking. It is recommended that the clinician elicit a portion of the CAPE-V stimulus list (sustained /a/ and all-voiced sentence

"We were away a year ago") *immediately prior to the onset of public speaking.* Thereby, the clinician can obtain a phonetically controlled speech sample under *maximum stress* that can be compared to baseline samples. The stressor proper is modeled after the Trier Social Stress Test (TSST; Kirschbaum et al., 1993) and involves an impromptu public speaking task performed under social-evaluative conditions and time pressure. The social-evaluative component is critical and should be created by the presence of an audience (at least one person in addition to the clinician) and concurrent videotaping. Ideally, an unfamiliar person trained in the protocol presents the stressor task to the client and stands in front of the client during the public speaking portion. We used a modified version of the original TSST in that we used only one stressor and by amending the setting and the instructions for the purpose of SEMG recordings. The full set of original instructions is available online at: http://www.macses.ucsf .edu/research/allostatic/challenge.php .

Instructions: (Take a stopwatch. Position a video camera in front of the client. Turn on the video camera. Position the client so that he or she looks straight ahead and sits in an upright position). *"The task we are going to have you do now is a speech task. Imagine you have applied for a job as a lawyer and you were invited to present yourself before a committee, which will evaluate you on the basis of your personal characteristics. Your task now is to convince the committee in a free speech that you are the best candidate for the vacant position. Following these instructions, you have 2 minutes to prepare for the speech. Please*

also note that you will be recorded by a video camera as well. We will record your speech for a subsequent voice frequency analysis to reveal any paraverbal signs of stress. The camera recording is used for later behavioral analysis. The members of the committee are trained in behavioral analysis and will take notes during your speech. Your speech is supposed to take 5 minutes. Do you have any questions?" (If question is asked regarding the type of lawyer, then respond: *"That's up to you."*)

(Check posture of the client: looking straight ahead, upright upper body.) *"Please start your preparation period and please keep as still as possible."*

(Start recording.)

(Clinician leaves the room or recording booth or stays out of sight and comes back 2 minutes later.) *"Please try to keep your head, arms and legs as still as possible."*

"First, please sustain 'a' for 3 to 5 seconds right now." (Time duration and move quickly to next instruction)

"Now, say the sentence: 'We were away a year ago.'" (Model the sentence with natural intonation and on one breath and move quickly to next instruction)

"Please begin your speech and speak for the entire period of 5 minutes and maintain eye contact with me."

(Start stopwatch.)

(Instructions for clinician who introduces the stress task: fake data protocol sheet on clipboard; take random notes; do not smile, do not laugh; maintain eye-contact.)

(Only after a pause of more than 10 seconds:) *"You still have time, please continue ..."*

Should it appear after another 10 seconds that the client has nothing further to say, then the clinician should ask questions until the end of the time period; the phrasing of these questions is left to the clinician's discretion, for example:

- *Why do you think that **you** are the best applicant for this position?*
- *What qualifies you in particular for this position?*
- *What other experiences have you had in this area?*
- *What about your studies identifies a special aptitude and motivation for this position?*
- *Where else did you apply? Why?*
- *What would you do, if your application here would not succeed?*

(After 5 minutes:) *"You can stop speaking now."*

4. Recovery

Instructions: *"Now we will have you rest quietly again for 7 minutes. Please try to keep your head, arms and legs as still as possible."* (Take video camera and leave the client behind.)

5. Repeated Baseline Speech

Follow instructions for baseline speech.

Other Measures

Other measures should be considered in order to study various aspects of psycho-logical, physiologic, and vocal function. The choice may depend on availability and clinical questions. Typical measures in psychophysiologic studies are psychological trait and state measures (e.g., scores on the NEO-Personality Inventory-Revised [NEO-PI-R; Costa & McCrae, 1992] and Positive and Negative Affect Scale-Expanded Form [PANAS-X; Watson & Clark, 1994]) and measures of autonomic nervous system function (blood pressure, heart rate, heart rate variability, skin conductance). The NEO-PI-R is based on a five-factor model of personality (neuroticism, extraversion, openness to experience, agreeableness, conscientiousness) and represents the current consensus in personality theory and research (John, Naumann, & Soto, 2008). Of note, the NEO-PI-R can be purchased by speech-language pathologists. With regard to voice measures, perceived vocal effort (e.g., direct magnitude estimation [DME, Colton, Casper, & Leonard, 2006; Wright & Colton, 1972]), and acoustic measures (voice fundamental frequency and intensity) easily can be added to the protocol by modifying the setup (headset microphone, audio recording synchronized with the EMG recordings). Discussion on the choice of measures can be found in the literature (Dietrich, 2008; Roy, Bless, & Heisey, 2000a, 2000b; van Mersbergen et al., 2008).

DATA ANALYSIS

Signal analysis for EMG can be as simple as visual inspection of the record, or as complex as quantitative analysis. Commonly used data analysis methods include calculation of the root mean square (RMS), spectral analysis, and integral averaging functions. Both RMS and integral averaging functions provide the user with an estimate of the amount of muscle energy expended, whereas spectral analyses characterize the component distribution of the muscles' energy. Although the specific details of these methods are beyond the scope of this chapter, the reader is referred to Cram and Kasman (1998) and Loeb and Gans (1986) for descriptions of some of these methods. Furthermore, the comparison and interpretation of the EMG signal, both within and between individuals, depends on normalization procedures. There is a constellation of factors that can influence and affect SEMG parametric values. Normalization of raw values for each individual allows for comparisons between muscle groups (e.g., due to muscle geometry), speakers (e.g., due to subcutaneous fat), and time points (Fridlund & Cacioppo, 1986; Lundberg, 2002). At this point, all records should be referenced back to the known value, that is, 50% RVC, and expressed as a percentage of it. The averaged middle portion of three trials of RVC should be used as reference (omit first and last second). It is up to the clinician to select adequate segments from the experimental phases for analyses. In order to perform comparisons between phases, the segments should be of similar length and pattern to ensure maximum comparability. For example, the all-voiced sentence, "We were away a year ago" can be analyzed with and without exposure to stress. With regard to spontaneous speech, only continuous, same-length portions of public speaking (e.g., including up to 2 seconds of speech pause) should be compared among individuals or between assessments (e.g., pre- and posttherapy). Finally, time courses can be evaluated, for example, with regard to the recovery phase.

NORMATIVE DATA

Normative data for extralaryngeal SEMG are not available for several reasons. The data from studies using SEMG are difficult to compare because of variability in the study sample and methodological differences. The comparison of SEMG raw values across individuals may be misleading, because: (1) individuals' anatomy of laryngeal muscles may differ, (2) the degree of fatty tissue overlying the muscles attenuates the signal (document body mass index), (3) the EMG signal is the summed activity of motor unit potentials across muscle groups, and (4) different instrumentation and procedures used across laboratories will introduce variability. However, instead of absolute values, ratios of muscle activity can be collected for database purposes (see normalization procedures). Following guidelines for obtaining extralaryngeal SEMG signals will increase the validity and reliability of SEMG data and their clinical and research utility. Publication standards for reporting EMG data should be followed, which have been put forth by the International Society of Electrophysiology and Kinesiology (Merletti, 1999).

CASE STUDIES

Two case studies are presented to illustrate differences in extralaryngeal behaviors between introverts and extraverts (cf. Dietrich, 2008). The first case study illustrates laryngeal behavior characteristics of an introverted individual. Mary was a 22-year-old female with good physical and mental health. She was a nonsmoker, and reported no voice problem. Her voice was judged as normal based on independent ratings by two certified speech-language pathologists. She was identified as a neurotic introvert based on scores on the Eysenck Personality Questionnaire-Revised (EPQ-R; Eysenck & Eysenck, 1994) and Multidimensional Personality Questionnaire-Brief Form (MPQ-BF; Patrick, Curtin, & Tellegen, 2002). She scored −0.91 SD below the norm on extraversion (EPQ-R), a *T* score of 45 on social potency (MPQ-BF), 1.70 SD above the norm on neuroticism (EPQ-R), and a *T* score of 71 on stress reaction (MPQ-BF). Her score on the Voice Handicap Index (Jacobson et al., 1997) was 28 (out of the maximum possible score of 120). During public speaking, her systolic blood pressure was on average 136 mm Hg. She reported twice as much vocal effort during public speaking as compared to a baseline comfortable amount of effort during speech (direct magnitude estimation). The pattern of Mary's SEMG results,

both submental (SM) and infrahyoid (IH) SEMG activity, is illustrated in Figure 15–2. During any phase, IH activity was greater than SM activity. The major difference between baseline speeches and speaking under stress was an increase in IH SEMG activity.

The pattern of findings for Mary was different compared to that of Jackie, a 28-year-old female extravert. Jackie also was in good physical and mental health, did not smoke, and reported no voice problem. Her voice was judged as normal. She was identified as a non-neurotic extravert. She scored 1.34 SD above the norm on extraversion (EPQ-R), a *T* score of 66 on social potency (MPQ-BF), −2.31 SD below the norm on neuroticism (EPQ-R), and a *T* score of 31 on stress reaction (MPQ-BF). Her score on the *Voice Handicap Index* was zero. During public speaking her systolic blood pressure on average was 145 mm Hg. She reported no perceived vocal effort during public speaking. The

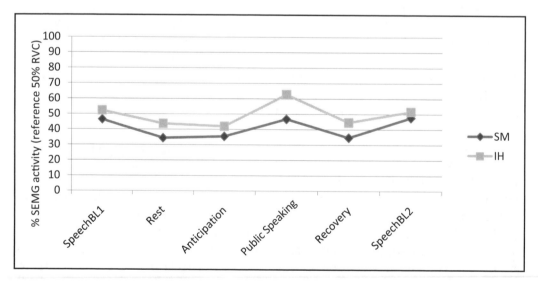

Figure 15–2. Case study Mary (introvert): Submental (SM) and infrahyoid (IH) surface electromyographic (SEMG) activity across phase expressed in percentage of normalized SEMG activity (50% reference voluntary contraction [RVC]).

pattern of Jackie's SEMG results is illustrated in Figure 15–3. During baseline speech, IH activity generally was lower than SM activity. The major difference between baseline speeches and speaking under stress was an increase in IH activity and, to a smaller extent, an increase in SM activity. However, IH activity did not rise above SM activity.

The comparison of the case studies reveals an interesting general imbalance between IH and SM activity during speech in the introvert, which was not evident in the extrovert. Furthermore, this imbalance became potentiated during perceived stress in the introvert. In the extravert, the general increase in SEMG activity during stress did not cause an imbalance between SM and IH activity. Moreover, the overall normalized magnitude of SEMG activity generally was lower in the extravert. The systolic blood pressure rose significantly in both individuals from a baseline state of normal blood pressure typical for this age

group. Yet, the final extralaryngeal behavior during public speaking was different for these two individuals. In addition, Jackie did not report an increase in general negative affect during public speaking (score 13 [general negative affect scale: minimum 10, maximum 50], PANAS-X) whereas Mary reported an increase (score 26).

In the greater psychophysiologic context, the introvert's results are interpreted as a reflection of behavioral inhibition, which was potentiated during exposure to a specific social-evaluative stressor, public speaking. Of clinical relevance is the notion that increased IH activity may lower the larynx or stiffen the laryngeal framework in light of concurrent SM activity during speech. Such imbalance may reduce laryngeal flexibility and contribute to inefficient laryngeal behavior and vocal fatigue typical of MTD. As shown in these case studies, introverted individuals may exhibit a disposition for this particular laryngeal behavior and their perceived

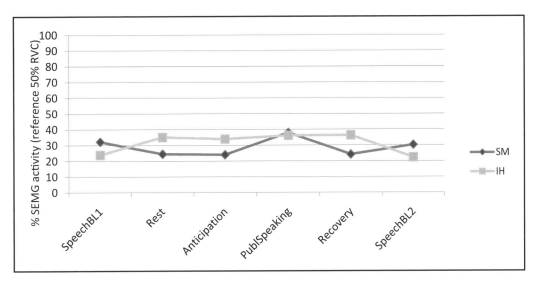

Figure 15–3. Case study Jackie (extravert): Submental (SM) and infrahyoid (IH) surface electromyographic (SEMG) activity across phase expressed in percentage of normalized SEMG activity (50% reference voluntary contraction [RVC]).

vocal effort may have an underlying physiologic source. Therefore, the clinical relevance of dispositional vocal behavior and its underlying psychophysiologic mechanisms deserve continued attention.

REFERENCES

Andrews, S., Warner, J., & Stewart, R. (1986). EMG biofeedback and relaxation in the treatment of hyperfunctional dysphonia. *British Journal of Disorders of Communication, 21,* 353–369.

Angsuwarangsee, T., & Morrison, M. (2002). Extrinsic laryngeal muscular tension in patients with voice disorders. *Journal of Voice, 16*(3), 333–343.

Aronson, A. E. (1990). *Clinical voice disorders: An interdisciplinary approach* (3rd ed.). New York, NY: Thieme.

Borden, G. J., Harris, K. S., & Raphael, L. J. (2003). *Speech science primer: Physiology, acoustics, and perception of speech* (4th ed.). Philadelphia, PA: Lippincott Williams & Wilkins.

Colton, R. H., Casper, J. K., & Leonard, R. (2006). *Understanding voice problems: A physiological perspective for diagnosis and treatment* (3rd ed.). Baltimore, MD: Lippincott Williams & Wilkins.

Costa, P. T., & McCrae, R. R. (1992). *Revised NEO Personality Inventory (NEO-PI-R) professional manual.* Odessa, FL: Psychological Assessment Resources.

Cram, J. R., & Kasman, G. S. (1998). *Introduction to surface electromyography.* Gaithersberg, MD: Aspen.

De Luca, C. J. (1997). The use of surface electromyography in biomechanics. *Journal of Applied Biomechanics, 13*(2), 135–163.

De Luca, C. J. (2002). *Surface electromyography: Detection and recording* [Electronic version]. Retrieved from http://www.delsys.com/Attachments_pdf/WP_SEMGintro.pdf

Dickerson, S. S., & Kemeny, M. E. (2004). Acute stressors and cortisol responses: A theoretical integration and synthesis of laboratory research. *Psychological Bulletin, 130,* 355–391.

Dietrich, M. (2008). *The effects of stress reactivity on extralaryngeal muscle tension in vocally normal participants as a function of personality.* Unpublished dissertation, University of Pittsburgh, Pittsburgh.

Eysenck, H. J., & Eysenck, S. B. G. (1994). *Manual of the Eysenck Personality Questionnaire.* San Diego, CA: EdITS.

Fairbanks, G. (1960). *Voice and articulation drillbook* (2nd ed.). New York, NY: Harper and Row.

Fridlund, A. J., & Cacioppo, J. T. (1986). Guidelines for human electromyographic research. *Psychophysiology, 23*(5), 567–589.

Goldstein, D. S. (2001). *The autonomic nervous system in health and disease.* New York, NY: Dekker.

Hočevar-Boltežar, I., Janko, M., & Žargi, M. (1998). Role of surface EMG in diagnostics and treatment of muscle tension dysphonia. *Acta Otolaryngologica, 118,* 739–743.

Jacobson, B. H., Johnson, A., Grywalski, C., Silbergleit, A., Jacobson, G., Benninger, M. S., . . . Newman, C. W. (1997). The Voice Handicap Index (VHI): Development and validation. *American Journal of Speech-Language Pathology, 6*(3), 66–70.

John, O. P., Naumann, L. P., & Soto, C. J. (2008). Paradigm shift to the integrative Big Five trait taxonomy. History, measurement, and conceptual issues. In O. P. John, R. W. Robins, & L. A. Pervin (Eds.), *Handbook of personality, theory and research* (3rd ed., pp. 114–158). New York, NY: Guilford Press.

Juul-Kristensen, B., Laursen, B., Pilegaard, M., & Jensen, B. R. (2004). Physical workload during use of speech recognition and traditional computer input devices. *Ergonomics, 47*(2), 119–133.

Kempster, G. B., Gerratt, B. R., Verdolini Abbott, K., Barkmeier-Kraemer, J., & Hillman, R. E. (2009). Consensus auditory-perceptual evaluation of voice: Development of a standardized clinical protocol. *American Journal of Speech Language Pathology, 18*(2), 124–132.

Kirschbaum, C., Pirke, K.-M., & Hellhammer, D. H. (1993). The "Trier Social Stress Test" — A tool for investigating psychobiological stress responses in a laboratory setting. *Neuropsychobiology, 28,* 76-81.

Koufman, J. A., & Blalock, P. D. (1982). Classification and approach to patients with functional voice disorders. *Annals of Otology, Rhinology, and Laryngology, 91,* 372-377.

LeVeau, B., & Andersson, G. (1992). Output forms: Data analysis and applications. In *Selected topics in surface electromyography for use in the occupational setting: Expert perspective.* (Vol. Publication No. 91-100, pp. 69-102). Bethesda, MD: U.S. Department of Health and Human Services (NIOSH).

Loeb, G. E., & Gans, C. (1986). *Electromyography for experimentalists.* Chicago, IL: University of Chicago Press.

Lundberg, U. (2002). Psychophysiology of work: Stress, gender, endocrine response, and work-related upper extremity disorders. *American Journal of Industrial Medicine, 41,* 383-392.

Luschei, E. S., & Finnegan, E. M. (2008). Electromyographic techniques for the assessment of motor speech disorders. In M. R. McNeil (Ed.), *Clinical management of sensorimotor speech disorders* (2nd ed., pp. 149-176). New York, NY: Thieme.

McNulty, W. H., Gevirtz, R. N., Berkoff, G. M., & Hubbard, D. R. (1994). Needle electromyographic evaluation of a trigger point response to a psychological stressor. *Psychophysiology, 31,* 313-316.

Merletti, R. (1999). Standards for reporting EMG data. *Journal of Electromyography and Kinesiology, 9*(1), III-IV.

Morrison, M. D., Nichol, H., & Rammage, L. A. (1986). Diagnostic criteria in functional dysphonia. *Laryngoscope, 96,* 1-8.

Morrison, M. D., & Rammage, L. A. (1993). Muscle misuse voice disorders: Description and classification. *Acta Oto-Laryngologica, 113,* 428-434.

Netsell, R. (1982). Speech motor control and selected neurologic disorders. In S. Grillner,

B. Lindblom, J. Lubker, & A. Persson (Eds.), *Speech motor control* (pp. 247-261). New York, NY: Pergamon Press.

Patrick, C. J., Curtin, J. J., & Tellegen, A. (2002). Development and validation of a brief form of the Multidimensional Personality Questionnaire. *Psychological Assessment, 14*(2), 150-163.

Redenbaugh, M. A., & Reich, A. R. (1989). Surface EMG and related measures in normal and vocally hyperfunctional speakers. *Journal of Speech and Hearing Disorders, 54,* 68-73.

Roy, N. (2003). Functional dysphonia. *Current Opinion in Otolaryngology and Head and Neck Surgery, 11,* 144-148.

Roy, N., & Bless, D. M. (2000). Toward a theory of the dispositional bases of functional dysphonia and vocal nodules: Exploring the role of personality and emotional adjustment. In R. D. Kent & M. J. Ball (Eds.), *Voice quality measurement.* San Diego, CA: Singular.

Roy, N., Bless, D. M., & Heisey, D. (2000a). Personality and voice disorders: A multitrait-multidisorder analysis. *Journal of Voice, 14,* 521-548.

Roy, N., Bless, D. M., & Heisey, D. (2000b). Personality and voice disorders: A superfactor trait analysis. *Journal of Speech, Language, and Hearing Research, 43,* 749-768.

Roy, N., Bless, D. M., Heisey, D., & Ford, C. N. (1997). Manual circumlaryngeal therapy for functional dysphonia: An evaluation of short- and long-term treatment outcomes. *Journal of Voice, 11,* 321-331.

Roy, N., & Leeper, H. A. (1993). Effects of the manual laryngeal musculoskeletal tension reduction technique as a treatment for functional voice disorders: Perceptual and acoustic measures. *Journal of Voice, 7,* 242-249.

Seifert, E., & Kollbrunner, J. (2005). Stress and distress in non-organic voice disorders. *Swiss Medical Weekly, 135,* 387-397.

Soderberg, G. L. (1992). Recording techniques. In *Selected topics in surface electromyography for use in the occupational setting: Expert perspectives* (Vol. Publication No. 91-100, pp. 23-41). Bethesda, MD: U.S.

Department of Health and Human Services (NIOSH).

Solomon, N. P. (2008). Vocal fatigue and its relation to vocal hyperfunction. *International Journal of Speech-Language Pathology, 10*(4), 259–266.

Stemple, J. C., Weiler, E., Whitehead, W., & Komray, R. (1980). Electromyographic biofeedback training with patients exhibiting hyperfunctional voice disorder. *Laryngoscope, 90*, 471–476.

Titze, I. R. (1995). *Workshop on acoustic voice analysis: Summary statement*. Iowa City, IA: National Center for Voice and Speech.

van Mersbergen, M., Patrick, C., & Glaze, L. (2008). Functional dysphonia during mental imagery: Testing the trait theory of voice disorders. *Journal of Speech, Language, and Hearing Research, 51*(6), 1405–1423.

Verdolini, K., Rosen, C. A., & Branski, R. C. (Eds.). (2005). *Classification manual for voice disorders-1*. Mahwah, NJ: Erlbaum.

Watson, D., & Clark, L. A. (1994). *The PANAS-X: Manual for the Positive and Negative Affect Schedule-Expanded form*. The University of Iowa.

Wright, H. N., & Colton, R. H. (1972). Some parameters of vocal effort. *Journal of the Acoustical Society of American, 51*(1A), 141.

Zemlin, W. R. (1998). *Speech and hearing science: Anatomy and physiology* (4th ed.). Needham Heights, MA: Allyn & Bacon.

APPENDIX 15-A

The Rainbow Passage

When the sunlight strikes raindrops in the air, they act as a prism and form a rainbow. The rainbow is a division of white light into many beautiful colors. These take the shape of a long round arch, with its path high above, and its two ends apparently beyond the horizon. There is, according to legend, a boiling pot of gold at one end. People look, but no one ever finds it. When a man looks for something beyond his reach, his friends say he is looking for the pot of gold at the end of the rainbow.

Throughout the centuries people have explained the rainbow in various ways. Some have accepted it as a miracle without physical explanation. To the Hebrews it was a token that there would be no more universal floods. The Greeks used to imagine that it was a sign from the gods to foretell war or heavy rain. The Norsemen considered the rainbow as a bridge over which the gods passed from Earth to their home in the sky. Others have tried to explain the phenomenon physically. Aristotle thought that the rainbow was caused by reflection of the sun's rays by the rain.

Since then physicists have found that it is not reflection, but refraction by the raindrops which causes the rainbows. Many complicated ideas about the rainbow have been formed. The difference in the rainbow depends considerably upon the size of the drops, and the width of the colored band increases as the size of the drops increases. The actual primary rainbow observed is said to be the effect of superimposition of a number of bows. If the red of the second bow falls upon the green of the first, the result is to give a bow with an abnormally wide yellow band, since red and green light, when mixed, form yellow. This is a very common type of bow, one showing mainly red and yellow, with little or no green or blue.

CHAPTER 16

Laryngeal Electromyography

WEN XU AND DEMIN HAN

PURPOSE

- To study laryngeal nerve and muscle functions in order to determine:
  - The cause (neuromuscular and/or mechanical) of vocal fold impairment.
  - The severity of the neuropathic laryngeal injuries.

INTRODUCTION

Laryngeal electromyography (LEMG) measures the electrical activities of the laryngeal nerves using electrodes. It is used to investigate the mobility of laryngeal muscles and to determine if nerve damage is the cause. LEMG assesses the physiologic characteristics of both the laryngeal nerves and laryngeal muscles (Carrat et al., 2000; Koufman et al., 2001; Mostafa et al., 2004; Munin, Murry, & Rosen, 2000; Sataloff, Mandel, Mann, & Ludlow, 2004; Sulica & Blitzer, 2004; Tellis, Rosen, Thekdi, & Sciote, 2004; Xu, Han, Hou, Zhang, & Zhao, 2007). LEMG has been used for many decades since the work of Faaborg-Andersen and Buchthal in the late 1950s (Buchthal, 1959; Faaborg-Andersen & Buchthal, 1956). Clinical diagnostic protocols for vocal fold immobility used to rely on medical history and physical examination of the larynx per se. LEMG allows a more accurate diagnosis in individuals with laryngeal neuromuscular disorders. An overview of the principles of LEMG can be found in a chapter by Sulica, Blitzer, and Meyer (2006).

EQUIPMENT AND MATERIALS

Recording System

The instruments generally used in conducting LEMG include electrodes, amplifiers, a display system, a loudspeaker, and data storage devices. This chapter describes a four-channel Nicolet Vikingquest Electromyographic system (Nicolet Biomedical, Madison, WI). The system uses one channel to connect with the EMG electrodes and another channel is connected to a microphone for recording acoustic signals synchronously (Figure 16-1).

Types of Electrode

Different electrode types (surface electrode or needle electrode) have been used in LEMG procedure to record muscle or nerve electrophysiologic activity (Hillel, 2001; Jacobs & Finkel, 2002; Koufman et al., 2001; Sataloff et al., 2004; Sataloff et al., 2010; Xu et al., 2007; Yin, Qiu, & Stucker, 1997). Surface electrodes, which are non-invasive, refer to electrodes placed on the skin over the target muscle and register summated electrical activities from the muscle group or nerve fibers. When surface electrodes are used, they can be susceptible to interference from nearby muscle activities and indeed small laryngeal muscles responses could not be identified individually using surface electrodes. Needle electrodes are inserted close to individual muscles and hence can discriminate individual muscle activities within a narrow radius from the recording tip. Needle electrodes are more precise and therefore are more appropriate for laryngeal examination. The choice of appropriate needle electrodes (from among concentric needle electrodes, bipolar concentric needle electrodes, monopolar needle elec-

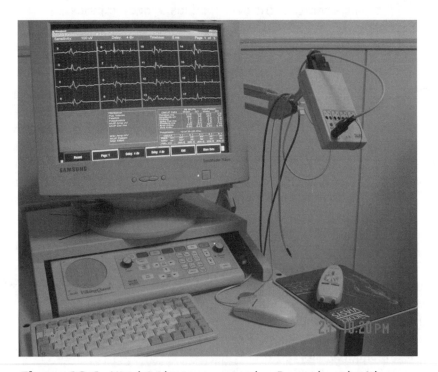

Figure 16–1. Nicolet electromyography. Reproduced with permission from Han, D., Sataloff, R. T., and Xu, W (Eds.). *Voice medicine* [in Chinese]. Beijing, China. People's Republic Publishing House. Copyright ©2007.

trodes, hooked-wire electrodes, or single fiber electrodes; see Figure 16–2) varies and depends on the clinical information required (Jacobs & Finkel, 2002; Koufman et al., 2001; Sataloff et al., 2004; Sataloff et al., 2010; Yin et al., 1997). Concentric needle electrodes often are the optimal choice for EMG study of laryngeal muscles (Hillel, 2001; Jacobs & Finkel, 2002; Xu et al., 2007; Yin et al., 1997). Single-fiber electromyography (SFEMG) is useful in the evaluation of disorders of neuromuscular transmission and the assessment of motor unit morphology. This type of electrode requires the skills of the examiner and the cooperation of the patient. Hence SFEMG often is not the choice of routine diagnostic tool for laryngeal nerve and muscle disorders. One can also choose a hooked-wire electrode (Hillel, 2001), which remains in place during vigorous activity but is more difficult to reposition and may cause more local trauma to muscle (Jaffe, Solomon, Robinson, Hoffman, & Luschei, 1998).

PROCEDURES

Laryngeal electromyographic evaluation is discussed under three sections in the present chapter: routine LEMG examination, laryngeal nerve conduction examination, and repetitive nerve stimulation test. LEMG data often are evaluated by both laryngologists and neurologists.

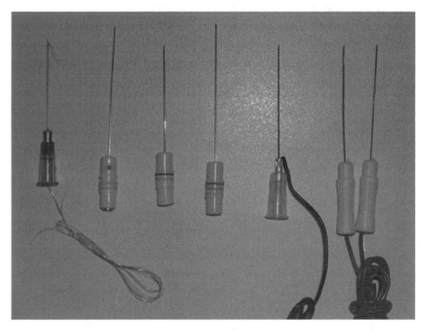

Figure 16–2. Different types of needle electrodes (*from left to right*: hooked-wire electrode, single fiber electrode, concentric needle electrode (35 mm), concentric needle electrode (45 mm), botulinum toxin injection needle electrode, monopolar needle electrodes). Reproduced with permission from Han, D., Sataloff, R. T., and Xu, W (Eds.). *Voice medicine* [in Chinese]. Beijing. China: People's Republic Publishing House. Copyright ©2007.

Routine LEMG Examination

During routine LEMG examination, four types of EMG activities are recorded: (1) needle insertional potentials, which are caused by the movement of the needle electrode in the laryngeal muscle; (2) nerve spontaneous potentials, which are the basal laryngeal muscle activity at rest with just the breathing and no other voluntary contraction; (3) motor unit potential, which are the individual discharges of motor neurons evoked during mild voluntary contraction; and (4) recruitment potentials, which are the maximum activity of voluntary muscle contraction (Figure 16-3).

The patient lies supine with the neck extended. A surface ground electrode is placed on the patient's sternum. Generally, local topical anesthetics are not necessary but, if required, it is recommended that

1 mL of 0.5% tetracaine hydrochloride be used through the cricothyroid membrane. Applying local anesthetics may be particularly useful for recording activities of the posterior cricoarytenoid muscle. In our clinic, concentric needle electrodes are placed percutaneously into the following muscles: the thyroarytenoid muscle, the posterior cricoarytenoid muscle, and the cricothyroid muscle (Figure 16-4). For the thyroarytenoid muscle, the needle is passed through the cricothyroid membrane in the midline and then continued superiorly and laterally to reach the thyroarytenoid muscle. For the posterior cricoarytenoid, the needle is passed through the cricothyroid membrane, then through the posterior lamina of the cricoid cartilage to the side reaching the posterior cricoarytenoid.

The accuracy of needle placement is confirmed by checking the insertional

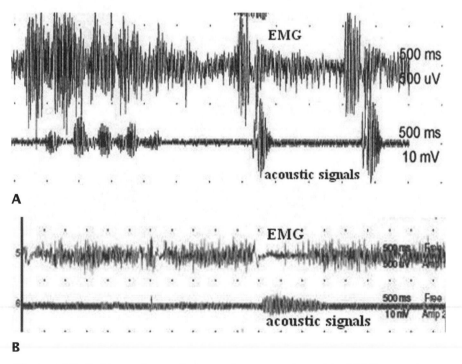

Figure 16–3. Normal recruitment electromyographic (EMG) pattern **A.** in thyroarytenoid muscle and **B.** posterior cricoarytenoid muscle.

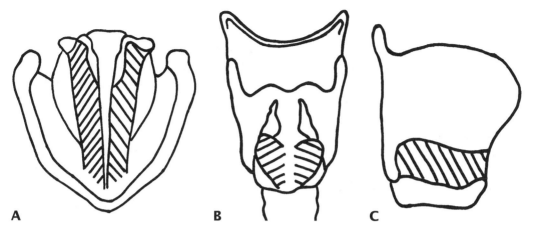

Figure 16–4. Laryngeal muscles (*shaded areas*). **A.** Superior view of larynx show-ing thyroarytenoid muscles. **B.** Posterior view of larynx showing posterior cricoarytenoid muscles **C.** Lateral view of larynx showing cricothyroid muscles.

potential activity during the procedure, anatomic landmarks used in needle insertion, and the relationship of the specific muscles with phonatory and respiratory tasks:

- The thyroarytenoid muscle functions as a primary adductor of the larynx. It should be active in all phonation tasks, coughing, or the Valsalva maneuver.
- The cricothyroid muscle is specifically active during efforts to increase pitch.
- The posterior cricoarytenoid muscle acts as a primary abductor. It demonstrates significant electrical activity during sniffing, rapid breathing but has little activity during phonation.

Laryngeal Nerve Conduction Examination

Laryngeal nerve conduction examination is useful in identifying and localizing the site of lesion. This procedure examines the electrical activities of the muscles supplied by the specific nerve that is stimulated during the examination procedure. The amplitude, duration and latency of compound evoked potentials are analyzed. For superior laryngeal nerve, which supplies the cricothyroid muscle, the *stimulation electrode is* inserted percutaneously between the greater cornu of the hyoid and the superior cornu of the thyroid cartilage. The recording electrode is inserted into the cricothyroid muscle. For the recurrent laryngeal nerve, which supplies the thyroarytenoid and posterior cricoarytenoid muscle, the *stimulation electrode* is inserted percutaneously lateral to trachea at the level of 2.0 to 2.5 cm below the cricoid cartilage. The recording electrode is inserted into thyroarytenoid or posterior cricoarytenoid muscle. The amplitudes, latency, duration, and waveforms of the response potentials from the cricothyroid, thyroarytenoid, and posterior cricoarytenoid muscle are evaluated. It has been suggested that the amplitude of evoked LEMG potentials relates to the function of the axon of the nerve, whereas the latency of the evoked potentials reflects the function of the medulla of the nerve (Kimaid et al., 2004). Thus, these two measures are useful indicators for the severity of the neuropathic laryngeal injury.

Repetitive Nerve Stimulation Test

Repetitive stimulation of peripheral nerves to detect neuromuscular transmission defects is a standard electrodiagnostic tests. Diagnosis of myasthenia gravis, a common neuromuscular junction disease, often is confirmed by using this test. Abnormal neuromuscular transmission in myasthenia gravis results in clinical fatigable weakness in specific striated muscle groups. The diagnosis of myasthenia gravis requires the presence of a combination of clinical manifestations, pharmacologic testing, and electrophysiologic study with EMG. The repetitive nerve stimulation test is the most important test in the diagnosis of myasthenia gravis (Carpenter, McDonald, & Howard, 1979; Juel & Massey, 2007; Nemoto et al., 2005). Ocular weakness with asymmetric ptosis and binocular diplopia are typical initial presentations of myasthenia gravis. Some experts have observed that some patients may have laryngeal symptoms as their initial symptoms of myasthenia gravis (Hartl, Leboulleux, Klap, & Schlumberger, 2007; Liu, Xia, Men, Wu, & Huang, 2007; Mao et al., 2001). In our clinic, we also found many individuals with myasthenia gravis exhibited asymmetry and abnormal findings on laryngeal electromyography (Xu, Han, Hou, Hu, & Wang, 2009).

The repetitive nerve stimulation test for the laryngeal muscle is performed using monopolar needle electrodes to repetitively stimulate the recurrent and superior laryngeal nerves at low frequency (1 Hz, 3 Hz). The percentage of reduction in the amplitude of the evoked potentials of the corresponding laryngeal muscles between the first and the fourth compound muscle action potential responses. A reduction of more than 10% in the amplitude of the evoked potentials is considered to be abnormal, and the muscle is considered to be involved in myasthenia gravis (Juel & Massey, 2007; Nemoto et al., 2005; Xu et al., 2009). We also found that the repetitive nerve stimulation test for the laryngeal muscles has a high sensitivity (87.5%) in identifying myasthenia gravis (Xu et al., 2009). In myasthenia gravis, the thyroarytenoid muscles, and in particular the cricothyroid muscles, are more likely to demonstrate abnormal repetitive nerve stimulation findings than other laryngeal muscles.

Precautions

The placement of needle electrodes into a compromised airway, as in bilateral vocal fold immobility, may present some risk if edema develops. Therefore, the presence of an otolaryngologist to take precautionary measures such as preparation for emergency tracheotomy or administration of corticosteroids to alleviate the edema is essential before or during LEMG procedure. There also are risks associated with the electrode placement. Laryngeal edema or bleeding is the most common complications. These problems may be alleviated by using hot packs and cold compression, use of corticosteroids, or topical vasoconstrictors. In children who require sedation or general anesthesia because of discomfort and fear of the use of needle placement (Jacobs & Finkel, 2002), the risks involved in the sedation or anesthetics also should be taken into consideration.

DATA INTERPRETATION

Normative data developed in our clinic are listed in Table 16-1 (Xu et al., 2007). Figure 16-5 illustrates the electrical activities

Table 16–1. Normative Data of Laryngeal Electromyography

Measures	Cricothyroid Muscle	Thyroarytenoid Muscle	Posterior Cricoarytenoid Muscle
Latent periods of evoked potentials	1.7±0.4 ms	1.7±0.3 ms	1.8±0.5 ms
Amplitudes of evoked potentials	4.9±4.3 mV	7.6±5.3 mV	4.4±3.3 mV

Source: Xu, W., Han, D., Hou, L., et al., Value of laryngeal electromyography in diagnosis of vocal fold immobility. *Annals of Otology, Rhinology, and Laryngology, 116,* 576–581. Copyright © 2007.

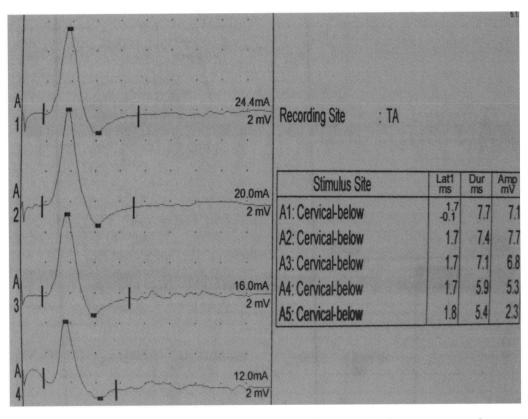

Figure 16–5. Recurrent laryngeal nerve evoked laryngeal electromyographic potentials of thyroarytenoid muscle.

of the thyroarytenoid muscle. Decreased evoked potentials were shown in patients with incomplete recurrent laryngeal nerve injuries with a delayed latency in the thyroarytenoid muscle (2.2 ms on average, and even up to 3.2 ms) and the posterior cricoarytenoid muscle (2.4 ms on average, and even up to 3.4 ms), and lower amplitude in the thyroarytenoid (from 0.2 to 1.6 mV) and posterior cricoarytenoid muscle (from 0.2 to 2.2 mV) (Xu et al., 2007). The increased latent period has been found to be indicative of nerve impairment, and the reduced amplitudes of evoked potentials is used to indicate the severity of impairment.

Immobility of the vocal folds may be of neuromuscular or mechanical origins. Mechanical problems such as cricoarytenoid joint dislocation or fixation or posterior glottic scarring generally yield normal LEMG findings. The recruitment potentials showed full interference patterns and are more active than in normal individuals. With increasing contractility, the amplitude and interference patterns increase greatly in compensation. The amplitude, duration, and latency of evoked LEMG signals also would be normal.

Denervation can be found in the intrinsic laryngeal muscles dominated by the troubled nerve in early stage. LEMG may appear as either fibrillation potentials or positive sharp waves. Our experience suggests that LEMG can be performed as early as 1 to 2 weeks after injury (Xu et al., 2007), although one has to caution against inaccuracy in determining the degree of injury using LEMG too early. A lacerated nerve completely cut through will demonstrate no electrical activities. Individuals with incomplete nerve injuries may demonstrate normal potentials at the same time with denervated potentials. Reduced recruitment activities will appear either as a simple pattern or a mixed pattern. The signals of evoked LEMG would decrease, with longer latency and lower amplitude (Figure 16–6). With time, reinnervation may occur. The signs of reinnervation

include motor unit potentials with larger amplitude firing at increased frequencies even at low-level muscle contraction. Another possible sign of reinnervation includes polyphasic motor unit potentials increase in amplitude and with a longer duration (see Figure 16–6).

In some cases of laryngeal nerve injury, through synchronous analysis of LEMG and laryngeal function activity, it is not uncommon to find the affected posterior cricoarytenoid muscle to be activated synchronously with the thyroarytenoid muscle during phonation or a cough (Figure 16–7). In some cases, the affected thyroarytenoid muscle would also be activated synchronously with the posterior cricoarytenoid on inspiration (see Figure 16–7). This phenomenon is called synkinesis, in which the regenerated axons are believed to grow in the direction to the motor end plates of antagonistic muscles, resulting in the antagonists' contracting synchronously. With laryngeal synkinesis, reinnervation of the adductor and abductor musculature of the larynx results in a simultaneous contraction of the abductor and adductor musculature of the vocal fold. Although synkinesis does not improve vocal fold movement, it can be useful in maintaining vocal fold tension and preventing vocal fold atrophy.

In summary, knowledge of changes in the characteristics of laryngeal behavior and LEMG performance and types of surgical nerve injuries is necessary to the diagnosis of laryngeal injuries. The differential diagnostic of vocal fold immobility should include a thorough history-taking, detailed physical examination including arytenoid palpation, and LEMG in order to arrive at an accurate diagnosis so that treatment or management can be appropriately planned.

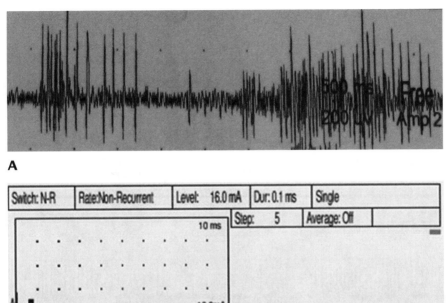

A

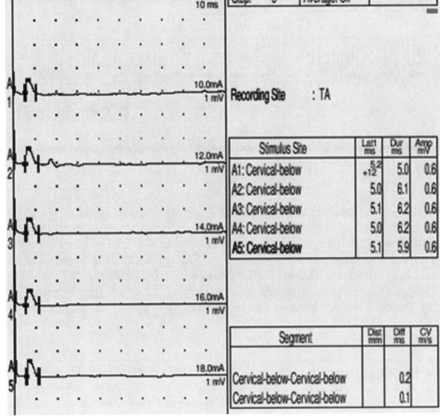

Switch: N-R	Rate:Non-Recurrent	Level: 16.0 mA	Dur: 0.1 ms	Single
		Step: 5	Average: Off	

Recording Site : TA

Stimulus Site	Lat1 ms	Dur ms	Amp mV
A1: Cervical-below	+12 5.2	5.0	0.6
A2: Cervical-below	5.0	6.1	0.6
A3: Cervical-below	5.1	6.2	0.6
A4: Cervical-below	5.0	6.2	0.6
A5: Cervical-below	5.1	5.9	0.6

Segment	Dist mm	Diff ms	CV m/s
Cervical-below-Cervical-below		0.2	
Cervical-below-Cervical-below		0.1	

B

Figure 16–6. Laryngeal electromygraphy of thyroarytenoid muscle with an incomplete recurrent laryngeal nerve injury. **A.** Simple and mixed recruitment pattern on involved side of thyroaryntenoid muscle. **B.** Reduced evoked muscle potential with delayed latency (5.0 ms) and lower amplitude (0.6 mV).Reproduced with permission from Xu, W., Han, D., Hou L, et al. Value of laryngeal myography in diagnosis of vocal fold immobility. *Annals of Otology, Rhinology and Laryngology, 116*, 576–581. Copyright © 2007.

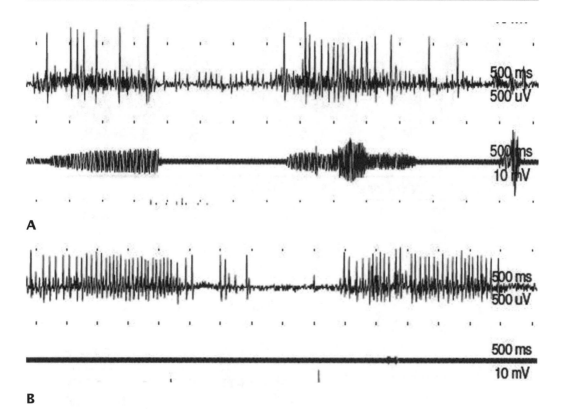

Figure 16–7. Laryngeal electromyography demonstrating synkinetic coactivation of the posterior cricoarytenoid muscle and thyroarytenoid muscles in an individual with recurrent laryngeal nerve injury: **A.** LEMG shows posterior cricoarytenoid activated on phonation. **B.** LEMG shows thyroarytenoid muscles activated on inspiration. Reproduced with permission from Xu, W., Han, D., Hou L, et al. Value of laryngeal myography in diagnosis of vocal fold immobility. *Annals of Otology, Rhinology and Laryngology, 116*, 576–581. Copyright © 2007.

CASE STUDY

A 26-year-old male college student suffered from dyspnea had a tracheotomy. He had a history of prolonged endotracheal intubation due to laryngeal fungal infection after bone marrow transplantation for treating leukemia. Previous stroboscopy showed bilateral vocal fold immobility and bilateral vocal fold paralysis was diagnosed initially (Figure 16-8). LEMG revealed, however, normal recurrent laryngeal and superior laryngeal nerve functions (see Figure 16-8). Further examination using arytenoid palpation under stroboscopy revealed interarytenoid fibrosis with a scar band. This suggested a very different treatment regime. For patients with suspected of bilateral vocal fold immobility, a thorough history-taking, careful local physical examination including arytenoid palpation, and LEMG are recommended examination procedures for making a proper diagnosis.

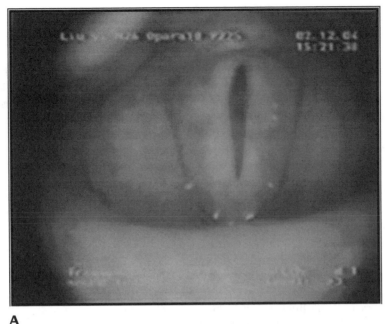

A

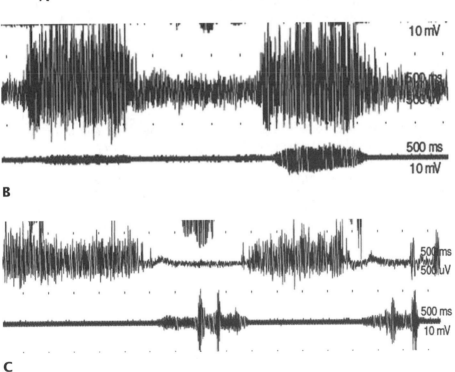

B

C

Figure 16–8. Stroboscopy and laryngeal electromyographic (LEMG) features of a 26-year-old patient with posterior glottic scarring: **A.** Stroboscopic view of bilateral vocal fold immobility during inspiration. **B.** LEMG demonstrated normal full interference pattern of recruitment on TA muscle. (Upper line = signal of LEMG. Lower line = signal of phonation). **C.** LEMG demonstrated normal full interference. Pattern of recruitment on PCA muscle. (Upper line = signal of LEMG. Lower line = signal of phonation).

REFERENCES

Buchthal, F. (1959). Electromyography of intrinsic laryngeal muscles. *Experimental Physiology, 44,* 137–148.

Carpenter, R. J., III., McDonald, T. J., & Howard, F. M., Jr. (1979). The otolaryngologic presentation of myasthenia gravis. *Laryngoscope, 89*(6), 922–928.

Carrat, X., Verhulst, J., Duroux, S., Pescio, P., Devars, F., & Traissac, L. (2000). Postintubation interarytenoid adhesion. *Annals of Otology, Rhinology and Laryngology, 109,* 736–740.

Faaborg-Andersen, K., & Buchthal, F. (1956). Action potentials from internal laryngeal muscles during phonation. *Nature, 177,* 340–341.

Hartl, D. M., Leboulleux, S., Klap, P., & Schlumberger, M. (2007). Myasthenia gravis mimicking unilateral vocal fold paralysis at presentation. *Journal of Laryngology and Otology, 121*(2), 174–178.

Hillel, A. D. (2001). The study of laryngeal muscle activity in normal human subjects and in patients with laryngeal dystonia using multiple fine-wire electromyography. *Laryngoscope, 111*(S97), 1–47.

Jacobs, I. N., & Finkel, R. S. (2002). Laryngeal electromyography in the management of vocal cord mobility problems in children. *Laryngoscope, 112*(7), 1243–1248.

Jaffe, D. M., Solomon, N. P., Robinson, R. A., Hoffman, H. T., & Luschei, E. S. (1998). Comparison of concentric needle versus hooked-wire electrodes in the canine larynx. *Otolaryngology-Head and Neck Surgery, 118*(5), 655–662.

Juel, V. C., & Massey, J. M. (2007). Myasthenia gravis. *Orphanet Journal of Rare Diseases, 2,* 1–13.

Kimaid, P. A., Crespo, A. N., Quagliato, E. M., Wolf, A., Viana, M. A., & Resende, L. A. (2004). Laryngeal electromyography: Contribution to vocal fold immobility diagnosis. *Electromyography and Clinical Neurophysiology, 44*(6), 371–374.

Koufman, J. A., Postma, G., N,, Whang, C. S., Rees, C. J., Amin, M. R., Belafsky, P. C., . . . Walker, F. O. (2001). Diagnostic laryngeal electromyography: The Wake Forest experience 1995–1999. *Otolaryngology-Head and Neck Surgery, 124*(6), 603–606.

Liu, W.-B., Xia, Q., Men, L.-N., Wu, Z.-K., & Huang, R.-X. (2007). Dysphonia as a primary manifestation in myasthenia gravis (MG): A retrospective review of 7 cases among 1520 MG patients. *Journal of the Neurological Sciences, 260*(1–2), 16–22.

Mao, V. H., Abaza, M., Spiegel, J. R., Mandel, S., Hawkshaw, M., Heuer, R. J., & Sataloff, R. T. (2001). Laryngeal myasthenia gravis: Report of 40 cases. *Journal of Voice, 15*(1), 122–130.

Mostafa, B. E., Gadallah, N. A., Nassar, N. M., Al Ibiary, H. M., Fahmy, H. A., & Fouda, N. M. (2004). The role of laryngeal electromyography in vocal fold immobility. *Journal of Oto-Rhino-Laryngology-Head and Neck Surgery, 66*(1), 5–10.

Munin, M. C., Murry, T., & Rosen, C. A. (2000). Laryngeal electromyography: Diagnostic and prognostic applications. *Otolaryngologic Clinics of North America, 33*(4), 759–770.

Nemoto, Y., Kuwabara, S., Misawa, S., Kawaguchi, N., Hattori, T., Takamori, M., & Vincent, A. (2005). Patterns and severity of neuromuscular transmission failure in seronegative myasthenia gravis. *Journal of Neurology, Neurosurgery and Psychiatry, 76,* 714–718.

Sataloff, R. T., Mandel, S., Mann, E. A., & Ludlow, C. L. (2004). Practice parameter: Laryngeal electromyography (an evidence-based review). *Otolaryngology-Head and Neck Surgery, 130*(6), 770–779.

Sataloff, R. T., Praneetvatakul, P., Heuer, R. J., Hawkshaw, M. J., Heman-Ackah, Y. D., Schneider, S. M., & Mandel. S. (2010). Laryngeal electromyography: Clinical application. *Journal of Voice, 24*(2), 228–234.

Sulica, L., & Blitzer, A. (2004). Electromyography and the immobile vocal fold. *Otolaryngologic Clinics of North America, 37,* 59–74.

Sulica, L., Blitzer, A., & Meyer, T. (2006). Laryngeal electromyography. In J. S. Rubin, R. T. Sataloff, & G. S. Korovin. (Eds.), *Diagnosis and treatment of voice disorders*. San Diego, CA: Plural Publishing.

Tellis, C. M., Rosen, C., Thekdi, A., & Sciote, J. J. (2004). Anatomy and fiber type composition of human interarytenoid muscle. *Annals of Otology, Rhinology and Laryngology, 113*(2), 97–107.

Xu, W., Han, D., Hou, L., Hu, R., & Wang, L. (2009). Clinical and electrophysiological characteristics of larynx in myasthenia gravis. *Annals of Otology, Rhinology and Laryngology, 118*(9), 656–661.

Xu, W., Han, D., Hou, L., Zhang, L., & Zhao, G.. (2007). Value of laryngeal electromyography in diagnosis of vocal fold immobility. *Annals of Otology, Rhinology and Laryngology, 116*(8), 576–581.

Yin, S. S., Qiu, W. W., & Stucker, F. J. (1997). Major patterns of laryngeal electromyography and their clinical application. *Laryngoscope, 107*(1), 126–136.

SECTION IV

Acoustics

CHAPTER 17

Multidimensional Analysis of Voice: Computerized Speech Lab

ADAM P. VOGEL

PURPOSES

- To provide acoustic assessment of voice quality across a variety of parameters.
- To provide a graphical and numerical objective representation of normal and pathological voices.

THEORETICAL BACKGROUND

Utilizing acoustic methods to assess voice quality provides the clinician or researcher with quantitative data on the client's performance. This in turn offers objective information on which to base decisions about the success or failure of treatment, whether an individual has changed as a function of a disease or condition, and for identification of deficits for differential diagnosis and characterization of pathol-

ogy. Vocal quality measurements based on acoustic data alone have clinical worth; however, their value is greater when combined with structured perceptual observation and instrumental assessment (e.g., laryngoscope) (Dejonckere et al., 2001). The limitations of acoustic analysis are often attributed to the occasional divergence between perceptual observations and their acoustic correlates (Martens, Versnel, & Dejonckere, 2007; Wolfe, Fitch, & Cornell, 1995). For example, pathological variation in broad measures like fundamental frequency (the acoustic correlate of pitch) are relatively easy to perceive both perceptually and identify acoustically (Maryn, Roy, De Bodt, Van Cauwenberge, & Corthals, 2009), yet variations in measures of perturbation (e.g., jitter, shimmer) documented acoustically can be difficult to perceive aurally, or may appear aberrant acoustically but appear within normal limits perceptually (Giovanni et al., 1996; Martin, Fitch, & Wolfe, 1995). This dichotomy can make judgments about client performance more complex than isolated methods or observations.

To limit the potential disconnection between single acoustic measures and perceptual observations, the Multi-Dimensional Voice Program (MDVP) of the KayPENTAX's computerized Speech Laboratory provides information on multiple acoustic constructs including fundamental frequency, frequency perturbation, amplitude perturbation, voice breaks, subharmonics and voice irregularity, spectral analysis, and tremor analysis. These parameters have been incorporated into voice quality investigations, with results varying as a function of disorder severity and population of interest (e.g., vocal fold nodules, dysarthria) (Campisi, Tewfik, Pelland-Blais, Husein, & Sadeghi, 2000; Cornwell, Murdoch, Ward, & Kellie, 2004). Some parameters provided by the MDVP are promoted as summative measures (e.g., soft phonation index (SPI) derived from the long-term average spectra [LTAS]) and aimed to offer quantitative information on vocal mechanisms like vocal fold closure (Roussel & Lobdell, 2006). LTAS provides objective information on intensity levels at various frequencies across the spectra (Lofqvist & Mandersson, 1987) and this information has been used in studies examining the role of vocal effort in shaping spectral energy (Fant, 1973; Fitch, 1989; Van Summers, Pisoni, Bernacki, Pedlow, & Stokes, 1988; Watson & Hughes,

2006), demonstrating that increases in loudness lead to decreases in the LTAS slope (Nordenberg & Sundberg, 2004; Sundberg & Nordenberg, 2006). Other measures derived from the LTAS, including the voice turbulence index (VTI) and the noise to harmonic ratio (NHR), have been shown to correlate with specific features of perceptual assessments (e.g., grade, roughness, breathiness, aesthenia, strain ([GRBAS]) including: *Grade* correlated with VTI, NHR, and SPI; *roughness* correlated with NHR only; and *breathiness* correlated with SPI only (Bhuta, Patrick, & Garnett, 2004).

DESCRIPTION

The MDVP is an optional component within KayPENTAX's Motor Speech Profile and Computerized Speech Laboratory (CSL). It forms part of a suite of software that aims to provide visual cueing and assessment of speech and voice performance. MDVP operates in a similar way to other KayPENTAX acoustic analysis products through the use of multiple visual windows and standard analysis settings (Figure 17–1). The software is available in two formats: a basic and an advanced version. Each version provides the same analysis facilities. However, the advanced format allows for investigations of individual acoustic measures. This functionality may be beneficial for users with an interest in studying a specific acoustic feature; however, the same results can be obtained using the basic program. This chapter focuses on the primary (basic) MDVP rather than the advanced version.

The MDVP has the capacity to provide data on 34 acoustic measures from a single voice sample. The output focuses on derivatives of amplitude and frequency

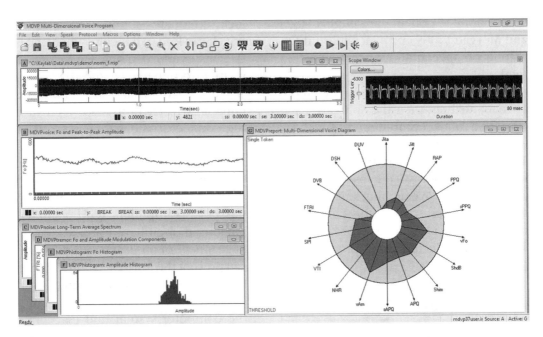

Figure 17–1. Main display screen following complete MDVP analysis.

variation and includes summative measures like the long-term average spectra (LTAS), jitter, shimmer, and a number of associated statistics such as noise-to-harmonic ratio and soft phonation index. This information combines to give a picture of vocal performance relating to vocal quality and is considered, by the manufacturers, to be more valuable than single metric descriptors such as jitter and shimmer alone.

EQUIPMENT AND MATERIALS

The equipment required to use the MDVP depends on the methods used to collect the voice samples. There are several references in the MDVP software instruction manual discussing the use of high-quality sound cards or specialized recording equipment when examining acoustic cor-

relates of vocal quality. These arguments are supported by several studies showing the variation in acoustic output that can occur depending on the recording configuration employed (Deliyski, Evans, & Shaw, 2005; Vogel & Maruff, 2008). The CSL-MDVP component has its own dedicated sound card. For the optimal results, voice samples should be acquired in a sound-treated room using a configuration that consists of a separate hard disk recorder, independent mixer, and high-quality microphone (Vogel & Morgan, 2009). If samples need to be recorded using a computer, the following issues need to be considered: noise of the computer, quality of the sound card, insulation of cabling, and quality of connection devices. Ideally, an audio interface could be used to act as an external sound card for the computer. This kind of device will provide a user with the capacity to attenuate the strength of the signal and the ability to use a high-quality microphone to collect the samples. Vogel and Morgan (2009) provides more information on speech and voice acquisition methods.

If the user is simply using the MDVP for data analysis, then the software itself (installed on a computer) is the only equipment necessary for acoustic analysis. The Multi-Speech program suite needs to be installed prior to MDVP installation as it functions as the overarching software program. Once these two features are established, the user is ready to record data and analyze the collected samples.

TEST PROCEDURES

General Guidelines

■ **Recording environment.** A quiet and sound treated recording environment is crucial for voice quality investigations. Deliyski, Shaw, and Evans (2005) suggest a minimum signal to noise ratio (SNR) of 42 is required when using KayPENTAX CSL in order to elicit accurate results. Some acoustic software programs appear to be more resistant to additive noise in the signal than others. However, ensuring the recording environment is free from extraneous noise is always desirable. This information is also relevant for the recording equipment itself. The MDVP manual warns users that virtually no generic computer sound cards in computers meet the minimum requirements stipulated by the National Center for Voice and Speech recommendations for acquisition performance used for voice measurements (Spielman, Staar, & Hunter, 2006). This is because personal computers often

lack adequate sound-level meters, which can lead to difficulty when one is flagging overloaded signal input. Issues relating to impedance and the loss of signal strength through loading and are limited by restrictions associated with the connector and wiring systems of the microphone in personal computers. Noise and interference produced inside the computer may result in a loss of dynamic range. Computer systems often possess preamplifiers with a limited range; and often have poor separation of channels for input and output, which can prevent the isolation of input signals from noise. Moreover, analog input signals can be corrupted as they enter the computer system, and inaccurate polarity can affect the pitch-extraction process (Vogel & Maruff, 2008).

■ **Recording time of day.** Although there is a lack of robust evidence documenting vocal variation in individuals over a single day, recent evidence from Vogel et al. (2011) suggests that small and systematic changes in the voice can occur in healthy adults over the course of a single day (i.e., between 09:00 and 17:00). These data indicate that recordings taken for the purpose of monitoring change over time (i.e., over several weeks) should be acquired at the same time each day, ensuring that intraindividual variation does not impact on any observed changes that may result from treatment or disease progression.

■ **Microphone selection and use.** In choosing a microphone for use in voice investigations, the user needs to consider a number of factors including the polar pattern, impedance, sensitivity, frequency response, power supply, conduction and wiring, and positioning. All these specifications influence the signal in different ways. Ideally, a high-quality microphone suited to voice acoustic analysis will be a head-mounted (position), condenser (power supply), cardioid (polar pattern) microphone with XLR connection (conduction and wiring), low impedance, sensitivity preferably ≥−60dB, and a wide frequency response (20 Hz to 20 kHz) (Vogel & Morgan, 2009). In a comparative study of microphones with diverse characteristics, Titze and Winholtz (1993) found that microphone sensitivity had the greatest effect on signal quality. However, the quality of acquired signals are duly affected by microphone distance (head-mounted microphones are ideal for voice quality investigations as they ensure a constant distance and angle between the mouth and microphone are maintained), polar pattern and angle of recording, as these features are all known to influence measures of perturbation, with smaller distances and cardioids microphones providing higher signal quality.

■ **Sample elicitation**. A study by Scherer and colleagues (1995) suggests that at least six productions are necessary to acquire a representative perturbation value in vocally healthy adults and up to 15 productions for voices with higher than average levels of instability. For studies looking at acoustic measures other than perturbation, (e.g., formant patterns), a minimum of two consecutive productions (one practice) appear to be necessary to acquire a stable production from a sustained vowel in vocally healthy adults (Vogel et al., 2011). For individuals with vocal pathology or motor speech disorder, more than two productions may be required to achieve a stable F0 and formant value.

Calibration

The MDVP software itself requires minimal calibration. There are **Capture** settings (under the **Options** tab of the menu bar), which allow the user to alter aspects of the recording process including sampling rate, input device, input channel, and the length of the sample (Figure 17–2). Once again, it is recommended that high-quality recording configurations are used to collect samples, as an alternative to computer acquired samples. However, if a computer is the only option, it is suggested that sampling rates remain high (e.g., 44.1 kHz) and a minimum of 3 seconds per sample are obtained. Samples can be saved either as WAV files (can be read by most software) or CSL signal files (*.NSP), which is a KayPENTAX specific file format.

There are a number of analysis settings for displaying and analyzing data once it has been acquired. Analysis settings are dependent on speaker characteristics and can be changed depending on the frequency profile of the sample (e.g., male, female). The CSL default settings are designed for use with most speakers (i.e., frequency ranges are set at 75 to 625 Hz); however, these settings may be inappropriate for samples that fall outside this range (e.g., speakers with low pitch, below 75 Hz). All display and analysis settings can be changed by selecting **MDVP** from the **Options** tab on the menu bar. Users will see that the majority of options available relate to the display rather than the analysis, making the process fairly straightforward for those without experience analyzing acoustic data. There are two preset frequency range options as well as the possibility of incorporating user-defined settings. If the user chooses to alter the frequency ranges, it is important to note that if the pitch floor is set too low, very fast

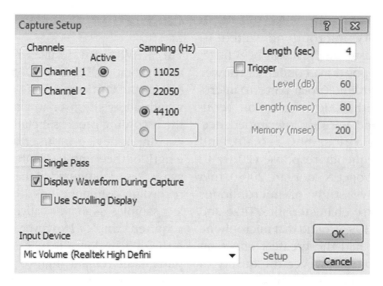

Figure 17–2. Capture settings.

F0 changes will be missed, and if it is set too high, low F0 values will be neglected (Vogel, Maruff, Snyder, & Mundt, 2009).

Recording

The quality of voice recordings is wholly determined by the quality of the acquisition configuration. Assuming that high-quality devices are employed to record samples, a configuration could include: a stand-alone hard disk recorder, an independent mixer to attenuate the incoming signal, and insulated wiring combined with a high-quality microphone in a sound-treated room. For samples acquired on a computer using the MDVP, users need to either rely on the established factory settings preset by the software or alter the settings according to their requirements. To record a sound, the user simply presses the **Record** shortcut button on the menu to commence and presses the **Stop** but-

tonat the bottom of the action window containing the preserved sound to stop. To save the file, the user can select the **Save as** option under the File menu. The file type can be determined at this stage and it is recommended that the .wav format is chosen over the CSL alternative given the limited use of NSP file types outside the KayPENTX software range.

> **Instructions:** *"Please speak at a pitch and volume that is appropriate for talking to one or two people in a quiet room. Can you say 'ah' for 5 seconds."* The recording process should then be repeated.

The utility of the MDVP depends on the needs of the user. If an evaluation of vocal quality is required, then eliciting a sustained vowel at the client's modal pitch is an appropriate candidate for post production analysis. If a basic description of F0 and frequency range is all that is needed, then connected speech samples can be analyzed (Yiu, Worrall, Longland, & Mitchell, 2000) (*Note:* Other KayPENTAX programs may be more suitable for this purpose, e.g., Multi Speech). For a more detailed list of voice tasks, including frequency range and intensity, see Chapter 19 by Ma in this edition on the Voice Range Profile.

Data Analysis

The strength of the MDVP lies in its analysis of sustained vowel samples. The speech and voice macros (under the **Macro** tab on the menu bar) provide a good starting point for new users. This facility lets you observe the various functions of the system without having to record your own data. Following the example provided in the "Voice Demo Macro—Normal Male," select a minimum of 3 seconds of the sample (preferably 1.5 seconds each side of the temporal midpoint). Specific parts of a sample can be selected by holding the **Shift** key down and pressing the left mouse button; this will prompt two blue lines to appear in the active window, one on top of the other. From here, click and drag one of the blue lines to the end of the desired selection. The time between each blue line will then be ready for analysis. In order to expand the analysis area, simply drag the blue lines to include the preferred section. The red and green (Ctrl and mouse) lines are not used in the analysis but allow the user to select specific sections of the sample for closer visual inspection (via the **View** tab). Once the preferred selection is identified within the blue lines, select the **ALL** shortcut tab, or press **F7**, or select the "Complete MDVP Analysis" option under the **Protocol** tab to initiate the whole battery of analysis

options. Once the analyses are complete, all active windows (i.e., A–G) will display information on specific acoustic parameters (e.g., C = LTAS; F = Amplitude Histogram; see Figure 17-1). Window "G" typically contains the graphical MDVP report and all summary information on the selected sample can be derived (Figure 17-3) from here. Right clicking the mouse within this window brings up a window with three useful options:

1. Information—provides data on the signal (e.g., length, sampling rate);
2. Statistics—provides all the acoustic information used to describe the sample (e.g., Average $f0$, Absolute Jitter) combined with normative data comparisons (cf. Figure 17-4);
3. Results—only works on individual active windows and provides a step-by-step breakdown of numerical information pertinent to specific analytical categories. This last option is useful for examining certain time points along the sample.

[*Note:* Titze (1995) recommends acoustic voice signals be classified into Type I (periodic or nearly periodic), Type II (signals with subharmonic frequencies that approach the fundamental frequency), and Type III (aperiodic) signals. He contends that performing acoustic perturbation analysis on Type III (aperiodic) signals gives inaccurate results and therefore is problematic. Caution should be exercised when using acoustic perturbation measures to quantify dysphonic voices, which are mostly aperiodic in nature (see Carding et al., 2004; Karnell, Chang, Smith, & Hoffman, 1997; Ma & Yiu, 2005; Titze, 1995; Yiu, 1999 for more detailed discussions)].

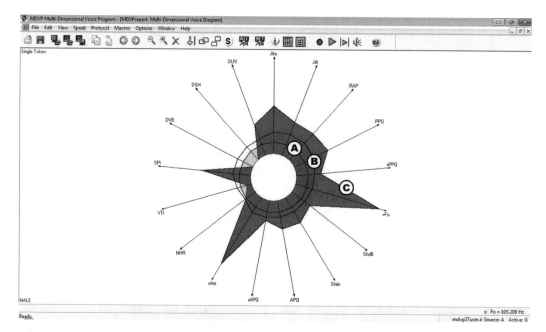

Figure 17–3. Example of graphical display of normative data versus patient data. *Note:* The circle A represents the normative data means for the parameters and circle B represents standard deviation around the norm means. The polygon C represents the patient's results. As illustrated in this figure, the patient's results of most parameters are outside norms, whereas the patient's result of the parameter VTI is inside the norm.

MDVPreport: Voice Report

Institution	University of Melbourne			Date	2010		Acc.#	
Name	M.S.			Gender	Male	Age 65	File	
Address				City	Melbourne		State	ZIP
Diagnosis	mixed spastic-ataxic dysarthria							
Comments								

Parameter	Name	Value	Unit	Norm(m)	STD(m)	Threshold
Average Fundamental Frequency	Fo	105.208	Hz	145.223	23.406	
Mean Fundamental Frequency	MFo	104.613	Hz	141.743	21.136	
Average Pitch Period	To	9.559	ms	7.055	1.052	
Highest Fundamental Frequency	Fhi	132.212	Hz	150.080	24.362	
Lowest Fundamental Frequency	Flo	94.985	Hz	140.418	23.729	
Standard Deviation of Fo	STD	7.612	Hz	1.349	0.675	
Phonatory Fo-Range in semi-tones	PFR	7		2.095	1.064	
Length of Analyzed Sample	Tsam	3.074	s	3.000	0.000	
Absolute Jitter	Jita	170.122	µs	41.663	36.481	83.200
Jitter Percent	Jitt	1.780	%	0.589	0.535	1.040
Relative Average Perturbation	RAP	1.056	%	0.345	0.333	0.680

Save As...
Print...
Info...
OK
Cancel

Figure 17–4. Selection of Voice Report including normative data derived from MDVP report. *Note:* A full report can be printed, including graphical display, by selecting the "print" option.

NORMATIVE DATA

Normative data are provided within the MDVP; however, these data are based on 15 normal voices. Figures 17-4 and 17-5 show tabulated data and a graphical representation of the relationship between analyzed and normative data. A number of other studies provide normative data on healthy adults (Gonzalez, Cervera, & Miralles, 2002), older adults (aged 70 to

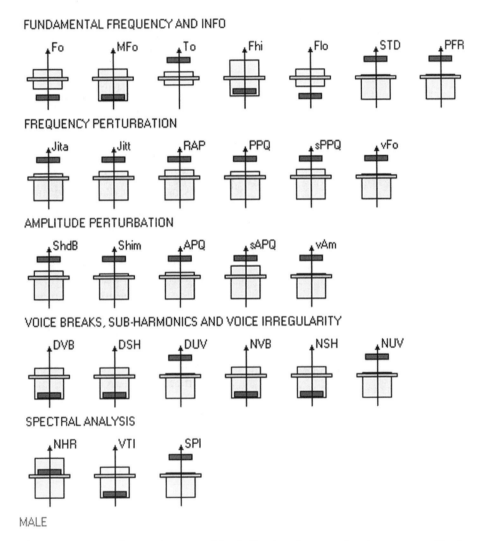

Figure 17-5. Alternative graphical display (normative bars—small) of MDVP report clearly showing aspects of sample falling outside norm mean range. *Note:* For each parameter, the longer line in the middle represents the normative data mean and the box represents the area of standard deviation around norm mean for that parameter. Patient's results are indicated by the shorter bars with the location of the bar illustrating whether patient data are inside or outside norms.

80 years) (Xue & Deliyski, 2001), aging (longitudinal data) (Verdonck-de Leeuw & Mahieu, 2004), and pediatric populations (Campisi et al., 2002).

CASE STUDY: PATIENT Z.T. (MIXED SPASTIC ATAXIC DYSARTHRIA)

Z.T. is a 42-year-old man with Friedreich ataxia, an autosomal recessive neurodegenerative disorder with progressive ataxia and dysarthria as primary outcomes of disease progression (Delatycki, Williamson, & Forrest, 2000). Perceptually, he presents with imprecise production of consonants, irregular articulatory breakdowns, intermittent distortion of vowels, harshness, pitch breaks, varied pitch and loudness, abnormal nasal resonance (typically hypernasal), and prolonged phonemes and intervals between words or syllables, manifesting in a slow rate of speech. The complete MDVP analysis was run over a sustained vowel produced by the patient (see Figures 17-3 through 17-5). The acoustic analysis indicated the following (compared to normative data provided within the MDVP):

■ Reduced average F0 and low basal F0—this is typically not a manifestation of dysarthria and simply may be the result of population variation.

■ Increased standard deviation of F0—in line with reduced control inherent in upper motor neuron disorders.

■ Above average frequency perturbation including absolute jitter, jitter percent, and F0 variation—common in spastic and ataxic dysarthrias.

■ Above average amplitude perturbation including shimmer in dB, shimmer per-

cent, and peak to peak amplitude variation—consistent with reduced motor control and perceptual observations,

■ Above average degree of voiceless (%) tokens—possibly indicative perceptual quality of "breathiness."

■ Above average soft phonation index taken from the LTAS—indicative of poor or incomplete vocal fold adduction (Mathew & Bhat, 2009; Roussel & Lobdell, 2006).

In this case study, the MDVP output was used to objectively characterize Z.T.'s vocal quality rather than as a means of acquiring pre/posttreatment data. Nevertheless, the areas of deficit identified using the program could serve as achievable therapeutic goals, assuming that all measures have practical perceptual correlates requiring remediation. Some appropriate treatment goals arising from data produced from the MDVP could focus on the impact of limited motor stability arising from cerebellar and upper motor neuron lesions. Perceptually, MDVP output relating to stability (i.e., frequency and amplitude perturbation) manifested in intermittent breaks in loudness and pitch during sustained vowels and connected speech. These difficulties are consistent with a diagnosis of mixed spastic-ataxic dysarthria and often affect the intelligibility and clarity of a patient's speech and voice, thus making them ideal candidates for intervention.

REFERENCES

Bhuta, T., Patrick, L., & Garnett, J. D. (2004). Perceptual evaluation of voice quality and its correlation with acoustic measurements. *Journal of Voice, 18*(3), 299–304.

Campisi, P., Tewfik, T. L., Manoukian, J. J., Schloss, M. D., Pelland-Blais, E., & Sadeghi, N. (2002).

Computer-assisted voice analysis: Establishing a pediatric database. *Archives of Otolaryngology-Head and Neck Surgery, 128*(2), 156–160.

Campisi, P., Tewfik, T. L., Pelland-Blais, E., Husein, M., & Sadeghi, N. (2000). MultiDimensional Voice Program analysis in children with vocal cord nodules. *Journal of Otolaryngology, 29*(5), 302–308.

Carding, P. N., Steen, I. N., Webb, A., Mackenzie, K., Deary, I. J., & Wilson, J. A. (2004). The reliability and sensitivity to change of acoustic measures of voice quality. *Clinical Otolaryngology and Allied Sciences, 29*(5), 538–544.

Cornwell, P. L., Murdoch, B. E., Ward, E. C., & Kellie, S. (2004). Acoustic investigation of vocal quality following treatment for childhood cerebellar tumour. *Folia Phoniatrica et Logopedica, 56*(2), 93–107.

Dejonckere, P. H., Bradley, P., Clemente, P., Cornut, G., Crevier-Buchman, L., Friedrich, G., … Woisard, V. (2001). A basic protocol for functional assessment of voice pathology, especially for investigating the efficacy of (phonosurgical) treatments and evaluating new assessment techniques. *European Archives of Oto-Rhino-Laryngology, 258*(2), 77–82.

Delatycki, M. B., Williamson, R., & Forrest, S. M. (2000). Friedreich ataxia: An overview. *Journal of Medical Genetics, 37*(1), 1–8.

Deliyski, D. D., Evans, M. K., & Shaw, H. S. (2005). Influence of data acquisition environment on accuracy of acoustic voice quality measurements. *Journal of Voice, 19*(2), 176–186.

Deliyski, D. D., Shaw, H. S., & Evans, M. K. (2005). Adverse effects of environmental noise on acoustic voice quality measurements. *Journal of Voice, 19*(1), 15–28.

Fant, G. (1973). *Speech sounds and features.* Cambridge, MA: MIT Press.

Fitch, H. (1989). Comments on "Effects of noise on speech production: Acoustic and perceptual analyses" [*J. Acoust. Soc. Am. 84,* 917–928 (1988)]. *Journal of the Acoustical Society of America, 86*(5), 2017–2019.

Giovanni, A., Robert, D., Estublier, N., Teston, B., Zanaret, M., & Cannoni, M. (1996). Objective evaluation of dysphonia: Preliminary results of a device allowing simultaneous acoustic and aerodynamic measurements. *Folia Phoniatrica et Logopaedia, 48*(4), 175–185.

Gonzalez, J., Cervera, T., & Miralles, J. L. (2002). Acoustic voice analysis: Reliability of a set of multi-dimensional parameters. *Acta Otorrinolaringologica Espanola, 53*(4), 256–268.

Karnell, M. P., Chang, A., Smith, A., & Hoffman, H. (1997). Impact of signal type of validity on voice perturbation measures. *NCVS Status and Progress Report, 11,* 91–94.

Lofqvist, A., & Mandersson, B. (1987). Longtime average spectrum of speech and voice analysis. *Folia Phoniatrica et Logopaedia, 39*(5), 221–229.

Ma, E. P.-M., & Yiu, E. M.-L. (2005). Suitability of acoustic perturbation measures in analyzing periodic and nearly periodic voice signals, *Folia Phoniatrica et Logopaedia, 57*(1), 38–47.

Martens, J. W., Versnel, H., & Dejonckere, P. H. (2007). The effect of visible speech in the perceptual rating of pathological voices. *Archives of Otolaryngology-Head and Neck Surgery, 133*(2), 178–185.

Martin, D., Fitch, J., & Wolfe, V. (1995). Pathologic voice type and the acoustic prediction of severity. *Journal of Speech and Hearing Research, 38*(4), 765–771.

Maryn, Y., Roy, N., De Bodt, M., Van Cauwenberge, P., & Corthals, P. (2009). Acoustic measurement of overall voice quality: A metaanalysis. *Journal of the Acoustical Society of America, 126*(5), 2619–2634.

Mathew, M. M., & Bhat, J. S. (2009). Soft Phonation Index—a sensitive parameter? *Indian Journal of Otolaryngology and Head and Neck Surgery, 61*(2), 127–130.

Nordenberg, M., & Sundberg, J. (2004). Effect on LTAS of vocal loudness variation. *Logopedics Phoniatrics Vocology, 29*(4), 183–191.

Roussel, N. C., & Lobdell, M. (2006). The clinical utility of the soft phonation index. *Clinical Linguistics and Phonetics, 20*(2–3), 181–186.

Scherer, R. C., Vail, V. J., & Guo, C. G. (1995). Required number of tokens to determine representative voice perturbation values. *Journal of Speech and Hearing Research, 38*(6), 1260–1269.

Spielman, J. L., Staar, A. C., & Hunter, E. J. (2006). *Recommendations for the creation of a recording laboratory.* Iowa City, IA: National Center for Voice and Speech.

Sundberg, J., & Nordenberg, M. (2006). Effects of vocal loudness variation on spectrum balance as reflected by the alpha measure of long-term-average spectra of speech. *Journal of the Acoustical Society of America, 120*(1), 453–457.

Titze, I. R. (1995). *Workshop on acoustic voice analysis: Summary statement.* Iowa City, IA: National Center for Voice and Speech.

Titze, I. R., & Winholtz, W. S. (1993). Effect of microphone type and placement on voice perturbation measurements. *Journal of Speech and Hearing Research, 36*(6), 1177–1190.

Van Summers, W. V., Pisoni, D. B., Bernacki, R. H., Pedlow, R. I., & Stokes, M. A. (1988). Effects of noise on speech production: Acoustic and perceptual analyses. *Journal of the Acoustical Society of America, 84*(3), 917–928.

Verdonck-de Leeuw, I. M., & Mahieu, H. F. (2004). Vocal aging and the impact on daily life: A longitudinal study. *Journal of Voice, 18*(2), 193–202.

Vogel, A. P., Fletcher, J., Snyder, P. J., Fredrickson, A., & Maruff, P. (2011). Reliability, stability and sensitivity to change and impairment in acoustic measures of timing and frequency. *Journal of Voice. 25*(2), 137–149.

Vogel, A. P., & Maruff, P. (2008). Comparison of voice acquisition methodologies in speech research. *Behavior Research Methods, 40*(4), 982–987.

Vogel, A. P., Maruff, P., Snyder, P. J., & Mundt, J. C. (2009). Standardization of pitch-range settings in voice acoustic analysis. *Behavior Research Methods, 41*(2), 318–324.

Vogel, A. P., & Morgan, A. T. (2009). Factors affecting the quality of sound recording for speech and voice analysis. *International Journal of Speech-Language Pathology, 11*(6), 431–437.

Watson, P. J., & Hughes, D. (2006). The relationship of vocal loudness manipulation to prosodic F0 and durational variables in healthy adults. *Journal of Speech, Language and Hearing Research, 49*(3), 636–644.

Wolfe, V. I., Fitch, J., & Cornell, R. (1995). Acoustic prediction of severity in commonly occurring voice problems. *Journal of Speech and Hearing Research, 38*(2), 273–279.

Xue, S. A., & Deliyski, D. D. (2001). Effects of aging on selected acoustic voice parameters: Preliminary normative data and educational implications. *Educational Gerontology, 27*(2), 159–168.

Yiu, E. M.-L. (1999). Limitations of perturbation measures in clinical acoustic voice analysis. *Asia Pacific Journal of Speech, Language and Hearing, 4*, 157–168.

Yiu, E. M.-L., Worrall, L., Longland, J., & Mitchell, C. (2000). Analysing vocal quality of connected speech using Kay's computerized speech lab: A preliminary finding. *Clinical Linguistics and Phonetics, 14*(4), 295–305.

CHAPTER 18

Acoustic Analysis Using Freeware: Praat

CATHERINE MADILL AND PATRICIA McCABE

PURPOSES

- To assess voice quality using acoustic analysis.
- To extract energy information pertaining to the glottal source and vocal tract resonances using spectrographic, frequency, and perturbation analysis.

INTRODUCTION

There are a number of acoustic analysis programs available. Each program provides a range of different analyses that can be performed on the recorded vocal signal. Some programs are specific in what features of the acoustic signal they analyze, whereas others are generic programs that analyze a range of acoustic features (e.g., Praat, KayPENTAX Computerized Speech Lab [CSL], Tiger's Dr Speech, CSpeech TF32). Different analysis programs use slightly different algorithms and signal analysis parameters. It therefore is recommended that the results be compared within programs, not between programs (Amir, Wolf, & Amir, 2009; Maryn, Corthals, De Bodt, Van Cauwenberge, & Deliyski, 2009).

Praat (Boersma & Weenink, 2008) has been used to describe the acoustic values present in voice samples of normal speakers (Brockmann, Storck, Carding, & Drinnan, 2008), the acoustic values of speakers with a range of voice disorders (Amir et al., 2009), and to evaluate treatment outcomes using acoustic analysis measures such as polyp removal (Stajner-Katusic, Horga, & Zrinski, 2008) and laryngeal manipulation therapy (Mathieson et al., 2009).

Unlike other generic acoustic analysis programs, Praat is freeware. It also can be configured using "scripts" to conduct analyses not set in the default program. Scripts allow a Praat user to automatically analyze specific features of a vocal signal, for example, pause time in connected speech, speech rate, or to evaluate higher formants on different speech samples. They also allow the user to automate processes, which would otherwise be time-consuming or repetitive. Scripts can be created for individual purposes or can be downloaded from various free Praat related Web sites. Some resources are listed at the end of this chapter to assist clincians find or write scripts using the Praat program.

DESCRIPTION

This chapter uses the Praat system (Version 5.1.21) to illustrate how to record and acoustically analyze the vocal signal, and how to interpret these analyses.

EQUIPMENT AND MATERIALS

- Software: Praat (download from http://www.Praat.org).
- Accessories for recording:
  - head-set microphone (e.g.,AKG Acoustics C420,Vienna,Austria).
  - high-quality digital interface or sound card (e.g., Edirol UA-25EX, Roland, U.S.).
  - ruler (for measuring mouth-to-microphone distance).
  - standard passage such as The Rainbow Passage (Fairbanks, 1960) or North Wind and the Sun (International Phonetic Association, 1999).
  - stopwatch to monitor the number of seconds in recording different tasks.

GENERAL GUIDELINES

Titze (1995) has developed a list of recommendations to assist clincans to standardize their recording and acoustic analysis techniques for comparison of results with other studies/colleagues. These recommendations can be found at the National Centre for Voice and Speech Web site (http://ncvs.org/museum-archive/downloadables.html) under the link *Workshop on Acoustic Voice Analysis: Summary Statement.* The most essential of these recommendations are summarized in the following sections.

Recording Environment

The recording should be carried out in a quiet environment with low ambient noise (less than 50 dB) (Deliyski, Shaw, & Evans, 2005a; Titze, 1995). Poor acoustic conditions can affect the validity of phonational intensity and frequency levels measured. This can compromise the accuracy of perturbation analyses from the recorded signal.

Recording Time-of-Day

There is clear evidence that time-of-day as well as vocal loading (voice use) influence a range of acoustic measures (Artkoski, Tommila, & Laukkanen, 2002; Rantala, Lindholm, & Vilkman, 1998; Rantala, Paavola, Korkko, & Vilkman, 1998). When recording and performing acoustic analysis on voice samples of the same individual across time, such as before and after voice treatment, it therefore is recommended that the recordings be carried out at approximately the same time-of-day and after equivalent vocal loadings as far as possible.

Mouth-to-Microphone Distance

The literature has documented the use of different mouth-to-microphone distances for voice recording. Titze (1995) recommends a microphone-to-mouth distance of less than 10 cm and preferably 3 to 4 cm for recording of prolonged vowels. For connected speech, the microphone-to-mouth distance should be longer to avoid air burst. The microphone should be positioned to the side of the mouth (45° to 90°) to reduce airburst from the mouth that may affect the quality of the recording. Throughout the recording, a constant mouth-to-microphone distance should be maintained and the use of head-set microphone is preferred, particularly for young children.

Sampling Rate

Praat, like other acoustic analysis programs, uses a default sampling rate of 44.1 kHz. A sampling rate of 50 kHz or above will ensure maximum accuracy (Deliyski, Shaw, & Evans, 2005b). However, the file size will be large for archive purposes. The literature suggests that 20 kHz is the minimum sampling rate for analyzing acoustic waveforms to incur only minimal error in the analysis of pertubation measures (Baken & Orlikoff, 2000; Titze, 1995).

Classifying the Vocal Signal Type

It is recommended that the recorded vocal signal be evaluated according to the periodicity of the vocal signal. Titze (1995) describes three types of voice signals: Type 1 signals, which are nearly periodic;

Type 2 signals, which contain strong subharmonic frequencies whose energies approach the energy of the fundamental frequency. Therefore, no obvious single fundamental frequency is present throughout the vocal signal; and Type 3 signals, which are chaotic and contain no periodic structure. Titze (1995) recommends that Type 1 signals are the only signal type suitable only for analyzing perturbation measures (e.g., shimmer, jitter, harmonics-to-noise ratio). Type 2 signals are suitable for spectrographic and other visual assessments. Type 3 signals are unsuitable for acoustic analysis of any form. Ma and Yiu (2005) provide examples of spectrograms of all three types of vocal signals.

Eliciting Habitual Pitch in Connected Speech

There is a large body of evidence indicating that habitual pitch varies across different tasks, contexts, and sample durations (Zraick, Birdwell, & Smith-Olinde, 2005; Zraick, Gentry, Smith-Olinde, & Gregg, 2006; Zraick, Skaggs, & Montague, 2000). It is recommended that habitual pitch be assessed across more than one task, or the results from two or three different tasks be averaged to determine a client's approximate habitual pitch level (Zraick et al., 2000).

Eliciting Habitual Pitch in a Prolonged Vowel

Awan (2001) describes a procedure to obtain the habitual pitch level using vowel prolongation. Under that procedure, the client is instructed to chant and count the numbers from one to four, then sustain the vowel /a/ for a few seconds. The middle 2-second stable phonation between the onset and the offset is to be used for fundamental frequency and perturbation analyses.

Analyzing the Vocal Signal

The basic Praat program has five analysis options: Spectrum, Pitch, Intensity, Formant, and Pulses. Each of the five analyses has a **Settings** option in the menu where the clinician can set the parameters of the analyses based on the individual vocal signal that is being analyzed. For example, the **Spectrum** setting of bandwidth will vary according to whether the clinician wants to produce a narrowband spectrogram or a wideband spectrogram. When selecting any of the five analysis options, the clinician will need to ensure that he or she selects the appropriate setting for the client and the type of analysis to be done. Guidelines for making these selections are available in the program manual, which can be found in the **Help** menu.

TEST PROCEDURES

Recording the Voice Signal

1. Before starting the recording process with the client, it is recommended that the clinician prepares the Praat windows for recording. To do so, double click on the **Praat** icon on the computer desktop. Two windows and a welcome screen will appear (Figure 18–1). The welcome screen should disappear after a few seconds. The welcome screen can also be closed manually. The other two windows are labeled **Praat Objects**

and **Praat Picture**. The **Praat Picture** window can then be closed.

2. Underneath the Praat Objects window in the top left-hand corner, click on **New** to reveal the dropdown menu. Select **Record mono Sound** if there is only one input (e.g., microphone). Select **Record stereo Sound** if there are two inputs (e.g., microphone and electroglottograph). A **Sound-Recorder** window will then be opened (Figure 18–2).

3. The **Mono** radio button is selected by default. Select the desired sampling rate from the list on the right hand side of the "pop-up" window by clicking on the radio button next to the sampling rate of choice. A sampling rate of 44.1 kHz is recommended (this is the default setting for the program).

4. It is recommended that the clinician tests the input from the microphone by doing a test recording before recording with the client. Click on **Record** on the bottom left hand side of the **SoundRecorder** window. As the voice is being recorded, a green column will appear in the "pop-up" window and blue bars will appear in the horizontal bar above the **Record** button. The column needs to remain green in color to avoid "clipping" of the vocal signal. Clipped vocal signals cannot be analyzed accurately as they do not contain all of the acoustic data in the original vocal signal. (**Trouble-shooting:** If the recording does not occur properly, check the computer **Sounds and Audio Devices** settings via the Microsoft Windows system **Control Panel** to ensure that the microphone is being detected by the computer internal sound card or the selected external sound card [whichever device the microphone is

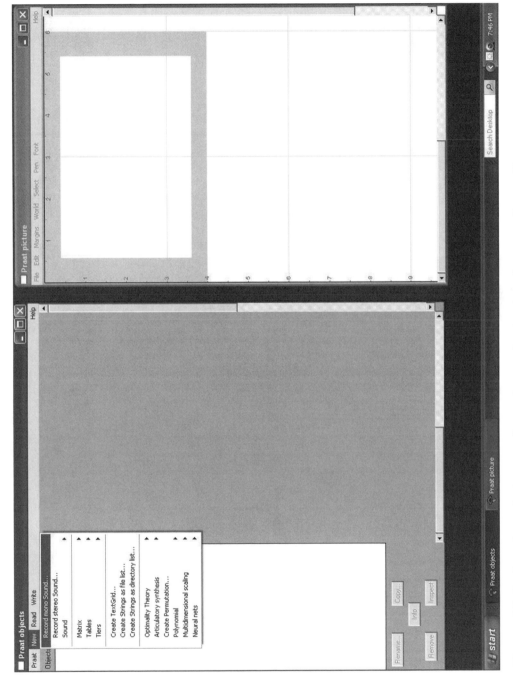

Figure 18–1. Opening window configuration and selecting the recording option.

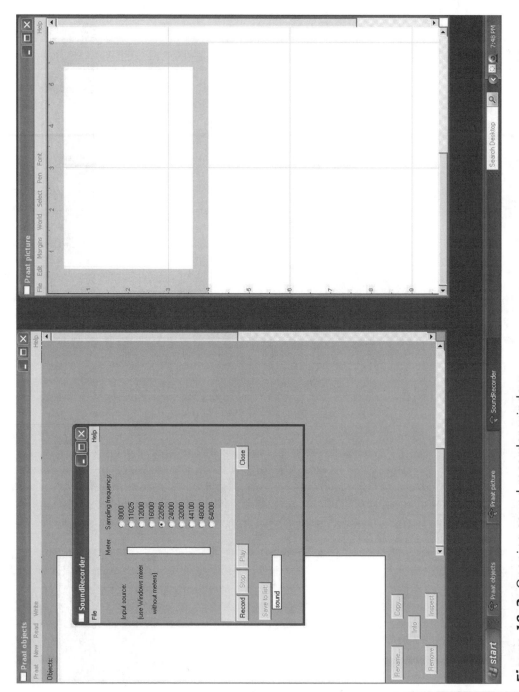

Figure 18-2. Opening sound recorder window.

plugged into]. This selection is made using the drop-down menu in the **Sound Recording** option.)

5. After doing a test recording, record the client's voice by repeating the procedures described in Step 4. To stop recording, click on the button click **stop**.

Saving the Vocal Signal

1. Once the recording of the vocal task has stopped, save the file by typing the file name (e.g., "test" or "JB21jan09") into the box next to **Name** in the

bottom right hand corner. If a script for analysis is used, then make sure the file name is no longer than eight characters and contains no spaces or punctuation. Click on **Save to list** to conduct an analysis on the file. Click on **Save to list & close** to save the file without analyzing the recorded sample. If the clinician does not want to save the file at all, click on **Close**.

2. If **Save to list** is clicked on, the file will appear in the **Praat Objects** window and can be analyzed from here (Figure 18–3). If the clinician wants to save the sound file to the computer or external storage, highlight the file

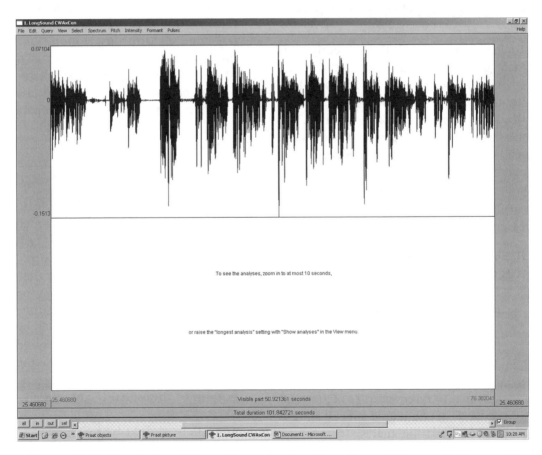

Figure 18–3. Vocal signal view after selecting from Praat Objects window and clicking on View.

name in the **Objects** list in the **Praat Objects** window. Then left click the mouse on the **write** menu in the top left hand side of the **Praat Objects** window. From the drop-down menu, select the format of sound file that you would like to save in (WAV is the most common form of sound file format).

3. It is recommended that the clinician opens and conducts a practice analysis on the test recording to ensure that the microphone and program settings are correct.

Loading and Viewing Prerecorded Files into Praat

To load prerecorded files directly into Praat, click the **Read** menu in the **Praat Objects** window (Figure 18–4). Select **Read from file** or **Open long sound file** to open the sound file into Praat. The file should then appear in the **Objects** list, ready for the clinician to analyze. Again, make sure the file name is no longer than eight characters with no punctuation if a script for analysis is used.

Instructional Steps for Recording

1. Fit the client with the head-mounted microphone to the side of the mouth (to minimize air burst noise).
2. Ask the client to produce a spontaneous speech sample. It is recommended that two to three samples of 30 to 60 seconds of connected speech should be obtained for analysis of average fundamental frequency (Zraick et al., 2006).

Instructions: *"We are going to assess your habitual pitch level in conversation. I want you to sit in front of the computer. Describe your daily voice usage using your most comfortable pitch, loudness, and rate. You will need to speak for 1 minute, and I will give you a hand signal to stop. Take breaths as you normally do. If you feel tired at any point during speaking, please let me know. You may start now."*

For young children and adults who are shy or find it difficult to think of sufficient things to say, cues such as, *"Tell me your favourite movie," "Tell me about your recent overseas trip"* and picture description, *"Tell me about this picture"* can be used. After the recording of the spontaneous speech sample is collected and saved, reassure the client and prepare the client for the next task, that is, to read aloud a standard passage such as The Rainbow Passage (Fairbanks, 1960), using his or her habitual voice.

(**Clinical Note:** It is advisable to view the waveform of the recorded file before moving on to the next task. If clipping of the signal has occurred (where the vocal signal is louder than the programme is set to capture), the frequency components at amplitude higher than the signal cutoff will be distorted and unable to be analyzed accurately. This will be apparent as the signal will have a flat line at the top and bottom of the signal [Figure 18–5].)

3. The client should be given time to familiarize him- or herself with any reading materials before recording.

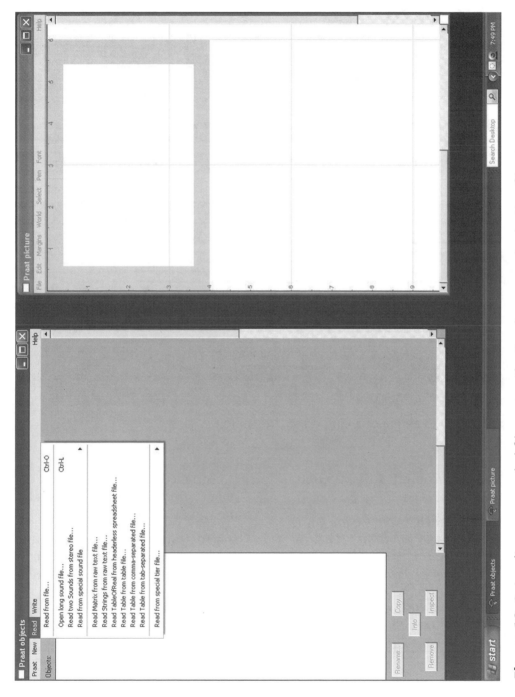

Figure 18–4. Loading prerecorded files using the Read menu and selecting files to open.

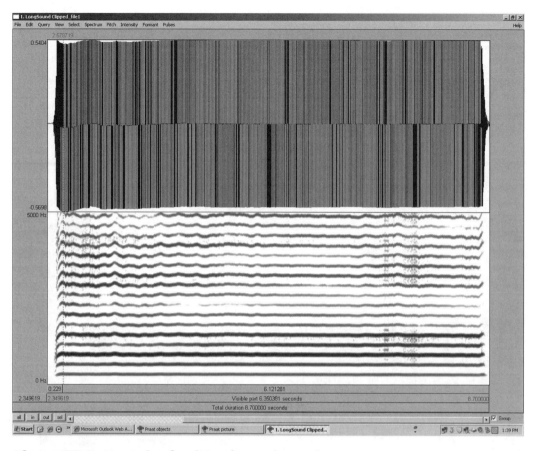

Figure 18–5. Example of a clipped sound sample.

The instructions below are given to the client:

Instructions: *"Now we are going to assess your habitual pitch level during reading. Please read aloud this passage at a comfortable volume as in your daily conversation. Spend some time now to get yourself familiarized with the passage. Please start when you are ready."*

4. The client will be asked to produce a prolonged vowel /a/ at his or her best habitual pitch level according to the procedure described by Awan (2001). In this procedure, the client is instructed to chant and count the number from one to four, then sustain the vowel /a/ for a few seconds.

Instructions: *"I want you to chant and count from one to four, then say 'ah' for about 8 seconds. I'll raise my hand to tell you when to stop."*

5. After the recording of the prolonged vowel sample is collected and saved, reassure the client that she or he has performed the task as per your instructions. Now, there should be three objects listed in the **Praat Objects** window for conducting acoustic analysis.

Data Analysis: Acoustic Signal Typing Using Spectrogram

1. Before conducting analysis of the vocal signal, it is essential to determine whether the signal type is suitable for acoustic analysis (Titze, 1995). To do this, highlight the prolonged vowel sample from the **Praat Objects** list. Then click on **Edit** in the menu on the right-hand side of the window. A new window will open with the waveform selected now visible.

2. Highlight the vocal signal (no longer than 10 seconds) by left clicking and dragging*. Select **Zoom to selection** from the **View** dropdown menu on the top right hand side of the sound file window or alternatively press **Cntrl + N**. The selected sample will now fill the window. Samples longer than 10 seconds can be analyzed, but the clinician needs to go to the **Show analyses** option in the **View** dropdown menu and manually adjust the length of the analysis.

3. Select **Show spectrogram** from the **Spectrogram** dropdown menu. The spectrogram of the acoustic signal will appear below the selected waveform section (Figure 18-6).

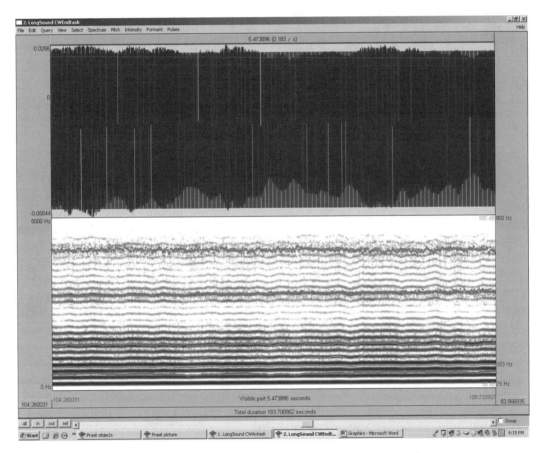

Figure 18-6. Prolonged vowel with spectrogram and formats for categorizing as Type 1, 2, or 3 signals.

4. To view the formants in the spectrogram, select **Show formants** in the **Formant** drop-down menu (see Figure 18–6). Formant settings can be changed manually using the **Formant settings** and **Advanced formant settings** options.

5. A visual interpretation of the periodicity of the vocal signal (Type 1, 2, or 3) can then be made. Note that this is a subjective process and, to date, there have not been any studies that reported on the reliability data.

Data Analysis: Voice Report

1. To generate a voice report including mean and median fundamental frequency (F0), shimmer, jitter, and harmonic-to-noise ratio (HNR), or noise-to-harmonic ratio (NHR), open the prolonged vowel sample from the **Objects** list in the **Praat Objects** window.

2. Highlight the middle stable portion of the signal. Zoom in to the selected section via the **View** drop-down menu or **Cntrl + N**.

3. Select **Pitch settings** from the **Pitch** drop-down menu. Praat sets a default setting of a minimum of 75 Hz and a maximum of 500 Hz. These values are respectively the lowest and the highest F0 values that can be analyzed. These values can be changed depending on the gender of the speaker and the type of voice signal, as the more fluctuations in periodicity in the signal, the greater the range will need to be. For example, Vogel, Maruff, Snyder, and Mundt (2009) recommend a minimum of 70 Hz and maximum of 250 Hz for male speakers and a minimum of 100 Hz and maximum of 300 Hz for female speakers. For severely pathologic voices or when

analysis errors occur (e.g., the program results indicate the sound is voiceless when it is audibly voiced), **Pitch Analysis** section under the **Help Manual FAQ** provides step-by-step instructions for adjusting pitch settings to allow analysis.

4. Select **Show pulses** from the **Pulses** drop-down menu—blue lines will appear on the waveform view to indicate the presence of periodic glottal components in the voice signal.

5. To produce a voice report, select the **Voice report** option from the **Pulses** drop-down menu. A **Praat: Info** window will open with the results of the analysis of the selected sample (Figure 18–7)

6. The spectrogram, pitch, intensity, and formant traces of the selected sample by choosing **Show analyses** from **View** dropdown menu and ticking each of the boxes (Figure 18–8). Mean values for pitch and intensity will appear on the right-hand side of the spectrogram next to the respective trace.

If there are any difficulties or errors in using the program, consult the program manual first. The easiest way to consult the Praat manual is to look under **Help** in the Praat program.

NORMATIVE DATA

Praat is increasingly being used to assess normal and disordered voices. Studies reporting typical voices only include those by Brockmann et al. (2008) who examined the effects of vocal loudness on jitter and shimmer values in healthy adults. Jitter and shimmer both increased significantly with decreasing loudness in both males and females.

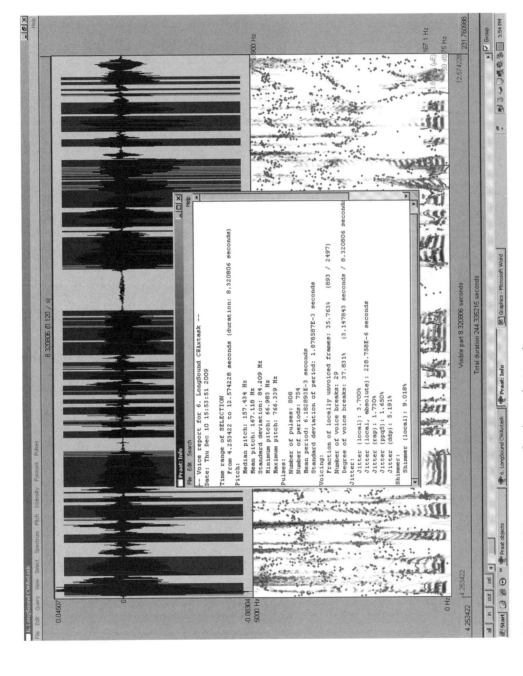

Figure 18–7. Voice report of selected signal.

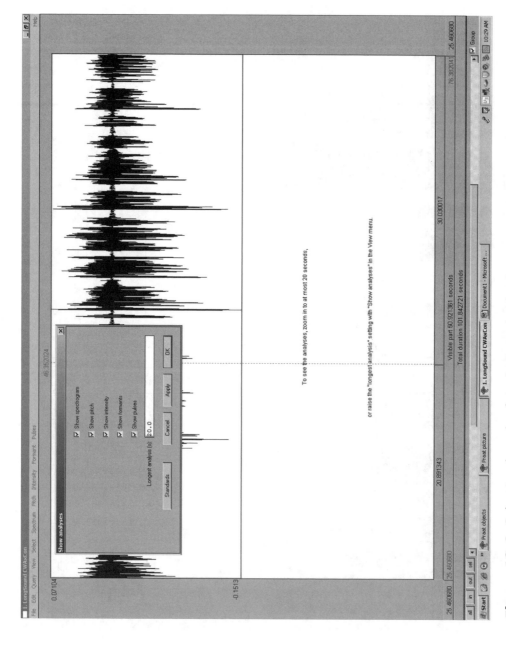

Figure 18–8. Selecting length of analysis and selecting spectrogram, pitch, intensity, formant, and pulses to appear on the analysis window view.

Oguz et al. (2007) reported Praat data of 72 healthy speakers and 18 individuals with unilateral vocal fold paralysis. Vogel et al. (2009) also used Praat to investigate the fundamental frequency of the voices of depressed but otherwise healthy adults. Mathieson et al. (2009) reported the spectrographic results of indivduals with muscle tension dysphonia undergoing laryngeal manual therapy. Stajner-Katusic et al. (2008) used Praat to investigate the acoustic charactersistics of individuals who had undergone surgical removal of a unilateral polyp.

There are also a number of papers that compare Praat to other acoustic analysis softwares. Within this research are notional normative values for Praat analyses for both typical and atypical voice profiles. For example, Amir et al. (2009) reported Praat analysis data for individuals with vocal nodules, polyps, cysts, and functional voice disorders. Maryn et al. (2009) reported collective results for various voice disorders in comparing Multi-Dimensional Voice Program (MDVP) and Praat. Caution should be exercised in using this information as normative data as the population and individuals may differ considerably across studies (Table 18–1).

CASE STUDY: PATIENT C.W. (BILATERAL VOCAL FOLD NODULES)

C.W., a 44-year-old female teacher, was referred to a speech pathologist. She was diagnosed as having bilateral vocal fold nodules. She reported that her voice had deteriorated over the past 3 months. Perceptually, her voice in daily conversation was described as having glottal fry, slightly low pitched with occasional periods of voice loss and monotone, and mildly breathy and hoarse. She reported loss of her upper vocal range, vocal fatigue, and a sore throat after long periods of use. Her medical history was unremarkable and she reported no significant psychological stress. C.W. was observed to use noticeable effort when speaking. Her voice was recorded and analyzed with Praat at the initial assessment (Table 18–2).

The pretreatment assessment results indicate that C.W. had:

■ Evidence of acoustic noise on the narrowband spectrogram. This was evident from the gray shading between the dark lines (harmonics) in the higher frequencies and the fact that the formant traces were not clearly defined (especially in the third and fourth formants) (Figure 18–9). This signal was classified as a Type 1 signal based on the description of Titze (1995).

■ Reduced mean and median pitch values for both reading passage and vowel samples when compared with normal values (see Table 18–2) (Oguz et al., 2007).

■ Increased values for shimmer and jitter indicating greater perturbation in the vibration of the true vocal folds, which correlates with perceived breathiness (Oguz et al., 2007).

■ Increased noise-to-harmonic ratio, which is correlated with the perceived hoarseness in her voice (Oguz et al., 2007).

Therapy to eliminate phonotraumatic adductory vocal behaviours were used to treat C.W. Release of laryngeal constriction exercises (Bagnall, 2007) and training in simultaneous and glottal stroke onsets (Harris, 1998) were introduced to C.W.

Table 18–1. Studies That Used Praat and Provide Normative Data

Authors (Year)	Participant Description	Number of Participants (Gender)	Acoustic Parameters
Amir et al. (2009)	Nodules Polyp Cyst Functional voice disorder	58 (all females)	F0 Jitter Shimmer NHR DUV
Brockmann et al. (2008)	Typical voice in soft, medium, and loud phonation	57 (28 females, 29 males)	F0 Jitter Shimmer
Mathieson et al. (2009)	Pre-post laryngeal manipulation therapy	10 (2 females, 8 males)	F0 Jitter Shimmer NHR
Oguz et al. (2007)	Typical voice Unilateral vocal fold paralysis	72 (48 females, 24 males) 18 (10 females, 8 males)	F0 Jitter Shimmer NHR Intensity
Stajner-Katusic et al. (2008)	Male pre-post polyp removal	5 (all males)	F0 Jitter Shimmer HNR DVB
Vogel et al. (2009)	Depressed but otherwise healthy adults	20 (10 females, 10 males)	F0

DUV: degree of unvoiceness; DVB: degree of voice breaks; F0: fundamental frequency; HNR: harmonic-to-noise ratio; NHR: noise-to-harmonic ratio.

Table 18–2. Praat Voice Report Values Pretreatment and Post-Treatment for C.W.

Acoustic Measure	Pretreatment Value	Post-Treatment Value
Pitch (The Rainbow Passage):		
Median pitch	157.43 Hz	176.30 Hz
Mean pitch	167.12 Hz	181.14 Hz
Standard deviation	84.21 Hz	47.38 Hz
Minimum pitch	66.98 Hz	81.51 Hz
Maximum pitch	766.34 Hz	628.66 Hz

Table 18–2. *continued*

Acoustic Measure	Pretreatment Value	Post-Treatment Value
Pitch (vowel):		
Median pitch	176.19 Hz	183.00 Hz
Mean pitch	176.30 Hz	181.1 Hz
Standard deviation	2.39 Hz	1.23 Hz
Minimum pitch	155.50 Hz	179.43 Hz
Maximum pitch	188.96 Hz	186.38 Hz
Pulses:		
Number of pulses	1422	1489
Number of periods	1418	1488
Mean period	5.8×10^{-3} seconds	5.46×10^{-3} seconds
Standard deviation of period	1.0×10^{-4} seconds	3.0×10^{-5} seconds
Voicing:		
Fraction of locally unvoiced frames	0.12% (3/2432)	0% (0/2440)
Number of voice breaks	1	0
Degree of voice breaks	0.29% (0.018/8.10 sec)	0% (0/8.13 sec)
Jitter:		
Jitter (local)	0.58%	0.29%
Jitter (local, absolute)	3.3×10^{-5} seconds	1.6×10^{-5} seconds
Jitter (rap)	0.32%	0.17%
Jitter (ppq5)	0.35%	0.17%
Jitter (ddp)	0.97%	0.5%
Shimmer:		
Shimmer (local)	2.19%	1.09%
Shimmer (local, dB)	0.198 dB	0.096 dB
Shimmer (apq3)	1.17%	0.60%
Shimmer (apq5)	1.36%	0.66%
Shimmer (apq11)	1.66%	0.80%
Shimmer (dda)	3.5%	1.8%
Harmonicity of the voiced parts only:		
Mean autocorrelation:	0.9904	0.9989
Mean noise-to-harmonics ratio:	0.0126	0.0011
Mean harmonics-to-noise ratio:	23.31 dB	29.97 dB

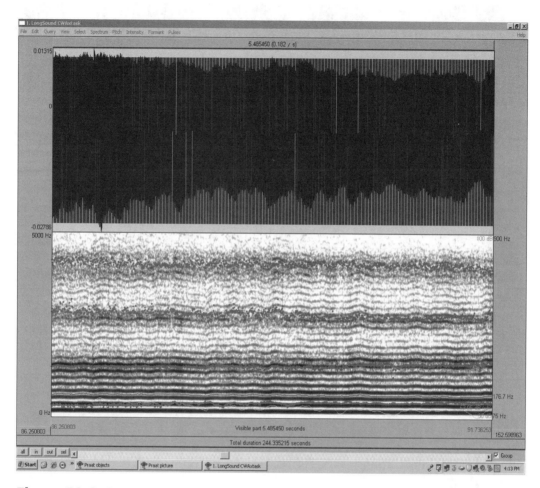

Figure 18–9. Pretreatment prolonged vowel. Note the acoustic noise around the third and fourth formant.

Perceptual training was also conducted to assist C.W. in raising her awareness of a clearer voice and effortless sensation of this new type of phonation. Exercises to enable mastery of a release of constriction postures in single sound, two to three-word phrases, and spontaneous speech were progressively mastered in seven sessions of therapy over 5 months. Otolaryngologist's review confirmed that her vocal nodules had fully resolved after five sessions over 4 months.

A comparison of pre- and post-treatment evaluation data (see Table 18–2) confirmed that C.W.'s voice had improved:

■ There was evidence of a reduction in the acoustic noise between the harmonics on the spectrogram. The formant traces were more clearly defined (Figure 18–10).

■ There was an increase in the mean and median pitch values for both reading passage and vowel samples (see Table 18–2).

■ There was a decrease in the values for shimmer and jitter indicating a reduction in the perturbation in the vibration of the true vocal folds, and greater stability of the mucosal wave and therefore the sound of the voice (see Table 18–2).

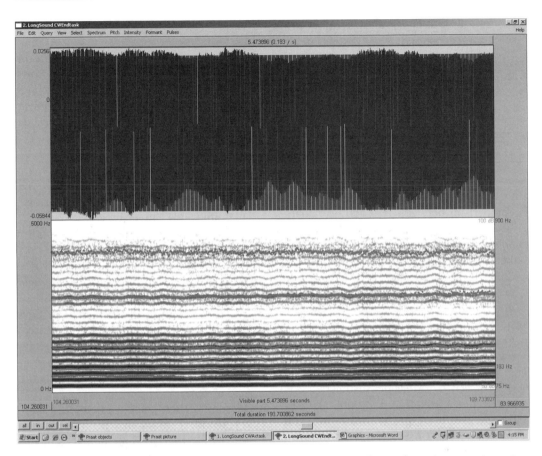

Figure 18–10. Post-treatment prolonged vowel. Note the reduced acoustic noise around the third and fourth formant when compared to that in Figure 18–9.

■ There was a decrease in the noise-to-harmonic ratio, which is correlated with the reduction in perceived hoarseness in her voice (see Table 18–2).

EXTRA RESOURCES

For more support in using Praat, see:

■ http://www.fon.hum.uva.nl/praat/This is the Praat home page for a range of tutorial and manuals for beginners.
■ http://Praatlanguagelab.com/ This Web site has video demonstrations for

recording, playing and saving voice signals onto Praat.

As Praat is an open source software, new modules and upgrades are constantly being developed. Examples of this include a script to detect syllable nuclei (De Jong & Wempe, 2009) and a suite of scripts from Georgia State University for automated analysis of amplitude, duration, formants, and so forth from multiple files (Owren, 2008). Before using Praat to analyze multiple acoustic files, it is recommended that users search the Internet for new scripts that will automate repetitive tasks such as formant analysis. The Praat home page provides a link to The Praat Users Groups (2009), where users of Praat discuss problems and solutions in the use of the software for specific projects and tasks.

REFERENCES

Amir, O., Wolf, M., & Amir, N. (2009). A clinical comparison between two acoustic analysis softwares: MDVP and Praat. *Biomedical Signal Processing and Control, 4,* 202–205.

Artkoski, M., Tommila, J., & Laukkanen, A.-M. (2002). Changes in voice during a day in normal voices without vocal loading. *Logopedics Phoniatrics Vocology, 27*(3), 118–123.

Awan, S. N. (2001). *The voice diagnostic protocol: A practical guide to the diagnosis of voice disorders.* Gaithersburg, MD: Aspen.

Bagnall, A. (2007). *Voicecraft workshop manual. Voicecraft*™. Adelaide, Australia.

Baken, R. J., & Orlikoff, R. F. (2000). *Clinical measurement of speech and voice* (2nd ed.). San Diego, CA: Singular.

Boersma, P., & Weenink, D. (2008). *Praat: Doing phonetics by computer* (Version 5.1.21) [Computer program]. Retrieved November 21, 2009, from http://www.Praat.org/.

Brockmann, M., Storck, C., Carding, P. N., & Drinnan, M. J. (2008). Voice loudness and gender effects on jitter and shimmer in healthy adults. *Journal of Speech, Language, and Hearing Research, 51,* 1152–1160.

De Jong, N. H., & Wempe, T. (2009). Praat script to detect syllable nuclei and measure speech rate automatically. *Behavior Research Methods, 41*(2), 385–390.

Deliyski, D. D., Shaw, H. S., & Evans, M. K. (2005a). Adverse effects of environmental noise on acoustic voice quality measurements. *Journal of Voice, 19,* 15–28.

Deliyski, D. D., Shaw, H. S., & Evans, M. K. (2005b). Influence of sampling rate on accuracy and reliability of acoustic voice analysis. *Logopedics, Phoniatrics, Vocology, 30,* 55–62.

Fairbanks, G. (1960). *Voice and articulation drillbook.* New York, NY: Harper and Row.

Harris, S. (1998). Speech therapy for dysphonia (pp. 139–206). In T. Harris, S. Harris, D. M. Howard, & J. S Rubin. *The voice clinic handbook.* London, UK: Whurr.

International Phonetic Association. (1999). *Handbook of the International Phonetic Association: A guide to the use of the International Phonetic Alphabet.* Cambridge, UK: Cambridge University Press.

Ma, E. P.-M., & Yiu, E. M.-L. (2005). Suitability of acoustic pertubation measures in analysing periodic and nearly periodic voice signals. *Folia Phoniatrica et Logopaedica, 57*(1), 38–47.

Maryn, Y., Corthals, P., De Bodt, M., Van Cauwenberge, P., & Deliyski, D. (2009). Perturbation measures of voice: A comparative study between Multi-Dimensional Voice Program and Praat. *Folio Phoniatrica et Logopaedia, 61,* 217–226.

Mathieson, L., Hirani, S. P., Epstein, R., Baken, R. J., Wood, G., & Rubin, J. S. (2009). Laryngeal manual therapy: A preliminary study to examine its treatment effects in the management of muscle tension dysphonia. *Journal of Voice, 23,* 353–366.

Oguz, H., Demirci, M., Safak, M. A., Arslan, N., Islam, A., & Kargin, S. (2007). Effects of unilateral vocal cord paralysis on objective voice measures obtained by Praat. *European Archives of Otorhinolaryngology, 264,* 257–261.

Owren, M. J. (2008). GSU Praat tools: Scripts for modifying and analysing sounds using Praat acoustics software. *Behavior Research Methods, 40,* 822–829.

Praat Users Groups. http://uk.groups.yahoo.com/group/praat-users/ Retrieved online on 12 November 2009.

Rantala, L., Lindholm, P., & Vilkman, E. (1998). F0 change due to voice loading under laboratory and field conditions. A pilot study. *Logopaedics, Phoniatrics, Vocology, 23,* 164–168.

Rantala, L., Paavola, L., Korkkö, P., & Vilkman E. (1998). Working-day effects on the spectral characteristics of teaching voice. *Folia Phoniatrica et Logopaedica*, *50*, 205–211.

Stajner-Katusic, S., Horga, D., & Zrinski, K. V. (2008). A longitudinal study of voice before and after phonosurgery for removal of a polyp. *Clinical Linguistics and Phonetics*, *22*(10–11), 857–863.

Titze, I. R. (1995). *Workshop on acoustic voice analysis: Summary statement.* Denver, CO: National Center for Voice and Speech.

Vogel, A. P., Maruff, P., Snyder, P. J., & Mundt, J. C. (2009). Standardization of pitch-range settings in voice acoustic analysis. *Behavior Research Methods*, *41*(2), 318–324.

Zraick, R. I., Birdwell K. Y., & Smith-Olinde, L. (2005). The effect of speaking sample duration on determination of habitual pitch. *Journal of Voice*, *19*, 197–201.

Zraick, R. I., Gentry, M. A., Smith-Olinde L., & Gregg, B. A. (2006). The effect of speaking context on elicitation of habitual pitch. *Journal of Voice*, *20*(4), 545–559.

Zraick, R. I., Skaggs, S. D., & Montague J. C. (2000). The effect of task on determination of habitual pitch. *Journal of Voice*, *14*, 484–489.

CHAPTER 19

Voice Range Profile: Phog

ESTELLA P.-M. MA

PURPOSES

- To assess vocal functions in terms of pitch and loudness production.
- To provide a visual representation of an individual's vocal performance in pitch and loudness range.

THEORETICAL BACKGROUND

The presence of laryngeal pathologies can lead to changes in vocal fold mass, length, and/or tension (Colton, Casper, & Leonard, 2006). This affects laryngeal aerodynamic functions including airflow and subglottal air pressure, which have an impact on phonational frequency and intensity measures. Voice range profile is a two-dimensional graphic display of an individual's minimum and maximum phonational intensity levels across his or her total phonational frequency range, with the intensity values plotted against the frequency values (Baken & Orlikoff, 2000; Coleman, 1993; Kent, Kent, & Rosenbek, 1987). The term "voice range profile" was officially

proposed by the Voice Committee of the International Association of Logopedics and Phoniatrics in 1992 (IALP, 1992). Alternative terms used in the literature include phonetogram (Airainer & Klingholz, 1993; Akerlund, Gramming, & Sundberg, 1992), phonetography (Heylen, Mertens, Pattyn, & Wuyts, 1996), voice profile (Bohme & Stuchlik, 1995), phonational profiles (Morris, Brown, Hicks, & Howell, 1995), voice area (Schutte & Seidner, 1983), and Stimmfeld (Hacki, 1988).

The shape of a typical voice range profile obtained from a vocally healthy individual takes the form of an oblique oval (Pabon, 1991) (Figure 19–1). The lower curve of the profile, or the lower intensity contour, reflects the minimum phonational intensity levels across the individual's total phonational frequency

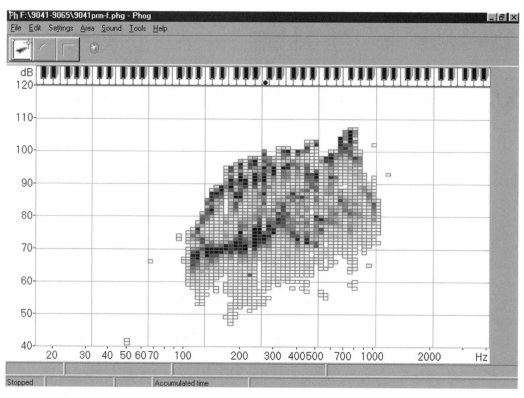

Figure 19–1. Sample voice range profile recorded from an individual with normal voice.

range. The upper curve of the profile, or the upper intensity contour, reflects the maximum phonational intensity levels across the individual's total phonational frequency range. The lower and the upper intensity contours join together at the minimum phonational frequency and the maximum phonational frequency values. Frequency measures (the maximum frequency, the minimum frequency, and frequency range) and intensity measures (the maximum intensity, the minimum intensity, and intensity range) can be analyzed from the voice range profile. The area of a voice range profile gives an indication of the individual's vocal capacity. Some authors (e.g., Heylen et al., 1998; Sulter, Schutte, & Miller, 1995) have also analyzed

the slope of the upper intensity contour and the slope of the lower intensity contour as indicators of vocal performance.

The voice range profile frequently has been used to differentiate dysphonia from healthy voices. In individuals with laryngeal pathologies, there may be:

■ A reduction of maximum frequency range, with more prominent reduction in high frequencies. The presence of laryngeal pathologies increases the vocal fold mass per unit length, which limits vocal folds vibrating at high frequencies. Also, the increase in vocal fold tension associated with the laryngeal pathologies leads to an increase in vocal fold stiffness and this prevents stretching vocal folds to phonate at high frequencies (Colton et al., 2006). The highest possible phonational frequency level is therefore reduced (Heylen et al., 1998; Heylen, Wuyts, Mertens, De Bodt, & van de Heyning, 2002; McAllister, Sederholm, Sundberg, & Gramming, 1994).

■ A reduction of maximum intensity range, with more prominent increase of minimum phonational intensities. The minimum intensity level reflects the phonatory threshold of an individual. When phonating with the minimal loudness level, the air-stream passing through the glottis would be very low. With the presence of laryngeal pathologies, the vocal fold mass per unit length increases and subsequently limits the flexibility of the vocal folds to set vocal folds into vibration at a very low airstream (Gramming & Akerlund, 1988). It therefore is not uncommon for dysphonic individuals to find it difficult to phonate at very low intensity levels as in the vocally healthy individuals.

■ A reduction of voice range profile area due to the reduced maximum frequency and intensity ranges.

Some authors adopt the concept of voice range profile to assess and display connected speech production using a two-dimensional graphic plot (Emerich, Titze, Svec, Popolo, & Logan, 2005; Ma et al., 2007; Ternstrom, Andersson, & Bergman, 2000). Such a speech range profile provides a functional analysis of an individual's vocal performance as in daily conversations. Ma and her colleagues (2007) recently evaluated the use of speech range profile measures in classifying females with dysphonia and healthy voices. They found that the combined use of only two measures of speech range profile (speaking frequency range and maximum speaking intensity level) could accurately classify 93.6% of the female individuals (117 out of 125 females).

DESCRIPTION

Several commercial systems are available for recording voice range profiles. These systems include the Swell's Phog from Hitech Development AB (http://www.savenhitech.no/eng/), Voice Profiler from Alphatron Medical Systems (http://www.alphatronmedical.nl), Voice Range Profile from KayPENTAX (http://www.kaypentax.com), and Phonetogram from Dr. Speech (http://www.drspeech.com). Among these systems, Phog and Voice Profiler claim to be sensitive to capturing connected speech range profiles.

This chapter uses the Phog system to illustrate how to assess voice range profile and speech range profile. Figure 19–2 shows the equipment setup of Swell's Phog and Figure 19–3 shows the main display screen of the Phog program.

EQUIPMENT AND MATERIALS

■ Recording software: Swell's Phog from Hitech Development AB.

■ Accessories for calibration: sound level meter, loudspeakers, ruler (for measuring mouth-to-microphone distance).

■ Accessories for recording: Head-set microphone (AKG c420), standard passage such as North Wind and the Sun (International Phonetic Association, 1999) or The Rainbow Passage (Fairbanks, 1960).

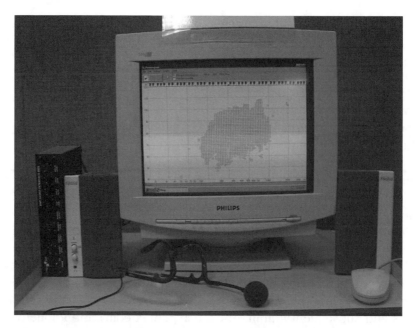

Figure 19–2. Equipment setup of the Swell's Phog.

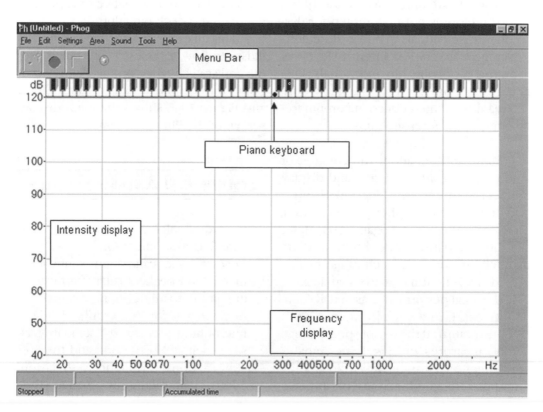

Figure 19–3. Main display screen of the Phog program.

TEST PROCEDURES

General Guidelines

▪ **Recording environment.** Poor acoustic conditions can affect the validity of phonational intensity levels measured. The recording should be carried out under a quiet environment with low ambient noise (less than 40 dB).

▪ **Recording time-of-day.** There is not enough evidence in the literature to suggest that different time-of-day has an effect on the recording of voice range profile (van Mersbergen, Verdolini, & Titze, 1999). However, when assessing voice range performance of the same individual across time, for example, before, during and after receiving voice treatment, it is recommended that all the recordings be carried out at the same time of day.

▪ **Mouth-to-microphone distance.** The literature has documented the use of different mouth-to-microphone distances for recording voice range profiles. The Union of European Phoniatricians (UEP) recommends the use of the 30-cm mouth-to-microphone distance for recording a voice range profile (Schutte & Seidner, 1983). Throughout the recording, a constant mouth-to-microphone distance should be maintained and the use of headset microphone is preferred.

▪ **Eliciting maximum phonational intensity range.** Throughout the recording, the clinician can provide the client with hand signals to encourage and prompt for the client's maximum intensity (Coleman, 1993). In addition, each testing tone should be repeated three times for more reliable recording of the softest and loudest phonations of the speaker (Sihvo, Laippala, & Sala, 2000).

▪ **Eliciting maximum phonational frequency range.** The maximum and minimum phonational frequencies should be elicited by a discrete-step task in the direction of mid (habitual)-basal-to-ceiling (Zraick, Nelson, Montague, & Monoson, 2000).

Calibration

The Phog system detects the speaker's phonation through a microphone. The corresponding phonational intensity level is then displayed on the computer screen. As the intensity level of the sound signal shown by the program depends on the microphone gain and also the microphone distance from the client's mouth, the system needs to be calibrated before recording. The following calibration procedure ensures that the microphone signal is based on sound pressure level at 30 cm microphone distance (the UEP-recommended distance):

1. Start the calibration procedure by clicking on **Settings** from the menu bar and then select **Calibration**. A calibration wizard will then appear on the computer screen (Figure 19–4). Then select the calibration tone source and method. In the following steps, the calibration tone **1kHz sinusoid from phonetograph** and calibration method **Ext. volume control** will be used for demonstration.

2. In the calibration wizard, input the distance that the microphone will be placed from the mouth during actual recording (the author recommends 5 cm) and type "30 cm" in the **. . . but pretend it is at** box.

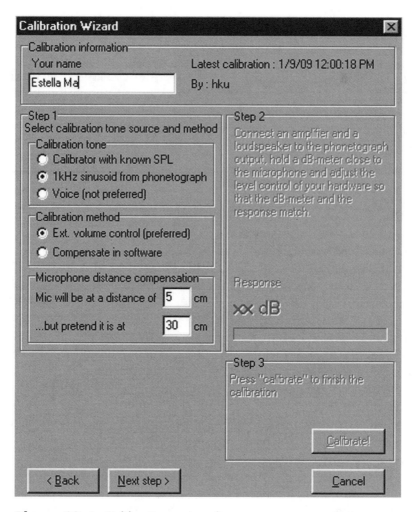

Figure 19–4. Calibration wizard.

3. When the button **Next step** is pressed, a high-frequency tone of 1 kHz will be generated by the Phog system and played through the loudspeaker. Hold the sound level meter and the microphone at the same distance away from the loudspeaker (the author recommends 30 cm which is the UEP-recommended distance for recording voice range profile; Figure 19–5). Measure the sound pressure level of the tone using the sound level meter.

4. Adjust the **MIC L/R LEVEL** knob of the DSP Mixer until the dB-level displayed on the computer screen matches that of the sound level meter within ± 0.5 dB. For example, the dB-level of the 1 kHz tone is 78.3 dB (see Figure 19–5), the dB-level shown by the Phog program on the computer screen should fall between 77.8 dB and 78.8 dB. Click on the button **Next step** once the two readings match and click on the button **Calibrate!** to complete the calibration process.

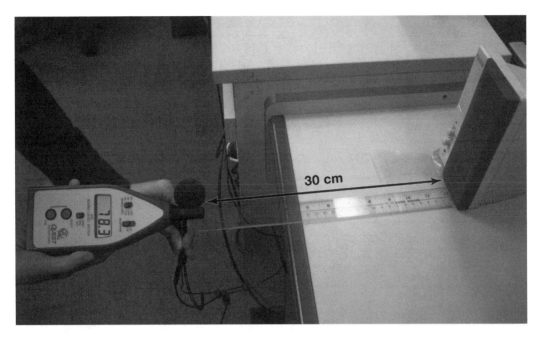

Figure 19–5. Calibration procedure: Hold the sound level meter close to the microphone. Adjust the level control of the DSP Mixer until the dB-level displayed on the computer screen matches that of the sound level meter.

Recording Voice Range Profile

1. Prior to the actual recording, ask the client to practice pitch gliding five times as a "warm-up" exercise to facilitate his or her maximum vocal performance (Coleman, 1993). This warm-up exercise also gives the clinician a general idea of the client's phonational frequency range.

   Instructions: *"We are going to assess your voice range. Let's do some warm-up exercises first by gliding up and down the pitch like this.* (The clinician then gives a full modeling of the gliding) *We will repeat this exercise five times."*

2. The clinician should then obtain an estimation of the client's habitual pitch level. This habitual pitch level will serve as the starting tone for recording voice range profile. Awan (2001) describes a procedure to obtain habitual pitch level. Under that procedure, the client is instructed to chant and count the number from one to four, then sustain the vowel /a/ for a few seconds. The corresponding frequency and intensity level will be registered simultaneously on the computer screen as a dot.

   Instructions: *"I want you to chant and count from one to four, then say 'ah' for 6 seconds."*

3. The recording begins with the lower intensity contour followed by the upper intensity contour to avoid vocal fatigue (Behrman, Agresti, Blumstein, & Sharma, 1996) (Figure 19-6). To record the lower intensity contour

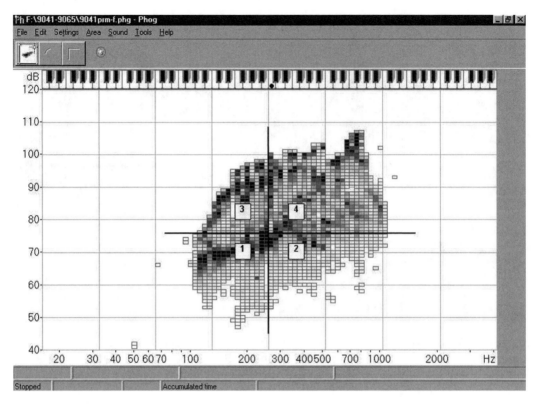

Figure 19–6. Sequence in eliciting a voice range profile.

(see sections 1 and 2 on Figure 19-6), the habitual pitch level obtained from the previous step should be presented by clicking on the corresponding musical note through the piano keyboard on the computer screen. The client is asked to produce the minimum intensity at that target tone. Give the instructions below to the client:

Instructions: *"I will now present a musical tone to you, please say 'ah' following that tone at your most comfortable loudness. Then gradually lower the loudness until it reaches your softest voice at that tone, but remember, do not whisper."*

4. Give positive reinforcement to the client and then proceed to a lower tone.

Each consecutive semitone should be tested in order to reveal whether there exists any phonation breaks which present as a gap within the client's voice range profile:

Instructions: *"Very good. This is exactly what I'd like and it records your minimum loudness at this tone. Now we are going to repeat this procedure at a lower tone. Here's the tone."* (click the next semitone on the piano keyboard).

5. The recording procedure should then be repeated by going down the musical notes one semitone at a time until the client cannot sustain his or her phonation at any lower pitch. Generally, it has been agreed that modal (or, chest) and falsetto (or, loft) register

phonations are accepted for voice range profile, but vocal fry (or, pulse) register phonations are not accepted (Baken & Orlikoff, 2000).

6. The recording procedure should be continued by going up the musical notes one semitone at a time from the client's habitual pitch level until he or she cannot sustain the phonation at any higher pitch. The lower intensity contour is collected. Clear instruction should be given:

   Instructions: *"OK, now, we are going to repeat the procedure at a higher tone. Here's the tone."*

7. The upper intensity contour (indicated as sections 3 and 4 in Figure 19-6) will be recorded starting from the client's habitual pitch level. The client is asked to produce the loudest voice at that target tone:

   Instructions: *"I will now present a musical tone to you, please say 'ah' following that tone at your most comfortable loudness. But this time, I want you to gradually raise the loudness until it reaches your loudest voice at that tone but remember, do not shout."*

8. The recording procedure then repeats with musical notes going down one semitone at a time on the piano scale until the client cannot sustain his or her phonation at any lower frequency. Give positive reinforcement. Provide the following instructions to the client:

   Instructions: *"Very good. This is exactly what I'd like and it records your maximum possible loudness at this tone. Now we are going to repeat this procedure at a lower tone. Here's the tone."*

9. The recording procedure then repeats with musical notes going up one semitone at a time on the piano scale starting from the client's habitual pitch level until he or she cannot sustain his or her phonation at any higher frequency.

   Instructions: *"OK, now, we are going to repeat this procedure at a higher tone. Here's the tone. You can use your falsetto voice, like this. (Give a model of falsetto voice)"*

Recording Speech Range Profile

The speech range profile is recorded by asking the client to read aloud a standard passage using his or her habitual voice. The client should be given time to familiarize him- or herself with the material before recording. Give the instructions below to the client:

Instructions: *"Please read aloud this passage comfortably as in your daily conversations. Spend some time now to get yourself familiarized with the passage."* (**Note:** For those clients who have limited reading ability such as young children, speech materials other than reading aloud a passage such as monologue: *"Tell me your favorite movie," "Tell me about your recent overseas trip"* and picture description: *"Tell me about this picture"* can be used.)

Data Analysis

1. Locate the voice range profile contour on the computer screen by clicking on the mouse cursor. The frequency

value (in hertz and semitone) and intensity value (in dB) will be detected automatically at the cursor by the program and displayed on the computer screen. It generally is recommended that clinician report the frequency range in semitones rather than hertz for standard comparison within and between clients. The conversion can be done easily with the algorithm: ($\log_{10}$ [The highest frequency in hertz ÷ The lowest frequency in hertz]) ÷ $\log_{10}2 \times 12$.

2. To obtain the voice profile area, place the mouse cursor over the profile and right click the mouse. The value of the area (in semitone dB) automatically will be displayed on the bottom left corner of the computer screen.

NORMATIVE DATA

Table 19-1 lists the means and standard deviations of voice limit measures as

Table 19–1. Normative Adult Female Data of Voice Limit Measures as Derived from Voice Range Profile (VRP) and Speech Range Profile (SRP) Reported in Ma et al. (2007)

Measures		Dysphonic (N = 90) Mean	(SD)	Normal Voice (N = 35) Mean	(SD)
Frequency measures					
Highest frequency (in hertz)	VRP	854.98	(251.25)	1232.85	(221.42)
	SRP	297.75	(50.00)	336.06	(51.07)
Lowest frequency (in hertz)	VRP	127.65	(20.99)	115.01	(12.00)
	SRP	130.65	(18.83)	134.89	(12.33)
Frequency range (in semitone)	VRP	32.36	(6.39)	40.89	(3.73)
	SRP	14.21	(3.07)	15.69	(2.48)
Intensity measures					
Maximum intensity (in dB)	VRP	109.28	(5.18)	105.66	(6.12)
	SRP	94.57	(5.55)	85.37	(3.52)
Minimum intensity (in dB)	VRP	60.64	(7.41)	48.91	(3.12)
	SRP	74.23	(6.12)	66.66	(3.31)
Intensity range (in dB)	VRP	48.63	(8.06)	56.74	(6.29)
	SRP	20.33	(3.23)	18.71	(3.30)
Profile areas (in dBA × semitones)	VRP	931.47	(266.31)	1421.80	(232.23)
	SRP	173.17	(41.28)	185.77	(45.26)

The intensity levels were measured at 30 cm.

derived from voice range profile (VRP) and speech range profile (SRP) in a group of Cantonese females. These figures were taken from a previous study by the author (Ma et al., 2007). The data were collected from 90 dysphonic females and 35 females with healthy voices. Table 19-2 lists the means and standard errors of voice limit measures from a group of children (Heylen et al., 1998).

CASE STUDY: PATIENT J.Y. (BILATERAL VOCAL FOLD NODULES)

J.Y., a 38-year-old female teacher, was referred to speech pathologist by an otolaryngologist. She was diagnosed as having bilateral vocal fold nodules. She reported that her voice had worsened significantly

Table 19-2. Normative Children Data of Voice Range Profile Measures Reported in Heylen et al. (1998)

Measures	Dysphonic children* (N = 136)		Normal children[†] (N = 94)	
	Mean	(SE)	Mean	(SE)
Frequency measures				
Lowest frequency (in Hz)	196.3	(2.5)	192.8	(2.5)
Highest frequency (in Hz)	550.0	(11.0)	857.0	(21.0)
Total frequency range (in Hz)	354.0	(13.0)	663.0	(22.0)
Number of semitone in modal register	13.8	(0.3)	18.0	(0.3)
Number of semitone in falsetto register	5.5	(0.4)	8.4	(0.4)
Total number of semitone	19.4	(0.5)	26.4	(0.5)
Intensity measures				
Lowest intensity (in dB)	52.4	(0.3)	48.2	(0.3)
Highest intensity (in dB)	95.2	(0.5)	98.0	(0.6)
Total intensity range (in dB)	42.7	(0.6)	49.7	(0.6)
Morphological measures				
Slope of the upper intensity contour (in dB/ST)	1.94	(0.08)	1.14	(0.04)
Slope of the lower intensity contour (in dB/ST)	0.91	(0.05)	0.623	(0.024)

[†]Vocally healthy group composed of 53 boys and 41 girls.
*Dysphonic group composed of 87 boys and 49 girls.
SE = standard errors.

over the past year. She complained of "cannot speak loud" and "cannot be heard against noisy environments." She also complained of "not able to sing high pitched notes." When speaking, J.Y. demonstrated reduced jaw movement and limited range of mouth movement. Her voice was noted to be effortful. Perceptually, her voice in daily conversations was described as low-pitched and moderately breathy and rough. Pitch variation and loudness variation were markedly reduced such that her voice was monotonous. The following measures (Table 19–3, Figure 19–7) were taken with the Phog system at the initial assessment:

The pretreatment assessment results indicate that J.Y. demonstrated:

- Reduced maximum frequency range with prominent reduction in high frequencies—This is consistent with her complaints of "not able to sing high pitched notes."
- Reduced maximum intensity range due to an increase in minimum phonational intensity and decrease in maximum phonational intensity—This suggests that J.Y. cannot phonate at very low intensity levels. The result is also consistent with the complaint of "cannot

Table 19–3. Voice Range and Speech Range Performance of J.Y.

Measures		Pre-treatment	Post-treatment
Frequency measures			
Highest frequency (in hertz)	VRP	622.3	987.8
	SRP	246.9	311.1
Lowest frequency (in hertz)	VRP	130.8	123.5
	SRP	130.8	138.6
Frequency range (in semitone)	VRP	28.0	37.0
	SRP	12.0	15.0
Intensity measures			
Maximum intensity (in dB)	VRP	104	115
	SRP	94	86
Minimum intensity (in dB)	VRP	70	62
	SRP	78	68
Intensity range (in dB)	VRP	34	53
	SRP	16	18
Profile areas (in dBA × semitones)	VRP	560.0	1290.0
	SRP	115.0	158.0

VRP, voice range profile; SRP, speech voice profile.

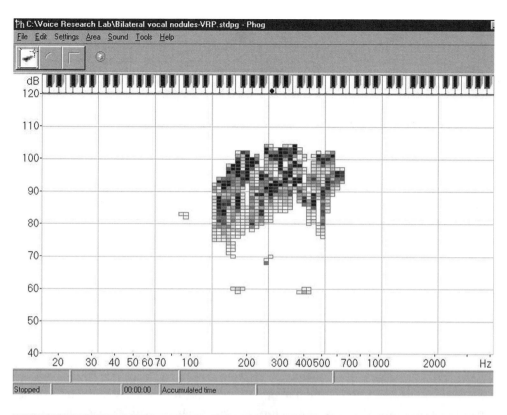

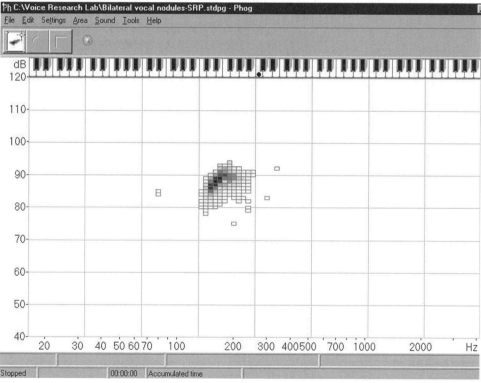

Figure 19–7. Voice range profile (*upper*) and speech range profile (*lower*) of J.Y. taken at the initial assessment.

speak loud" and "cannot be heard against noisy environments."

■ Reduced vocal capacity due to the reduced maximum frequency and intensity range.

■ Increased maximum speaking and minimum speaking intensity levels—This is consistent with the effortful speech judged by the clinician.

■ Reduced speech range profile area due to the reduced speaking frequency and intensity range—This is consistent with the clinical observation of monotonous voice.

The Lessac-Madsen Resonant Voice Therapy (LMRVT) (Verdolini-Marston, Burke, Lessac, Glaze, & Caldwell, 1995) was introduced to J.Y. with the aim to produce a clear and strong voice with minimal likelihood of phonotrauma. Moreover, chewing technique with a focus on an open mouth speaking (Ma, 2008) was introduced to J.Y.. The exercise promotes jaw movement, which results in increased oral cavity space, and stronger oral resonance during speaking. J.Y. received 10 sessions of voice therapy over the course of 3 months. Post-treatment evaluation data (see Table 19–3) suggested that J.Y. benefited from the voice therapy:

■ There was an increase in the highest phonational frequency and maximum frequency range.

■ There was an increase in the maximum intensity level and a decrease in the minimum intensity level.

■ The area of voice range profile increased significantly, suggesting an increase in vocal capacity.

■ The area of speech range profile also increased significantly, suggesting an increase in speaking variability.

REFERENCES

Airainer, R., & Klingholz, F. (1993). Quantitative evaluation of phonetograms in the case of functional dysphonia. *Journal of Voice*, 7(2), 136–141.

Akerlund, L., Gramming, P., & Sundberg, J. (1992). Phonetogram and averages of sound pressure levels and fundamental frequencies of speech: Comparison between female singers and nonsingers. *Journal of Voice*, 6(1), 55–63.

Awan, S. N. (2001). *The voice diagnostic protocol: A practical guide to the diagnosis of voice disorders*. Gaithersburg, MD: Aspen.

Baken, R. J., & Orlikoff, R. F. (2000). *Clinical measurement of speech and voice* (2nd ed.). San Diego, CA: Singular.

Behrman, A., Agresti, C. J., Blumstein, E., & Sharma, G. (1996). Meaningful features of voice range profiles from patients with organic vocal fold pathology: A programming study. *Journal of Voice*, 10, 269–283.

Bohme, G., & Stuchlik, G. (1995). Voice profiles and standard voice profile of untrained children. *Journal of Voice*, 9(3), 304–307.

Coleman, R. F. (1993). Sources of variation in phonetograms. *Journal of Voice*, 7(1), 1–14.

Colton, R. H., Casper, J. K., & Leonard, R. (2006). *Understanding voice problems: A physiological perspective for diagnosis and treatment* (3rd ed.). Philadelphia, PA: Lippincott Williams & Wilkins.

Emerich, K. A., Titze, I. R., Svec, J. G., Popolo, P. S., & Logan, G. (2005). Vocal range and intensity in actors: A studio versus stage comparison. *Journal of Voice*, 19(1), 78–83.

Fairbanks, G. (1960). *Voice and articulation drillbook*. New York, NY: Harper and Row.

Gramming, P., & Akerlund, L. (1988). Nonorganic dysphonia: Phonetograms for normal and pathological voices. *Acta Otolaryngo (Stockholm)*, 106, 468–476.

Hacki, T. (1988). Die Beurteilung der quantitativen Sprechstimmleistungen. Das Sprechstimmfeld im Singstimmfeld. *Folia Phoniatrica, 40*, 190-196.

Heylen, L., Mertens, F., Pattyn, J., & Wuyts, F. L. (1996). Phonetography in voice diagnoses. *Acta Oto-Rhino-Laryngologica Belgica, 50*, 299-308.

Heylen, L., Wuyts, F. L., Mertens, F., De-Bodt, M., Pattyn, J., Croux, C., & van de Heyning, P. H. (1998). Evaluation of the vocal performance of children using a voice range profile index. *Journal of Speech, Language, and Hearing Research, 41*(2), 232-238.

Heylen, L., Wuyts, F. L., Mertens, F., De Bodt, M., & van de Heyning, P. H. (2002). Normative voice range profiles of male and female professional voice users. *Journal of Voice, 16*(1), 1-7.

IALP. (1992). International Association of Logopedics and Phoniatrics (IALP) voice committee discussion of assessment topics. *Journal of Voice, 6*, 194-210.

International Phonetic Association. (1999). *Handbook of the International Phonetic Association: A guide to the use of the International Phonetic Alphabet*. Cambridge, UK: Cambridge University Press.

Kent, R. D., Kent, J. F., & Rosenbek, J. C. (1987). Maximum performance tests of speech production. *Journal of Speech and Hearing Disorders, 52*, 367-387.

Ma, E. (2008). Chewing technique: Speak with an "Open Mouth." In A. Behrman & J. Haskell (Eds.), *Exercises for voice therapy* (pp. 85-86). San Diego, CA: Plural Publishing.

Ma, E., Robertson, J., Radford, C., Vagne, S., El-Halabi, R., & Yiu, E. (2007). Reliability of speaking and maximum voice range measures in screening for dysphonia. *Journal of Voice, 21*(4), 397-406.

McAllister, A., Sederholm, E., Sundberg, J., & Gramming, P. (1994). Relations between voice range profiles and physiological and perceptual voice characteristics in ten-year-old children. *Journal of Voice, 8*(3), 230-239.

Morris, R. J., Brown, W. S., Hicks, D. M., & Howell, E. (1995). Phonational profiles of male trained singers and nonsingers. *Journal of Voice, 9*, 142-148.

Pabon, J. P. H. (1991). Objective acoustic voice-quality parameters in the computer phonetogram. *Journal of Voice, 5*(3), 203-216.

Schutte, H. K., & Seidner, W. (1983). Recommendation by the Union of European Phoniatricians (UEP): Standardizing voice area measurement/Phonetography. *Folia Phoniatrica, 35*, 286-288.

Sulter, A. M., Schutte, H. K., & Miller, D. G. (1995). Differences in phonetogram features between male and female subjects with and without vocal training. *Journal of Voice, 9*, 363-377.

Sihvo, M., Laippala, P., & Sala, E. (2000). A study of repeated measures of softest and loudest phonations. *Journal of Voice, 14*(2), 161-169.

Ternstrom, S., Andersson, M., & Bergman, U. (2000). An effect of body massage on voice loudness and phonation frequency in reading. *Logopedics Phoniatrics Vocology, 25*(4), 146-150.

van Mersbergen, M. R., Verdolini, K., & Titze, I. R. (1999). Time-of-day effects on voice range profile performance in young, vocally untrained adult females. *Journal of Voice, 13*(4), 518-528.

Verdolini-Marston, K., Burke, M. K., Lessac, A., Glaze, L., & Caldwell, E. (1995). Preliminary study of two methods of treatment for laryngeal nodules. *Journal of Voice, 9*(1), 74-85.

Zraick, R. I., Nelson, J. L., Montague, J. C., & Monoson, P. K. (2000). The effect of task on determination of maximum phonational frequency range. *Journal of Voice, 14*(2), 154-160.

SECTION V

Resonance

CHAPTER 20

Nasometry in the Evaluation of Resonance Disorders

ALICE LEE AND TARA L. WHITEHILL

PURPOSE

■ To provide a quantitative measure of the balance of oral and nasal resonance during speech.

THEORETICAL BACKGROUND

Resonance is a term derived from the physics of sound that is applied in speech science to refer to the vibratory response of air in the vocal tract set in motion by a source of phonation (Crystal, 2003). The vocal tract extends inferiorly from the vocal folds to the opening of the mouth and the nose and consists of three main resonating cavities: the pharynx, the oral cavity, and the nasal cavity (Kent & Read, 2002). The pharynx and oral cavity are the main vocal tract airway. The nasal cavity can be considered as a side branch or additional acoustic system that can be coupled to the main vocal tract (Stevens, 2000). The coupling between the two cavities is regulated by the velopharyn-

geal port, which includes the velum, the lateral pharyngeal walls, and the posterior pharyngeal wall. In theory, velopharyngeal closure occurs during the production of nonnasalized vowels and nonnasal or oral consonants, whereas the velopharyngeal port remains open during the production of nasal sounds (see Peterson-Falzone, Hardin-Jones, & Karnell, 2009, for details on the velopharyngeal valving mechanism). Any disturbance to velopharyngeal structures or functions will affect the balance of oral and nasal resonance, and may lead to resonance disorders.

There are some controversies regarding whether resonance should be considered as within the scope of voice. Many experts now believe that, as resonance does not generate at the laryngeal level but rather concerns the modulation of acoustic energy created at the laryngeal level, and involves a distinct physiologic control mechanism, resonance disorders, therefore, should be distinguished from voice disorders (e.g., Riski & Verdolini, 1999). However, other researchers consider voice as the output of the respiration, phonation and resonance subsystems (e.g., Boone, 2004). Regardless of one's viewpoint on this issue, a clear understanding of resonance disorders and the terminology of resonance and its disorders is necessary for those who work within the broad field of voice disorders.

Resonance disorders include hypernasality, hyponasality, mixed resonance disorder, and cul-de-sac resonance. *Hypernasality* refers to the perception of excessive nasal resonance when producing vowels, voiced oral consonants, or both (Kent, 1999). It usually is observed in speakers with velopharyngeal dysfunction (VPD) due to anatomic or physiologic deficiencies (see Kummer, 2008). *Hyponasality* refers to reduced normal nasal resonance during speech, particularly during the production of nasal consonants (Kummer, 2008). Although hyponasality usually is associated with blockage in the nasopharynx or nasal cavity, it also can be caused by neurological impairment. *Mixed resonance* is a combination of hypernasality and hyponasality that occurs when there is a VPD as well as a blockage at the nasal airway (Kummer, 2008). It also may occur in individuals with inappropriate timing of velopharyngeal movement during speech due to oral-motor disorders (Kummer, 2008; Netsell, 1969). *Cul-de-sac resonance* occurs when the acoustic energy transmitted into the vocal tract is trapped by a blind pouch and speech sounds muffled (Kummer, 2008). It can occur when there is VPD in addition to anterior blockage in the nasal cavity.

It is important to differentiate between hypernasality and nasal emission. Nasal emission is characterized by an inappropriate release of air pressure through the nares during consonant production. Although both nasal emission and hypernasality are associated with VPD, nasal emission is considered an articulation disorder, rather than a resonance disorder (Kummer, 2008). Phoneme-specific nasal emission, where speakers show nasal emission for certain pressure consonants but can achieve adequate velopharyngeal closure when producing other consonants and vowels, is considered a learned disorder and is not associated with VPD (Kummer, 2008; Peterson-Falzone et al., 2009).

It is important to have methods of assessing resonance disorders that are both reliable and valid, to document severity and change over time. Perceptual judgment of resonance disorders is considered as the gold standard, as resonance disorders by definition are a perceptual phenomenon (Moll, 1964). However, perceptual judgment of nasality has been associated with poor reliability (e.g., Kent, 1999; Lee, Whitehill, & Ciocca, 2009; Lewis, Watterson, & Houghton, 2003), and typically does not provide much insight into the cause of the problem. Hence, researchers have sought to develop instrumental measures to evaluate velopharyngeal structure and movement, or the sequelae of velopharyngeal function. Although instrumental measures do not measure hypernasality per se, they can supplement the perceptual evaluation of resonance disorders, as discussed below (for a review, see Kuehn & Moller, 2000; Peterson-Falzone et al., 2009).

Instrumental procedures for evaluating velopharyngeal function can be categorized into direct and indirect measures (Dalston & Warren, 1985; Kuehn & Dalston,

1988). Direct measures, such as videofluoroscopy, nasendoscopy, ultrasound, and magnetic resonance imaging (MRI), allow visual inspection of velopharyngeal movement during speech production. Indirect measures evaluate the consequences of velopharyngeal dysfunction. These include acoustic analyses (spectrography and nasometry), accelerometry, aerodynamic measures, photodetection, and electromyography. Each instrumental measure offers different information regarding velopharyngeal function and each has its strengths and drawbacks. For example, videofluoroscopy allows the examiner to determine the cause of VPD and the size, location, and shape of the velopharyngeal gap, which is important for deciding the type of treatment (Kummer, 2008). However, it involves a small amount of radiation exposure. Although nasendoscopy does not involve radiation exposure, the insertion of a flexible endoscope into the nostril is an invasive procedure that may cause a certain level of discomfort to some clients. Most indirect measures are noninvasive and can be used for documenting treatment outcome. However, they give very little information on the associated cause of VPD. Therefore, the choice of instrumental measure(s) should be made depending on the type of information needed, the availability of particular equipment, and client characteristics (e.g., whether they can tolerate the evaluation procedure).

This chapter focuses on using nasometry, which is probably the most frequently used indirect measure of velopharyngeal function in both research and clinical settings (Kuehn & Moller, 2000; Zajac, 2008). It often has been used to assess individuals with resonance disorders due to cleft palate but has also been employed to evaluate resonance in professional voice users (e.g.,

Jennings & Kuehn, 2008). Details of the above mentioned instrumental measures are available from a number of sources (e.g., Bzoch, 2004; Kuehn & Moller, 2000; Kummer, 2008; Peterson-Falzone et al., 2009; Whitehill & Lee, 2008).

Nasometry involves the use of a computer-based device to record separately the acoustic energy emitted from the nose and the mouth, for calculating an index called the nasalance score. The nasalance score is the ratio of nasal acoustic energy to the sum of oral and nasal acoustic energy, expressed as a percentage. It ranges from 0 to 100%. Theoretically, the higher the perceived nasality, the higher the nasalance score. However, practically it is not possible to obtain 0% nasalance even during the production of nonnasal sounds because transpalatal acoustic transmission occurs and the oral acoustic energy emitted can reach the nasal microphone (Gildersleeve-Neumann & Dalston, 2001). In addition, nasalance scores may vary by about 3 to 5 percentage points across repeated readings within the same session (i.e., subject performance variability) or when the headset is removed and replaced (e.g., Seaver, Dalston, Leeper, & Adams, 1991; Watterson, Lewis, & Brancamp, 2005). The test-retest variability has been shown to be greater in speakers with hypernasality than in individuals with normal resonance (Watterson & Lewis, 2006).

Nasometric evaluation is quick and easy to administer and the procedure is noninvasive. The equipment is commercially available at a relatively low cost. However, users must understand that the nasalance score can be affected by co-occurring articulation errors and/or voice disorders. For example, the nasalance may be elevated if the speaker also has nasal emission; an individual with mixed resonance may have a nasalance score within the normal limit; and the presence of breathiness or low volume may reduce the nasalance score (Kummer, 2008). Nasometric evaluation should not be used as the sole resonance assessment procedure. The results should be interpreted together with perceptual judgments. In the case of discrepancies between perceptual and nasometric findings, users should check and ensure no procedural errors have occurred. Further investigations or considerations of the problem are warranted before making a diagnosis or treatment plan (see the Case Study for an example).

DESCRIPTION

Currently, there are three commercially available systems for nasometric evaluation: the Nasometer II (KayPENTAX, Lincoln Park, NJ), the NasalView (Tiger Electronics, Seattle, WA), and the NAS System[1] (Glottal Enterprises Inc., Syracuse, NY). The Nasometer is based on an earlier instrument called TONAR (The Oral-Nasal Acoustic Ratio; Fletcher & Bishop, 1970). All three systems measure nasalance in a similar manner but the handling of the audio signal differs between the systems. For example, the signal is bandpass-filtered in the Nasometer II and the NAS System but there is no bandpass-filtering for the NasalView (see Bressmann, 2005, for details). A number of studies have com-

pared the nasalance scores obtained using these different systems (e.g., Bressmann, 2005; Bressmann, Klaiman, & Fischbach, 2006; Lewis & Watterson, 2003). Significant differences in the nasalance scores were reported and the authors cautioned that scores from the different devices are not interchangeable. In addition, Watterson et al. (2005) compared the older Nasometer 6200 and the relatively new Nasometer II 6400 and found significant differences in nasalance score between the two models. Thus, care should be exercised when comparing nasalance scores between these two versions (Watterson et al., 2005). As the NasalView and the NAS System are not as widely used as the Nasometer and there are no normative data for these systems (Bressmann, 2005; Kummer, 2008), the rest of this chapter focuses on the materials and procedure for the Nasometer II only.

EQUIPMENT AND MATERIALS

■ The hardware of the Nasometer II includes a headset where two directional microphones are mounted on either side of a sound separation plate to collect acoustic signals emitted from the nose and mouth, respectively. The headset is connected to the Nasometer II external module, which is then linked to a personal computer (Figure 20–1). The Nasometer II 6400 comes with a specific sound card (Santa Cruz Sound Card) and software to be installed in

---

[1]Glottal Enterprises Inc. also manufactures a product called NVS (Nasality Visualization System), which combines the NAS system with another function for assessing nasal emission called the NEM (Nasal Emission Visualization) System. The NAS system measures nasalance using either a dual-chamber OroNasal mask or a hand-held partition handle for separation of oral and nasal sound. The equipment that Bressmann (2005) used in his study was the NAS system with the speech signals captured using the OroNasal mask. He referred to the setup as the OroNasal System.

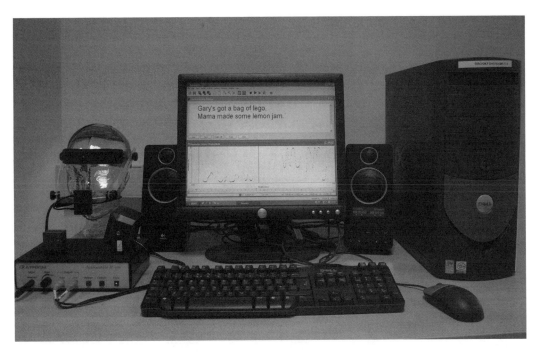

Figure 20–1. Equipment setup of the Nasometer II 6400. The Nasometer headset appears in the left upper portion of the photo, on a separately purchased head stand; the Nasometer II external module appears in the left lower portion of the figure.

the computer. A laptop is not recommended for use due to the wide variability of sound card performance and specifications in laptops. The newest version, the Nasometer II 6450 (Kay-PENTAX, Lincoln Park, NJ), uses a built-in sound chip installed in the Nasometer II hardware, which connects to the computer via USB interface; a laptop now can be used and this adds portability to the equipment.

- The software, the Nasometer II program, can be used for both assessment and treatment purposes. The application window of the program is made up of two windows: a stimulus display window on the top that shows picture or sentence stimuli and a data window below, which shows the nasometric data (or nasogram) when the speaker

produces the stimuli. The nasalance results may be displayed as a contour quantifying nasality on a time line (i.e., contour display mode), as a bar graph for an individual frame of data (i.e., bar display mode), or the data may be collected but hidden (i.e., empty display mode). Figure 20–2 shows the Nasometer II program with nasograms for two sentences (one loaded with non-nasal consonants and the other with nasal consonants) produced by a typical English-speaking adult.

- Standardized speech materials for nasometric evaluation have been developed for various languages (see Dalston, 2004; Kummer, 2008) and these should be used to compare the client's performance to the normative data for the purpose of diagnosis. The Nasometer II

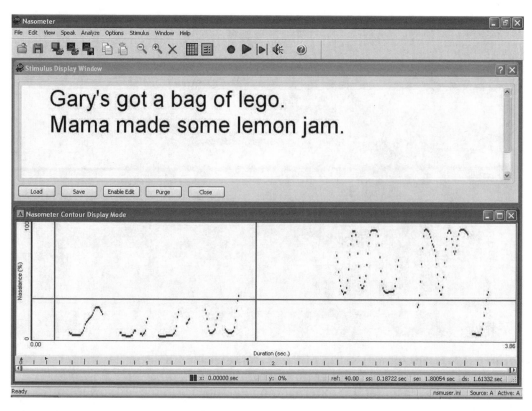

Figure 20–2. The Nasometer II program, with the speech stimuli displayed in the top window and the nasalance data of a typical English-speaking adult in contour display mode shown in the bottom window. The first nasogram, as marked by two vertical cursors, corresponds to the first sentence which is a nonnasal sentence. The nasal sentence has a higher mean nasalance score (64%) than the nonnasal sentence (12%). The horizontal line across the data window is a reference line (and is discussed further in the treatment section of this chapter).

software contains the following standardized speech materials: (1) the Zoo Passage (Fletcher, 1972), (2) the Rainbow Passage (Fairbanks, 1960), (3) the Nasal Sentences (Fletcher, 1978), (4) the Ball Passage (Fletcher, 1972), (5) the Susie Passage (MacKay & Kummer, 1993), and (6) the revised Simplified Nasometric Assessment Procedures (SNAP Test-R; Kummer, 2005; MacKay & Kummer, 1994) for children. The first three stimuli have been used most frequently in research studies. The Zoo Passage is a paragraph that is devoid of nasal phonemes. It allows the examiner to determine whether an individual is able to achieve and maintain adequate velopharyngeal closure during speech (Kummer, 2008). The Rainbow Passage is a paragraph that contains both nasal and nonnasal phonemes; 11.5% of the consonants are nasal consonants, which is representative of the frequency of occurrence of nasals in English. Therefore, it is useful for evaluating the impact of VPD in normal conversation (Dalston,

2004). The Nasal Sentences are heavily loaded with nasal phonemes. It usually is used to assess nasal obstruction (Kummer, 2008). The Ball Passage is loaded with bilabial stops (mostly /b/); whereas the Suzie Passage is embedded with fricatives (mostly /s/) and thus may be sensitive to phoneme-specific nasal emission. The SNAP Test-R contains speech materials (e.g., syllable repetitions, picture-cued sentences, and syntactically and semantically easier passages) that have been developed specifically for assessing children (see Kummer, 2008).

■ A number of other speech materials have been developed for use with the Nasometer. For example, the Turtle Passage (a nonnasal passage, similar to the Zoo Passage) and the Mouse Passage (which contains 11% nasal phonemes and thus is similar to the Rainbow Passage) are semantically and syntactically simpler passages designed to minimize reading difficulties in very young children (Watterson, Hinton, & McFarlane, 1996). The Turtle Passage does not have significantly different nasalance scores when compared to the Zoo Passage and there was a significant correspondence between nasalance results obtained using the Turtle Passage and perceptual rating of hypernasality (Watterson et al., 1996). Nonnasal sentences loaded with high-pressure consonants (e.g., stops and fricatives) and those loaded with low-pressure consonants (e.g., approximant /w/) have been used as well to explore the effect of co-occurring nasal emission on nasalance results (Sweeney, Sell, & O'Regan, 2004). A difference in nasalance score between the high-pressure consonant sentences and low-pressure consonant sentences may indicate the presence of nasal emission

that could sometimes be inaudible to the examiner. These passages and sentences are not available with the Nasometer II program but users can add them to their evaluation protocol; see "Creating a Stimulus File" described in the following section.

TEST PROCEDURES

General Guidelines

■ **Recording environment.** Speech recording should take place in a quiet environment, as advocated by many researchers (e.g., Bressmann, 2005).

■ **Client characteristics.** On the day of data collection, ensure that the client does not have a cold or other condition that can cause temporary nasal obstruction, as this may influence the nasalance score, preventing a valid assessment. To work with young children, play therapy may be needed before the nasometric evaluation to help desensitize the children to putting on the Nasometer headset. The examiner may call the headset a "superhero" mask, so to make the evaluation procedure more interesting to the child (Kummer, 2008). With adult clients, the examiner can explain why two microphones are needed, so they have a better understanding of the evaluation procedure; this can also facilitate clinician-client rapport.

■ **Placement of headset.** Clean the sound separation plate of the headset with antiseptic wipe or alcohol before placing the headset onto the client and after the evaluation procedure. Place the headset over the client's head and fit it by adjusting the top adjustment band and the Velcro strip at the back. The sound separation plate should be placed between the nose and the mouth and it should be perpendicular to the face of the speaker (Figure 20–3). The two microphones should be directly in front of the nose and the mouth. It is stated that an angle of more than 15 degrees from perpendicularity in either direction can affect the accuracy of the data (Kay Elemetrics, 2003). Once the plate is in proper position, the top and bottom adjustment knobs can be tightened to keep the plate in place. Make sure the headset is not too tight, which may cause discomfort and/or affect articulation, or too loose, which could affect the stability of the plate.

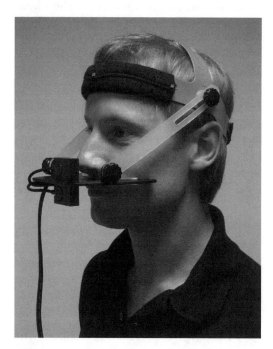

Figure 20–3. Placement of the Nasometer headset on a speaker. The sound separation plate is placed between the nose and the mouth, at 90 degrees to the face.

■ **Loading a Stimulus File.** Click the **Load** button in the stimulus display window.

■ **Creating a Stimulus File.** Users can edit existing stimulus files or create new stimulus files. Save a set of speech materials, such as oral sentences, onto a single stimulus file and make sure all stimuli can be viewed in a single window. This is because the software does not allow the users to scroll down within the stimulus window when it is on recording mode. To create a new stimulus file, click **Purge** in the stimulus window to clear it. Then click **Enable Edit** and enter the stimuli there, or copy/paste the stimuli from a word processing file. After that, click on **Disable Edit** and then **Save** to store the file. The size of the font can be adjusted by clicking the **Stimulus** menu and choosing **Adjust Text Font Size**.

■ **If the client makes an error in production,** the clinician may point this out to the client and ask them to read the sentence again. Make sure the previous sentence is erased by pressing the **F2** key from the keyboard; otherwise, the new sentence simply will be added to the previous error sentence. Some very young children or adults with neurological impairment may not be able to read text. In this case, the clinician may ask the client to repeat after him or her (Kay Elemetrics, 2003).

■ **Saving the data.** The speech data may be saved as stereo signal data in CSL signal file format (with an NSP file extension) or in wave audio file format (with a WAV file extension). The CSL signal format can only be read by the Nasometer software but the wave audio file format can be played by other computer programmes, such as Windows Media

Player and QuickTime Player. It may be convenient to save data in WAV format if the speech samples will be used in teaching or presentations. However, the quality of the playback is considered poorer as the speech signal is bandpass filtered with a low cutoff frequency of 300 Hz and high cutoff frequency at 750 Hz (Kay Elemetrics, 2003, p.3).

Calibration

The Nasometer II headset microphones should be calibrated before its first use and periodically thereafter, to ensure valid data collection and analysis (Kay Elemetrics, 2003; Kummer, 2008). Calibration is also recommended in the following situations: (1) have not used the device for some time (e.g., one month or more); (2) only connect the device every time before use; or (3) the device is moved to another location for data collection. Figure 20–4 shows the setup for calibration. The side of the headset plate that contains a notch should be inserted into the mounting bracket on the top of the Nasometer II external module, so that the two microphones are facing the calibration speaker and are equidistant from it. Place the headband of the headset directly behind the sound separation plate to reduce the effect of any sound reflections from the calibration tone during calibration. Next, set the **Line input** gain for the sound card

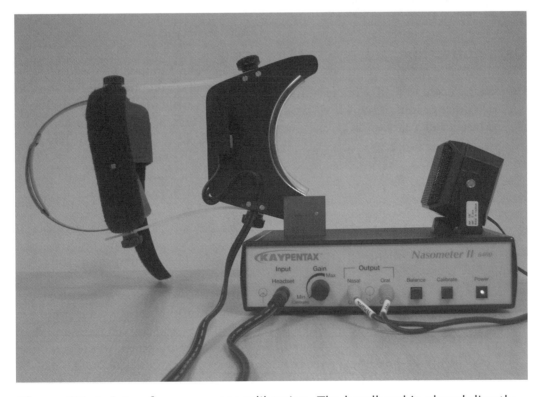

Figure 20–4. Setup for nasometer calibration. The headband is placed directly behind the sound separation plate and the Gain on the Nasometer II external module is set to minimum.

to maximum and the **Gain** on the Nasometer II external module to minimum. Switch on the external module and open the Nasometer II program. On the Toolbar of the program, click **Options** and select **Calibrate Nasometer Headset**. A blue progress meter will be shown in the application window and a message box reports "Calibrating Nasometer input audio . . . ". Press the **Calibrate** button on the external module and the speaker will produce a series of pulses directed toward the headset microphones. An Audio Calibration message box will appear after a short while and this reports the new calibration value, which will be saved and accessed by the Nasometer II program each time it is run. Press the **Calibrate** button again to turn off the pulses and close the Audio Calibration message box by clicking **OK**.

Data Collection

1. Ask the client to read over the stimuli, to familiarize him or herself with the materials before recording.

   Instructions: *"Please take a look at these sentences (or this paragraph) and let me know if you have any questions."*

2. Ask the client to read aloud the stimuli in his or her habitual voice. Tell him or her that he or she can start reading aloud the stimuli after the **Record** button at the Toolbar on the computer monitor or the **F12** key is pressed. When recording is finished, press the **space bar** to stop recording. Select **Save Signal Data** from the **File** menu, or press <Ctrl+S> keys. Make sure clients understand what

they are required to do before starting data collection.

Instructions: *"We are going to record your voice now. Please read aloud these sentences (or this paragraph) in your usual voice. You may start reading the sentences (or paragraph) after I have pressed this button. Is that clear?"*

3. Give positive reinforcement to the client and proceed to the next set of speech materials.

   Instructions: *"Very good. That is exactly what I want you to do. Now, let's look at some other sentences and I'll record your voice when you're ready."*

Data Analysis

1. To obtain the nasalance score, go to the Analyze menu on the Toolbar and select **Compute Result Statistics**, or press <Alt+S> keys. A window summarizing the statistics of the nasometric results will appear (Figure 20–5). The item, "Mean (%)," in the summary is the mean nasalance score for the entire file. The "Min (%)" and "Max (%)" are the lowest and highest values in the data, respectively.

2. It also is possible to measure the nasalance score of a selected sentence. Use the mouse to place a cursor at the start of the sentence; then press the **Shift** key and use the mouse to drag the cursor to the end of the sentence. Release the mouse click and the **Shift** key. There will be a red and blue vertical lines marking the selection (see also Figure 20–5). Press <Alt+S>

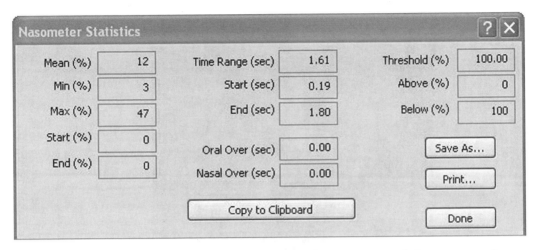

Figure 20–5. A pop-up window summarizing the statistics of the nasometric results of the nonnasal sentence shown in Figure 20–2.

to obtain the nasalance score. To remove the selection, click **View** and **Remove Selection Cursors**, or press **<Shift+Del>**.

Treatment

Decision regarding treatment should be made on the basis of the underlying cause(s) of the resonance problems. Generally speaking, speech therapy may work for clients whose resonance disorders are due to mislearning or those who show borderline or inconsistent velopharyngeal closure. Speech therapy is not appropriate if the resonance problem is due to structural defect or neuromuscular impairment (for a fuller discussion of this issue, see Kummer, 2008). In speech therapy, the Nasometer can be used as a tool for providing real-time visual feedback to help the clients to improve their resonance or to get rid of mislearned nasal emission. A green reference line can be placed on the nasogram in the data window to mark

the treatment goal for a particular session or task. For example, a short-term goal may be to achieve a mean nasalance score of less than 30% when producing nonnasal stimuli. The green reference line would be set at 30% and the client is instructed to try to achieve and maintain the nasalance contour below the reference line (see Figure 20-2). The reference line can be inserted by clicking **Options** menu and then **Select Nasometer Options . . .** ; select **Reference** and enter the target value in the Reference Cursor edit box or use the slide control to adjust the current cursor location; click **Apply** button. To make the treatment activity more interesting for children, clinicians may use the graphic reward function provided by the software (press **F8**, or select **Display Sprite** from the **Stimulus** menu) or the Nasometer games. Figure 20-6 shows one of the Nasometer games where a picture of a zoo is shown if the child can read aloud the Zoo Passage without excessive nasal resonance (again, a client-appropriate reference level can be selected by the

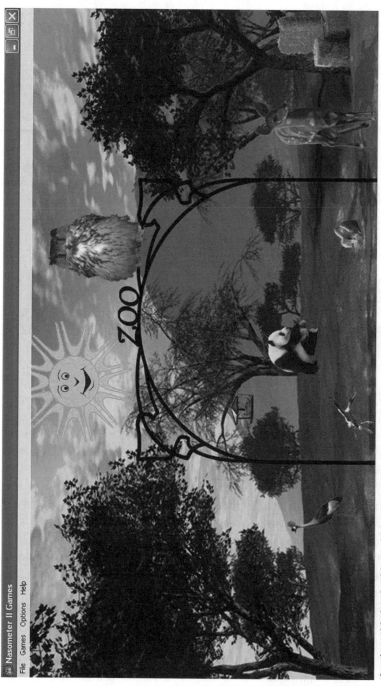

Look at this book with us. It's a story about a zoo. That is where bears go.

Today it's very cold out of doors, but we see a cloud overhead that's a pretty white fluffy shape.

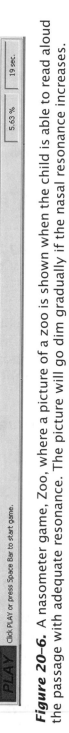

Figure 20–6. A nasometer game, Zoo, where a picture of a zoo is shown when the child is able to read aloud the passage with adequate resonance. The picture will go dim gradually if the nasal resonance increases.

clinician, on the basis of individual factors and baseline data; see Kummer, 2008). It should be noted that the current evidence regarding the Nasometer as a biofeedback tool in treatment is based on expert opinions (e.g., Kay Elemetrics, 2003; Kummer, 2008). There are few, if any, published studies on the results of speech therapy using nasometry.

NORMATIVE DATA

Normative nasalance data have been published for a number of languages; reviews or bibliographies of the findings are available from several sources, for example, Brunnegård and van Doorn (2009), Ibrahim (2009), Kummer (2008), and the KayPENTAX Web site (http://www.kayelemetrics.com). There have been numerous studies investigating the effects of language/dialect, age, and gender on nasalance scores. Overall, the findings are inconclusive (see Brunnegård & van Doorn, 2008). For example, Van Lierde, Wuyts, De Bodt, and Van Cauwenberge (2001) showed that Flemish-speaking females had significantly higher nasalance scores than male speakers on an oronasal passage (containing 11.67% nasal consonants) and a nasal passage. In contrast, Sweeney et al. (2004) reported no significant difference in nasalance scores between male and female Irish English-speaking individuals, on all stimuli. Previous studies also have reported the influence of the phonemic content of the speech stimuli on the nasalance scores. For example, speakers usually show higher nasalance scores for stimuli that are heavily loaded with high vowels (Lewis, Watterson, & Quint, 2000) and those that contain higher proportion of nasal phonemes (Watterson et al., 1996). The nasalance scores also may vary depending on the feature of voicing for consonants; there is no nasal resonance for voiceless consonants, whereas there is variable nasalance for voiced sounds (Kummer, 2008). Therefore, clinicians are advised to use the standardized speech stimuli for assessment and, if possible, to compare their clients' nasalance scores to normative scores that have been collected from control speakers of the same gender, from the same age range, using the same speech stimuli.

The normative data reported in previous studies usually include the mean, standard deviation, and range of nasalance scores, for each stimulus type and for male and/or female speakers (Table 20–1). Clinicians can compare the clients' scores to the mean, standard deviation, and range to determine if the clients' results are within normal limits, or how much the scores deviate from the mean. Various cutoff scores have been suggested to differentiate normal resonance and hypernasality (e.g., for nonnasal stimuli: 32%, Dalston, Warren, & Dalston, 1991; 26%, Hardin, Van Demark, Morris, & Payne, 1992), but there is no consensus. As general guidelines for differentiating normal resonance from hypernasality, Kummer (2008) suggested that, for nonnasal speech stimuli, nasalance scores below 20% indicate no hypernasality, scores within the range of 20 to 30% suggest borderline performance, and scores above 30% indicate excessive nasal resonance. These are in congruence with the guidelines suggested by Dalston (2004). In addition, users should also interpret the nasometric evaluation results with test-retest variability in mind. That is, a difference of 5% or less may not reflect a true or significant change or difference in resonance.

Table 20–1. Selected Normative Nasalance Scores (mean, standard deviation, and range) for Cantonese, English, and Spanish

Language	Age	Gender	N	Stimulus	Nasalance score (%) Mean	SD	Range
Cantonese[1]	18–33	Female	118	Oral sentences	16.79	5.99	8.00–38.24
			89	Nasal sentences	55.67	7.38	34.17–70.95
			117	Oral-nasal passage	35.46	6.22	19.09–54.28
English, North America[2]	16–63	Both	148	Oral passage (Zoo)	16	7	—
				Nasal sentences	62	6	—
				Oral-nasal passage (Rainbow)	36	6	—
Spanish, Puerto Rican[3]	21–43	Female	40	Oral passage	21.95	8.69	7.12–42.48
				Nasal sentences	62.07	7.77	37.51–78.71
				Oral-nasal passage	36.02	7.05	23.30–49.57

1 = Whitehill (2001); 2 = Seaver et al. (1991); see this article for the nasalance scores broken down by different geographic regions of North America; 3 = Anderson (1996).

CASE STUDY: PATIENT W.H. (REPAIRED LEFT UNILATERAL CLEFT LIP AND PALATE)

W.H. is an 11-year-old Cantonese-speaking boy with a repaired left unilateral cleft lip and palate. He had surgical repair of the lip at age 3 months and palate closure at 18 months. He was evaluated by a specialist speech-language pathologist on a multidisciplinary cleft palate team and was diagnosed as having mild hypernasality and compensatory misarticulations, characterized by glottal productions for voiced stops, fricatives, and affricates. Nasometric evaluation revealed a nasalance score of 37% for the Cantonese oral passage (Whitehill, 2001), which appeared consistent with the perceptual judgement of mild hypernasality. Speech therapy targeting the compensatory errors was given to W.H. His speech was assessed again posttherapy and the results were that his articulation was now normal but he had moderate hypernasality. A second nasometric evaluation showed a mean nasalance score of 49% for the same oral passage. He was then referred for videofluoroscopy and nasendoscopy examinations. The lateral view of videofluoroscopy showed a short velum relative to the posterior pharyngeal wall, resulting in velopharyngeal insufficiency (VPI). Both examinations showed incomplete velopharyngeal closure during pressure consonants. It is likely that W.H. had learned to use glottal productions as a strategy to attempt to reduce acoustic energy from entering the nasal cavity through the velopharyngeal gap. Thus, nasal resonance increased once the correct place of articulation was used. W.H. received secondary surgery (pharyngoplasty) for treating the VPI. Perceptual judgment, conducted 3 months postsurgery, showed adequate resonance. The nasometric evaluation showed a nasalance score of 19%, which is within normal limits, according to the normative nasalance data for Cantonese (Whitehill, 2001).

REFERENCES

Boone, D. R. (2004). G. Paul Moore Lecture: Unifying the disciplines of our voice smorgasbord. *Journal of Voice, 18*, 375–386.

Bressmann, T. (2005). Comparison of nasalance scores obtained with the Nasometer, the NasalView, and the OroNasal System. *Cleft Palate-Craniofacial Journal, 42*, 423–433.

Bressmann, T., Klaiman, P., & Fischbach, S. (2006). Same noses, different nasalance scores: Data from normal subjects and cleft palate speakers for three systems for nasalance analysis. *Clinical Linguistics and Phonetics, 20*(2–3), 163–170.

Brunnegård, K., & van Doorn, J. (2009). Normative data on nasalance scores for Swedish as measured on the Nasometer: Influence of dialect, gender, and age. *Clinical Linguistics and Phonetics, 23*(1), 58–69.

Bzoch, K. R. (2004). *Communicative disorders related to cleft lip and palate* (5th ed.). Austin, TX: Pro-Ed.

Crystal, D. (2003). *A dictionary of linguistics and phonetics*. Oxford, UK: Blackwell.

Dalston, R. M. (2004). The use of nasometry in the assessment and remediation of velopharyngeal inadequacy. In K. R. Bzoch (Ed.), *Communicative disorders related to cleft lip and palate* (5th ed., pp. 493–516). Austin, TX: Pro-Ed.

Dalston, R. M., & Warren, D. W. (1985). The diagnosis of velopharyngeal inadequacy. *Clinics in Plastic Surgery, 12*, 685–695.

Dalston, R. M., Warren, D. W., & Dalston, E. T. (1991). Use of nasometry as a diagnostic tool for identifying patients with velopharyngeal impairment. *Cleft Palate-Craniofacial Journal, 28*, 184–188; discussion 188–189.

Fairbanks, D. (1960). *Voice and articulation drill book.* New York, NY: Harper and Row.

Fletcher, S. G. (1972). Contingencies for bioelectronic modification of nasality. *Journal of Speech and Hearing Disorders, 37,* 329–346.

Fletcher, S. G. (1978). *Diagnosing speech disorders from cleft palate.* New York, NY: Grune & Stratton.

Fletcher, S. G., & Bishop, M. E. (1970). Measurement of nasality with TONAR. *Cleft Palate Journal, 7,* 610–621.

Gildersleeve-Neumann, C. E., & Dalston, R. M. (2001). Nasalance scores in noncleft individuals: Why not zero? *Cleft Palate-Craniofacial Journal, 38,* 106–111.

Hardin, M. A., Van Demark, D. R., Morris, H. L., & Payne, M. M. (1992). Correspondence between nasalance scores and listener judgments of hypernasality and hyponasality. *Cleft Palate-Craniofacial Journal, 29,* 346–351.

Ibrahim, H. M. (2009). *Nasality in the Malay language—Development of an assessment protocol for Malay-speaking children with cleft of the lip and/or palate.* Unpublished doctoral dissertation, University of Melbourne, Melbourne, Australia.

Jennings, J. J., & Kuehn, D. P. (2008). The effects of frequency range, vowel, dynamic loudness level, and gender on nasalance in amateur and classically trained singers. *Journal of Voice, 22,* 75–89.

Kay Electronics. (2003). *Nasometer II Model 6400. Installation, operations, and maintenance manual.* Lincoln Park, NJ: Kay-PENTAX.

Kent, R. D. (1999). Improving the sensitivity and reliability of auditory-perceptual assessment. *American Speech-Language-Hearing Association: Special Interest Division 5, 9*(1), 12–15.

Kent, R. D., & Read, C. (2002). *The acoustic analysis of speech* (2nd ed.). New York, NY: Singular.

Kuehn, D. P., & Dalston, R. M. (1988). Cleft palate and studies related to velopharyngeal function. In H. Winitz (Ed.), *Human communication and its disorders: A review* (Vol. 2, pp. 1–107). Norwood, NJ: Ablex.

Kuehn, D. P., & Moller, K. T. (2000). Speech and language issues in the cleft palate population: The state of the art. *Cleft Palate-Craniofacial Journal, 37,* 348–383.

Kummer, A. W. (2005). The MacKay-Kummer SNAP Test-R: Simplified nasometric assessment procedures. Available from KayPENTAX Web site: http://www.kayelemetrics.com

Kummer, A. W. (2008). *Cleft palate and craniofacial anomalies: Effects on speech and resonance* (2nd ed.). Clifton Park, NY: Delmar Cengage Learning.

Lee, A., Whitehill, T. L., & Ciocca, V. (2009). Effect of listener training on perceptual judgement of hypernasality. *Clinical Linguistics and Phonetics, 23,* 319–334.

Lewis, K. E., & Watterson, T. (2003). Comparison of nasalance scores obtained from the Nasometer and the NasalView. *Cleft Palate-Craniofacial Journal, 40,* 40–45.

Lewis, K. E., Watterson, T. L., & Houghton, S. M. (2003). The influence of listener experience and academic training on ratings of nasality. *Journal of Communication Disorders, 36,* 49–58.

Lewis, K. E., Watterson, T., & Quint, T. (2000). The effect of vowels on nasalance scores. *Cleft Palate-Craniofacial Journal, 37,* 584–589.

MacKay, I. R. A., & Kummer, A. W. (1993). Nasometric evaluation of velopharyngeal function in non-literate subjects. *Journal of the Acoustical Society of America, 93,* (4), 2337–2338.

MacKay, I. R. A., & Kummer, A. W. (1994). Simplified nasometric assessment procedures. In Kay Elemetrics Corp. (Ed.), *Instruction manual: Nasometer Model 6200-3* (pp. 123–142). Lincoln Park, NJ: Kay Elemetrics Corp.

Moll, K. L. (1964). "Objective" measures of nasality. *Cleft Palate Journal, 1,* 371–374.

Netsell, R. (1969). Evaluation of velopharyngeal function in dysarthria. *Journal of Speech and Hearing Disorders, 34,* 113–122.

Peterson-Falzone, S. J., Hardin-Jones, M. A., & Karnell, M. P. (2009). *Cleft palate speech* (4th ed.). St. Louis, MO: Mosby.

Riski, J. E., & Verdolini, K. (1999). Is hypernasality a voice disorder? *ASHA, 41*(1), 10–11.

Seaver, E. J., Dalston, R. M., Leeper, H. A., & Adams, L. E. (1991). A study of nasometric values for normal nasal resonance. *Journal of Speech and Hearing Research, 34,* 715–721.

Stevens, K. N. (2000). *Acoustic phonetics.* Cambridge, MA: M.I.T. Press.

Sweeney, T., Sell, D., & O'Regan, M. (2004). Nasalance scores for normal-speaking Irish children. *Cleft Palate-Craniofacial Journal, 41,* 168–174.

Van Lierde, K. M., Wuyts, F. L., De Bodt, M., & Van Cauwenberge, P. (2001). Nasometric values for normal nasal resonance in the speech of young Flemish adults. *Cleft Palate-Craniofacial Journal, 38,* 112–118.

Watterson, T., Hinton, J., & McFarlane, S. (1996). Novel stimuli for obtaining nasalance measures from young children. *Cleft Palate-Craniofacial Journal, 33,* 67–73.

Watterson, T., & Lewis, K. E. (2006). Test-retest nasalance score variability in hypernasal speakers. *Cleft Palate-Craniofacial Journal, 43,* 415–419.

Watterson, T., Lewis, K., & Brancamp, T. (2005). Comparison of nasalance scores obtained with the Nasometer 6200 and the Nasometer II 6400. *Cleft Palate-Craniofacial Journal, 42,* 574–579.

Whitehill, T. L. (2001). Nasalance measures in Cantonese-speaking women. *Cleft Palate-Craniofacial Journal, 38,* 119–125.

Whitehill, T. L., & Lee, A. S.-Y. (2008). Instrumental analysis of resonance in speech impairment. In M. J. Ball, M. R. Perkins, N. Müller, & S. Howard (Eds.), *Handbook of clinical linguistics* (pp. 332–343). Oxford, UK: Blackwell.

Zajac, D. J. (2008). Translating principles of speech science to clinical practice: Current and future trends in craniofacial disorders. *Perspectives on Speech Science and Orofacial Disorders, 18*(1), 31–40.

SECTION VI

Auditory-Perceptual Evaluation

CHAPTER 21

Perceptual Assessment of Voice Quality: Past, Present, and Future

JODY KREIMAN AND BRUCE R. GERRATT

PURPOSE

■ To provide a theoretical framework on perceptual voice assessment for:
  - ■ Measuring what a voice sounds like.
  - ■ Tracking changes in voice quality with treatment.
  - ■ Understanding the underlying physical problems that cause the perceived voice quality disorder.

THEORETICAL BACKGROUND

Measurement of voice quality is at the heart of clinical assessment of voice disorders. It is usually the most relevant aspect of voice to patients, who typically do not consider themselves improved until their voices sound better. Quality also is the most accessible vocal attribute, and can be assessed continuously by the patient, the clinician, or by anyone who hears the voice. Quality measures thus are ideal for documenting treatment progress and assessing treatment efficacy. In fact, they arguably are better for this purpose than other kinds of measures because they directly address the issue that led the patient to seek treatment in the first place.

It therefore is not surprising that the study of vocal quality has a very long history, dating back at least to the Romans. In the oldest and most common approach to quality measurement, a listener rates the voice of interest on a set of scales that measure the listener's auditory impressions. This approach is familiar, easy to apply, and easy to understand. As Table 21-1 shows, the scales used in such evaluation

Table 21–1. Selected Venerable and Modern Labels for Vocal Quality

Julius Pollux (Second Century AD; Austin, 1806)	Moore (1964)	Gelfer (1988)
Brassy	Brassy, metallic	Metallic
Brilliant	Brilliant, bright	Bright, vibrant
Clear	Clear, white	Clear
Deep	Deep	Resonant, low
Dull	Dull, dead	Dull
Harsh	Harsh, strident	Harsh
Shrill, sharp	Shrill, sharp	Shrill, sharp
Thin	Thin	Thin

protocols are deeply ingrained in Western culture, and have changed very little in 2000 years. Familiar terms like harsh, clear, bright, smooth, weak, shrill, deep, dull, thin, hoarse, and metallic can be found in Roman writings on oratory (Austin, 1806), and also in modern studies of voice quality (e.g., Gelfer, 1988; Karnell et al., 2007). Some differences do exist between venerable and modern descriptive terminology. For example, antique descriptive schemes included terms related to the personality and emotional state of the speaker (confused, doleful) and terms related to articulation and rhetorical ability (articulate, distinct). More modern compendia include terms like "breathy" and "nasal" that are commonly used in the study of vocal pathology. However, similarities among traditions far outweigh differences, and many labels have been in consistent use for centuries. The weight of this long tradition gives such scales a ring of truth that reinforces the widespread belief in their validity.

A number of rather similar protocols for voice evaluation based on such scales have been proposed over the years. Scales have varied slightly from instrument to instrument, but the methods are all nearly identical: A listener hears a voice sample and rates it on a set of scales for specific vocal qualities. For example, users of the CAPE-V (Consensus Auditory-Perceptual Evaluation–Voice) protocol (Kempster, Gerratt, Verdolini Abbott, Barkmeier-Kraemer, & Hillman, 2009; Figure 21–1) rate voices on visual analog scales for overall severity, roughness, breathiness, strain, pitch, and loudness, and on any additional scales the clinician may wish to add. The GRBAS protocol (Isshiki, Okamura, Tanabe, & Morimoto, 1969) assesses voices on scales for essentially the same qualities (grade [equivalent to overall severity], roughness, breathiness, asthenicity [weakness], and strain), but uses four-point scales instead of marks on a line. The Stockholm Voice Evaluation Consensus Model, or SVEC (Hammarberg, 1997), includes judgments

---

Consensus Auditory-Perceptual Evaluation of Voice (CAPE-V)

Name:_____   Date:_____

The following parameters of voice quality will be rated upon completion of the following tasks:
1. Sustained vowels, /a/ and /i/ for 3-5 seconds duration each.
2. Sentence production:
    a.   The blue spot is on the key again.
    b.   How hard did he hit him?
    c.   We were away a year ago.
    d.   We eat eggs every Easter.
    e.   My mama makes lemon muffins.
    f.   Peter will keep at the peak.
3. Spontaneous speech in response to: "Tell me about your voice problem." or "Tell me how your voice is functioning."

> Legend: C = Consistent   I = Intermittent
> MI = Mildly Deviant
> MO = Moderately Deviant
> SE = Severely Deviant

SCORE

Overall Severity _____ C   I   ____/100
                    MI   MO   SE

Roughness _____ C   I   ____/100
             MI   MO   SE

Breathiness _____ C   I   ____/100
               MI   MO   SE

Strain _____ C   I   ____/100
          MI   MO   SE

Pitch   (Indicate the nature of the abnormality): _____
          _____ C   I   ____/100
             MI   MO   SE

Loudness   (Indicate the nature of the abnormality): _____
             _____ C   I   ____/100
                MI   MO   SE

_____   _____ C   I   ____/100
             MI   MO   SE

_____   _____ C   I   ____/100
             MI   MO   SE

COMMENTS ABOUT RESONANCE: NORMAL   OTHER (Provide description):_____
_____

ADDITIONAL FEATURES (for example, diplophonia, fry, falsetto, asthenia, aphonia, pitch instability, tremor, wet/gurgly, or other relevant terms):

Figure 21–1. The CAPE-V assessment protocol (Kempster et al., 2009).

of roughness and breathiness, but discards grade, asthenicity, and strain in favor of aphonia, tenseness, laxness, creakiness, grating, instability, voice breaks, and diplophonia. The superficial similarity of these different assessment tools is undermined somewhat by differences in the meaning given to the different scales in the different systems. For example, in the GRBAS protocol, breathiness is defined as a dry, hard, excited, pointed, cold, choked, rough, cloudy, sharp, poor, and bad vocal quality (Isshiki et al., 1969), whereas in the Stockholm consensus model, breathiness is associated with wheezing, lack of timbre, moments of aphonia, huskiness, and lack of creak (Hammarberg, Fritzell, Gauffin, Sundberg, & Wedin, 1980). However, few clinicians are aware of these differences in the psychometrics underlying various rating instruments, without which the protocols are very similar indeed to the scales described in the second century AD by Julius Pollux.

The resemblances among voice assessment protocols and the lack of change over decades have sometimes created the impression that the major issues surrounding quality measurement have been solved, and that clinicians and researchers have agreed on the best way to measure quality in the clinic. Use of the name "consensus model" in the Stockholm and CAPE-V protocols enhances this impression. However, this apparent agreement also can be viewed as a failure to move beyond the familiar descriptive framework provided by the ancients. By conducting research using terminology and concepts derived from tradition and not from a theory or model of voice quality, users are left with no basis for answering some rather fundamental questions governing the selection and interpretation of scales. For example, which scales should be included (or excluded) and why? How are scales related to underlying acoustic variables, and what is the relationship of one scale to the others (correlated? independent? interacting?). Behind these issues lurks the larger problem of the ontologic status of a protocol for assessing voice quality.

Rating scale protocols for quality assessment have never been based on a model of voice quality, and because the construct being measured is not well defined, it is not possible to determine that a given set of scales or acoustic measurements is the "correct" one for measuring it. This fundamental problem of validity, what we are really measuring, and why, has continuously plagued attempts to make clinically meaningful measures of voice quality; but without a clear delimitation of the thing being measured, this problem will never be solved because it is impossible to determine that any proposed scale or set of scales is either necessary or sufficient.

One solution to this problem may lie in the American National Standards Institute (ANSI) definition of quality as those attributes of a sound other than its pitch and loudness that allow a listener to judge that two sounds are the same or different (ANSI, 1960). This definition implies that the goal of a quality assessment protocol is to quantify not a set of specific vocal attributes, but instead the complete sound of a voice, the speaker's integral, overall, personal vocal quality. By applying this definition, it becomes possible to evaluate the adequacy of a quality assessment tool: To the extent that a set of ratings or acoustic measures combine with measures of pitch and loudness to precisely specify the overall, integral quality of the target stimuli (and not just a subset of specific features), that assessment protocol is a valid measure of quality. Existing rating scale protocols cannot meet this standard. A set of GRBAS or CAPE-V ratings (or any other set of ratings) gives users no idea whatsoever about the personal quality of the voice being measured (nor were they intended to). Because the thing being measured is unspecified in such protocols, it is difficult to imagine how this limitation can be overcome without abandoning rating scales altogether in favor of a different measurement approach targeting overall quality, as advocated in this chapter.

One attempt to apply a more theoretically motivated approach to quality assessment resulted in Voice Profile Analysis (e.g., Laver, Wirz, Mackenzie, & Hiller, 1981), which translates the problem of measuring quality from the perceptual into the physical realm. In Voice Profile Analysis, features for voice quality are defined in terms of the manner in which the sound was produced, resulting in features for labial configuration, jaw position, velopharyngeal function, laryngeal mode, and so on (Figure 21–2). By describing voice production in terms specified by phonetic theory, this analysis produces a kind of recipe for the resultant sound quality.

	FIRST PASS		SECOND PASS						
	Neutral	Non-neutral	SETTING	moderate			extreme		
				1	2	3	4	5	6
A. VOCAL TRACT FEATURES									
1. Labial			Lip rounding/protrusion						
			Lip spreading						
			Labiodentalization						
			Minimised range						
			Extensive range						
2. Mandibular			Close jaw						
			Open jaw						
			Protruded jaw						
			Extensive range						
			Minimised range						
3. Lingual tip/blade			Advanced tip/blade						
			Retracted tip/blade						
4. Lingual body			Fronted tongue body						
			Backed tongue body						
			Raised tongue body						
			Lowered tongue body						
			Extensive range						
			Minimised range						
5. Pharyngeal			Pharyngeal constriction						
			Pharyngeal expansion						
6. Velopharyngeal			Audible nasal escape						
			Nasal						
			Denasal						
7. Larynx height			Raised Larynx						
			Lowered Larynx						
B. OVERALL MUSCULAR TENSION									
8. Vocal tract tension			Tense vocal tract						
9. Laryngeal tension			Tense larynx						
			Lax larynx						
C. PHONATION FEATURES									

		Present		Scalar Degree					
	SETTING	Neutral	Non-neutral	Moderate			Extreme		
				1	2	3	4	5	6
10. Voicing type	Voice								
	Falsetto								
	Creak								
	Creaky								
11. Laryngeal frication	Whisper								
	Whispery								
12. Laryngeal irregularity	Harsh								
	Tremor								

Figure 21–2. Laver's Voice Profile Analysis (Laver et al., 1981). *continues*

			Neutral	SETTING	moderate			extreme		
					1	2	3	4	5	6
D. PROSODIC FEATURES										
13.Pitch	Mean			High						
				Low						
	Range			Minimised range						
				Extensive range						
	Variability			High						
				Low						
14. Loudness	Mean			High						
				Low						
	Range			Extensive range						
				Minimised range						
	Variability			High						
				Low						
E. TEMPORAL ORGANIZATION										
15. Continuity				Interrupted						
16. Rate				Fast						
				Slow						
F. OTHER FEATURES										
17. Respiratory support				Adequate						
				Inadequate						
18. Dyplophonia				Absent						
				Present						

Figure 21–2. *continued*

Unfortunately, comprehensiveness in terms of describing voice production does not translate easily into a psychoacoustic model of the necessary and sufficient set of scales for quality assessment, because a production model does not predict what features are perceptually salient under which circumstances. In other words, voice profile analysis specifies where information about quality *might* be, but does not actually model listeners' behavior. The system works as a model of quality only with the added assumptions that each included physiologic parameter is perceptually significant, and that listeners can separate the different scales perceptually. However, evidence against both these assumptions exists (see Kreiman, Vanlancker-Sidtis, & Gerratt, 2005, for review).

An additional lingering, long-standing problem is the issue of rating reliability in quality assessment protocols. Scale reliability in the traditional statistical sense has very little meaning in clinical settings because it measures the likelihood that a new random sample of raters would produce the same mean rating as the group studied, averaged across all the voices studied. This is seldom what we want to know in the clinic or the lab, where the interesting question is the likelihood that two individual raters will produce the same rating for a given voice sample: the probability of listener agreement. These two approaches are quite different from each other and therefore can lead to very different conclusions about reliability. Table 21–2 compares values of conventional reliability statistics (the commonly-used intraclass correlation and Cronbach's alpha) to the likelihood that two raters will agree exactly in their ratings of a voice, for three different sets of published data. Table 21–2 shows that, even when conventional reliability statistics suggest data sets are completely reliable, the like-

Table 21-2. Interlistener Reliability and Agreement for Three Previously Published Data Sets

Traditional Reliability Statistics	Probability of Exact Agreement Between Two Listeners	Reference
Intraclass correlation = 0.99 α = 0.99	p (exact) = 0.32	Kreiman et al. (1993)
Intraclass correlation = 0.93 α = 0.97	p (exact) = 0.21	Kreiman et al. (1994)
Intraclass correlation = 0.89 α = 0.90	p (exact) = 0.26	Kreiman & Gerratt (1996)

lihood of listener agreement can still be very poor, sometimes failing to reach even chance levels in the midrange of the rating scale (Kreiman & Gerratt, 1998), arguably the range of voice quality deviation most commonly seen in the clinic.

Clinicians and researchers have suggested a number of solutions to the "unreliable rater" problem, implying that listeners' unreliable auditory perceptual systems are the inherent causes of poor listener agreement for voice quality judgments. One of these (proposed by Shrivastav, Sapienza, & Nandur, 2005) involves averaging ratings to achieve a reliable mean, based on the assumption that rating variability across and within raters is mostly random. We present evidence below that challenges this assumption. Other proposed statistical approaches include assessing reliability using rank-order correlations for four raters on one out of four scales (Karnell et al., 2007), Pearson's *r* or kappa (Maryn, Corthals, van Cauwenberge, Roy, & de Bodt, 2010), or by measuring correlations among average ratings (Shrivastav & Camacho, 2010). These approaches based on correlation can indicate that different listeners tend to give scores of similar rela-

tive magnitude to the stimuli, but do not reflect the extent to which absolute scores are comparable (so that good "reliability" scores may occur when one listener hears all stimuli as severely pathologic, whereas another hears them all as mildly deviant). Other researchers have suggested training listeners to increase the extent to which they share common standards for different qualities (e.g., Chan & Yiu, 2006; Shewell, 1998); using fewer scale values, as the GRBAS protocol does (which increases agreement but also increases the likelihood of chance agreement (e.g., De Bodt, Wuyts, Van de Heyning, & Croux, 1997; Webb et al., 2004); and applying anchored protocols with comparison stimuli to which the target voices are compared (thereby, hypothetically, reducing reliance on internal standards for different qualities) (e.g., Awan & Lawson, 2008; Chan & Yiu, 2002; Gerratt, Kreiman, Antoñanzas-Barroso, & Berke, 1993). Some authors also have suggested giving up and simply asking patients about satisfaction with their voices or voice-related quality of life, without attempting a detailed or quantitative assessment of quality (e.g., Hogikyan & Sethuraman, 1999; Hogikyan, Wodchis,

Terrell, Bradford, & Esclamado, 2000; see Franco & Andrus, 2009, who argue that patient surveys may be superior to other methods of evaluating surgical outcomes). This last approach is useful in that it helps clinicians to gauge the overall success of a treatment approach; but satisfaction ratings do not provide insight into why the treatment succeeds or fails with individual patients or about which physical changes actually modified the resultant sound.

Another popular solution to the problem of rater (un)reliability is to substitute aerodynamic, electroglottographic, or especially acoustic measures of vocal signals for subjective assessments of voice quality. These approaches are discussed elsewhere in this book. Knowledge of what physical and acoustic changes actually cause which variations in quality (and vice versa) would provide a basis for analysis protocols that help clinicians understand the reasons for success and failure in clinical cases, greatly enhancing their ability to focus and evaluate treatment. Current protocols do not meet this standard, again because they are not linked to any model of vocal quality so that changes in a measure are not easily understood in terms of changes in the sound of the voice. Briefly, systems for making acoustic measures of voice include the Dysphonia Severity Index (Wuyts et al., 2000), the Hoarseness Diagram (Frohlich, Michaelis, Strube, & Kruse, 2000), and the Multi-Dimensional Voice Program (MDVP; Kay Elemetrics, 1993). These systems are popular, presumably because the acoustic signal evokes a listener's perception of voice quality. However, despite occasional findings of moderate to high correlations among some acoustic measures and quality labels, the perceptual salience of the parameters measured is most often unknown, or is known to be very limited; for example,

listeners apparently are quite insensitive to changes in jitter and shimmer (Kreiman & Gerratt, 2005). In contrast, many classic psychoacoustic studies underlie our understanding of how changes in intensity and fundamental frequency (and other factors) form our impressions of loudness and pitch (see, e.g., Gescheider, 1985; or Fastl & Zwicker, 2007, for review). Virtually no such psychometric work has been undertaken to establish the relationship between voice quality and acoustic measures like (to name a few) cepstral peak prominence (Hillenbrand, Cleveland, & Erikson, 1994), amplitude differences between the first harmonic and the first or second formant (H1-A1 or H1-A2; Hanson, 1997), or the soft phonation index (Roussel & Lobdell, 2006), other than reports of varying correlations between an acoustic measure and some voice quality. Just as loudness and pitch do not exist without the listener, vocal quality is an acoustic-*perceptual* phenomenon, and we cannot evaluate the usefulness of an instrumental measure of quality without assessing quality as part of that process. For this reason, objective voice analyses do not solve the problem of rater unreliability or rating scale insufficiency, but rather introduce new questions about their own validity because their status as measurements of quality perception derives solely from correlations rather than actual psychoacoustic evidence.

In contrast to these approaches, we envision modeling quality psychoacoustically as a set of acoustic parameters that combine nonredundantly to capture the complete voice pattern, the way a person sounds. To derive such a model, we first must develop a reliable and valid method of measuring listeners' perceptions as we manipulate acoustic parameters to establish valid links between vocal acoustics and perceived quality. Instead of attempting to average away listener disagreement, we must find the sources of variability in listeners' judgments of quality in rating protocols, to guide development of alternative measurement tasks that are specifically designed to facilitate agreement among listeners.

We have made progress on this front in recent years. The literature provides evidence for four factors that introduce variability into measurements of quality: instability of internal standards for different qualities; difficulties isolating individual attributes in complex acoustic voice patterns; measurement scale resolution; and the magnitude of the attribute being measured (see Kreiman, Gerratt, & Ito, 2007, for review). To determine the extent to which these factors can explain listener variability, we manipulated four experimental factors corresponding to the four theoretical factors (Table 21–3; Kreiman et al., 2007). Our hypotheses were straightforward: These factors should account for most of the variability in agreement levels and listeners should agree best when all factors are controlled and worst when nothing is controlled.

Results indicated that these four factors accounted for 84.2% of the variance in the likelihood that listeners would agree exactly in their ratings. As hypothesized, the probability that any two raters will agree exactly in their ratings of a voice was nearly perfect (96% exact agreement) when all factors were controlled. The most important of the theoretical factors responsible for this level of agreement was the ease or difficulty of isolating a dimension in a complex pattern (the pathologic voice), represented in the experiment by use of matched versus unmatched anchor stimuli. When anchor stimuli acoustically matched the target voices except for the dimension of interest, rater agreement more than doubled. Interestingly, providing listeners with anchors that did not match the target stimuli resulted in worse agreement than did rating voices without any anchors at all (Table 21–4). These findings indicate that listeners can more accurately assess an acoustic attribute of a voice pattern in the context of the pattern itself. The findings also suggest that an ideal quality assessment protocol would: (1) not depend on selection/definition of labels for quality dimensions; (2) avoid

Table 21–3. Source of Rater Variability in Perceptual Voice Evaluation

Theoretical Source of Rater Variability	*Experimental Factor*
Instability of internal standards for different qualities	Presence or absence of comparison stimuli
Difficulties isolating individual attributes in complex acoustic voice patterns	Matched versus unmatched comparison stimuli
Measurement scale resolution	Visual analog scale versus 6-point scale
The magnitude of the attribute being measured	The mean rating for the voice

Table 21–4. The Average Probability of Exact Agreement Between Two Listeners in Six Different Experimental Conditions. (Standard deviations are listed in parentheses)

Comparison Stimulus Condition	Continuous Scale	Six-Point Scale
Custom comparison stimuli	0.96 (0.12)	0.63 (0.13)
Generic comparison stimuli	0.42 (0.11)	0.28 (0.08)
No comparison stimuli	0.53 (0.14)	0.30 (0.14)

Source: Data from Kreiman et al., 2007.

reliance on internal standards and help listeners focus attention; and (3) have fine scale resolution.

An analysis-by-synthesis approach to measuring quality meets these criteria. In this approach, listeners assess voice quality by adjusting the parameters of a speech synthesizer until the synthetic voice sample they create exactly matches the natural target voice being modeled. This approach does not depend on selection or definition of labels for quality dimensions, because quality is modeled as an integral pattern. The method also avoids reliance on internal standards for qualities because listeners perceptually compare the natural token to the synthetic copy while they manipulate acoustic parameters. At the same time, the technique helps listeners focus attention on specific acoustic dimensions: When listeners adjust an acoustic parameter, they can hear the result of the change immediately, and being able to hear ongoing quality changes in this manner brings the dimension under study to the foreground (in the same way that a camouflaged object or animal becomes visible when it moves). Scale resolution in the synthesizer can be matched to listeners' sensitivity to individual parameters. Finally, this method demonstrates actual causation between acoustic attributes and the perceived quality they evoke, avoiding correlative techniques. By controlling the sources of variability in quality assessment, the analysis-by-synthesis approach provides a tool for measuring quality reliably and validly.

In practice, this tool may not be easily translated into a practical clinical application, but it does facilitate assessment of the perceptual importance of putative acoustic antecedents of voice quality. By determining which parameters evoke perceptible changes, we can identify a set of acoustic measures of voice quality that are perceptually valid, in the same way that the decibel is a perceptually valid acoustic measure of sound intensity by virtue of its well-defined relationship to perceived loudness. Using this process, we can ultimately derive a truly psychoacoustic model of voice quality that specifies a set of acoustic measures that combine to quantify the sound of an individual voice (and not just the magnitude of certain attributes). Such a model could eliminate the need for subjective quality measures (including verbal scale ratings) because the perceptual importance of each acoustic parameter can be established; interactions among parameters can be modeled; and the composite set of parameters can be selected to specify voice quality. In other words, in the context of a model of quality, the parameters are not arbitrary; they are not redundant; and they are all perceptually valid.

Thus, our studies suggest that rater variability is not random, but largely predictable and therefore avoidable using suitable measurement instruments. This should not be surprising when we consider the long evolutionary history of voice use and the wide range of communicative functions subserved by voice quality (expression and perception of age, sex, reproductive status, personal identity, emotional status, and so on, in birds, reptiles, and a huge array of other vertebrate species; see Kreiman & Sidtis, 2011, for extended review). In this broader context, it seems counterintuitive that perceptual systems would incorporate large amounts of random variability (consistent with near-chance levels of interrater agreement) and that the important cognitive processes involved in voice perception would vary widely across individuals. Such large-scale variability would undermine the communicative efficiency of a signaling system with deep evolutionary roots, one that has contributed to the success of many species. It seems far more likely that the poor reliability and agreement levels observed in past rating studies are a product of the protocols themselves rather than of inherent differences in listeners' perceptual and cognitive functions (although learning can influence perception; see, e.g., Krishnan, Xu, Gandour, & Cariani, 2005, for discussion of neuroplastic effects of language learning on auditory perception). It then follows that future voice studies should focus on developing an overall model of voice quality that leads to valid measures resulting in good agreement levels, as suggested earlier in this chapter.

FUTURE DEVELOPMENT: TOWARD A COMPREHENSIVE THEORY OF VOICE

How might one go about deriving such a measurement instrument? If we assume that listeners pay more attention to attributes that vary substantially from voice to voice than to those that remain relatively constant, we can begin by first identifying acoustic attributes that best differentiate voices, and then testing the perceptual significance of these parameters. When we have identified a set of parameters for which listeners can hear small differences in a variety of contexts, we can apply speech synthesis to determine whether those parameters, plus pitch and loudness, are adequate to capture the quality of an individual's voice. Through iterations of this process, we can identify parameters that are redundant or that interact with each other perceptually. For example, the perceptual importance of spectral noise depends on the amount of harmonic energy present in the higher part of the spectrum: the more harmonic energy is present, the more change in inharmonic energy is needed before listeners can hear a difference (Gerratt & Kreiman, 2001, Shrivastav et al., 2005). Thus, a perceptually valid scale for spectral noise levels will need to correct for this interaction, in the same way that measures of loudness correct for perceptual interactions with frequency via "equal loudness" curves (Fletcher, 1934).

The ultimate goal of these psychoacoustic modeling efforts is a small set of acoustic parameters that are necessary and sufficient to precisely reproduce the overall, integral quality of voices and are therefore suitable to evaluate changes in voice quality in the clinic. Such measures would constitute a valid assessment tool because they are objective measures whose relationship to quality is understood theoretically and whose relevance to quality is demonstrated unequivocally by psychoacoustic evidence. This would allow clinicians to interpret changes in these acoustic measures in terms of their associated perceptual analog, in the same way that the sone relates loudness and sound intensity (Stevens, 1936) and the mel relates acoustic frequency and perceived pitch (Stevens, Volkmann, & Newman, 1937). Once this goal is achieved, we can consider the even more ambitious goal of a comprehensive theory of voice that relates changes in vocal physiology to the resultant changes in voice quality, and conversely maps changes in quality to the physical changes that caused them. Such a model would provide a theoretical basis for clinical assessment because it would specify causal links from laryngeal physiology, to voice acoustics, to quality, and back. We submit that development of such a comprehensive theory should be the primary goal of voice research.

In conclusion, the last 2000 years have produced awareness and descriptions of the importance of voice and its uses, but previous work has not led to very much theoretical understanding of the "whys" of quality. This has resulted in virtually no foundation of psychoacoustic evidence for the development or validation of measurement techniques. Voice quality has never been studied as part of a broader theory that encompasses the whole speech chain, so we cannot predict changes in the sound of a voice with changes in vocal fold vibrations, or interpret a change in the sound of a voice when one occurs. However, we may be nearing a solution to the long-term problem of generating reliable and valid measures of voice, whose derivation will make it possible to address other critical, basic questions that await our attention in the future.

Acknowledgments. A preliminary version of this paper was presented at the 2009 American Speech-Language-Hearing Association annual convention. The research described was supported by grant DC01797 from the National Institutes on Deafness and Other Communication Disorders.

REFERENCES

ANSI. (1960). *Acoustical terminology. ANSI S1.1.12.9.* New York, NY: Author.

Austin, G. (1806). *Chironomia*. London, UK: Cadell and Davies. Reprinted by Southern Illinois University Press, Carbondale, IL, 1966.

Awan, S. N., & Lawson, L. L. (2008). The effect of anchor modality on the reliability of vocal severity ratings. *Journal of Voice, 23,* 341–352.

Chan, K. M.-K., & Yiu, E. M.-L. (2002). The effect of anchors and training on the reliability of perceptual voice evaluation. *Journal of Speech, Language, and Hearing Research, 45,* 111–126.

Chan, K. M.-K., & Yiu, E. M.-L. (2006). A comparison of two perceptual voice evaluation training programs for naïve listeners. *Journal of Voice, 20,* 229–241.

De Bodt, M. S., Wuyts, F. L., Van de Heyning, P. H., & Croux, C. (1997). Test-retest study of the GRBAS scale: Influence of experience and professional background on perceptual rating of voice quality. *Journal of Voice, 11,* 74–80.

Fastl, H., & Zwicker, E. (2007). *Psychoacoustics: Facts and models* (3rd ed.). Berlin, Germany: Springer-Verlag.

Fletcher, H. (1934). Loudness, pitch, and the timbre of musical tones and their relation to the intensity, the frequency, and the overtone structure. *Journal of the Acoustical Society of America, 6,* 59-69.

Franco, R. A., & Andrus, J. G. (2009). Aerodynamic and acoustic characteristics of voice before and after adduction arytenopexy and medialization laryngoplasty with Gore-Tex in patients with unilateral vocal fold immobility. *Journal of Voice, 23,* 261-267.

Frohlich, M., Michaelis, D., Strube, H. W., & Kruse, E. (2000). Acoustic voice analysis by means of the hoarseness diagram. *Journal of Speech, Language, and Hearing Research, 43,* 706-720.

Gelfer, M. P. (1988). Perceptual attributes of voice: Development and use of rating scales. *Journal of Voice, 2,* 320-326.

Gerratt, B. R., Kreiman, J., Antoñanzas-Barroso, N., & Berke, G. S. (1993). Comparing internal and external standards in voice quality judgments. *Journal of Speech and Hearing Research, 36,* 14-20.

Gescheider, G. A. (1985). *Psychophysics: Method, theory, and application.* Hillsdale, NJ: Lawrence Erlbaum Associates.

Hammarberg, B. (1997). Perceptual evaluation of dysphonic voices. In *Proceedings of larynx '97.* Marseille, France, June 16-18, pp. 11-18.

Hammarberg, B., Fritzell, B., Gauffin, J., Sundberg, J., & Wedin, L. (1980). Perceptual and acoustic correlates of abnormal voice qualities. *Acta Otolaryngologica (Stockholm), 90,* 441-451.

Hanson, H. M. (1997). Glottal characteristics of female speakers: Acoustic correlates. *Journal of the Acoustical Society of America, 101,* 466-481.

Hillenbrand, J., Cleveland, R. A., & Erickson, R. L. (1994). Acoustic correlates of breathy vocal quality. *Journal of Speech and Hearing Research, 37,* 769-778.

Hogikyan, N. D. & Sethuraman, G. (1999). Validation of an instrument to measure voice-related quality of life (V-RQOL). *Journal of Voice, 13,* 557-569.

Hogikyan, N. D., Wodchis, W. P., Terrell, J. E., Bradford, C. R., & Esclamado, R. M. (2000). Voice-related quality of life (V-RQOL) following type I thyroplasty for unilateral vocal fold paralysis. *Journal of Voice, 14,* 378-386.

Isshiki, N., Okamura, H., Tanabe, M., & Morimoto, M. (1969). Differential diagnosis of hoarseness. *Folia Phoniatrica, 21,* 9-19.

Karnell, M. P., Melton, S. D., Childes, J. M., Coleman, T. C., Dailey, S. A., & Hoffman, H. T. (2007). Reliability of clinician-based (GRBAS and CAPE-V) and patient-based (V-RQOL and IPVI) documentation of voice disorders. *Journal of Voice, 21,* 576-590.

Kay Elemetrics. (1993). Multi-Dimensional Voice Program (MDVP). [Computer program]. Pine Brook, NJ: Author.

Kempster, G. B., Gerratt, B. R., Verdolini Abbott, K., Barkmeier-Kraemer, J., & Hillman, R. E. (2009). Consensus auditory-perceptual evaluation of voice: Development of a standardized clinical protocol. *American Journal of Speech Language Pathology, 18,* 124-132.

Kreiman, J., & Gerratt, B. R. (1996). The perceptual structure of pathologic voice quality. *Journal of the Acoustical Society of America, 100,* 1787-1795.

Kreiman, J., & Gerratt, B. R. (1998). Validity of rating scale measures of voice quality. *Journal of the Acoustical Society of America, 104,* 1598-1608.

Kreiman, J., & Gerratt, B. R. (2005). Perception of aperiodicity in pathological voice. *Journal of the Acoustical Society of America, 117,* 2201-2211.

Kreiman, J., Gerratt, B. R., & Berke, G. S. (1994). The multidimensional nature of pathologic vocal quality. *Journal of the Acoustical Society of America, 96,* 1291-1302.

Kreiman, J., Gerratt, B. R., & Ito, M. (2007). When and why listeners disagree in voice quality assessment tasks. *Journal of the Acoustical Society of America, 122,* 2354-2364.

Kreiman, J., Gerratt, B. R., Kempster, G. B., Erman, A., & Berke, G. S. (1993). Perceptual evaluation of voice quality: Review, tutorial, and a framework for future research. *Journal of Speech and Hearing Research, 36,* 21-40.

Kreiman, J., & Sidtis, D. (2011). *Foundations of voice studies: An interdisciplinary approach to voice production and perception*. Boston, MA: Wiley-Blackwell.

Kreiman, J., Vanlancker-Sidtis, D., & Gerratt, B. R. (2005). Perception of voice quality. In D. B. Pisoni & R. E. Remez (Eds.), *Handbook of speech perception* (pp. 338-362). Walden, MA: Blackwell.

Krishnan, A., Xu, Y., Gandour, J., & Cariani, P. (2005). Encoding of pitch in the human brainstem is sensitive to language experience. *Cognitive Brain Research, 25*, 161-168.

Laver, J., Wirz, S., Mackenzie, J., & Hiller, S. M. (1981). A perceptual protocol for the analysis of vocal profiles. *Edinburgh University Department of Linguistics Work in Progress, 14*, 265-280.

Maryn, Y., Corthals, P., van Cauwenberge, P., Roy, N., & de Bodt, M. (2010). Toward improved ecological validity in the acoustic measurement of overall voice quality: Combining continuous speech and sustained vowels. *Journal of Voice, 24*, 540-555.

Moore, P. (1964). *Organic voice disorders*. Englewood Cliffs, NJ: Prentice-Hall.

Roussel, N. C., & Lobdell, M. (2006). The clinical utility of the soft phonation index. *Clinical Linguistics and Phonetics, 20*, 181-186.

Shewell, C. (1998). The effect of perceptual training on ability to use the Vocal Profile Analysis scheme. *International Journal of Language and Communication Disorders, 33*, 322-326.

Shrivastav, R., & Camacho, A. (2010). A computational model to predict changes in breathiness resulting from variations in aspiration noise level. *Journal of Voice, 24*, 395-405.

Shrivastav, R., Sapienza, C. M, & Nandur, V. (2005). Application of psychometric theory to the measurement of voice quality using rating scales. *Journal of Speech, Language, and Hearing Research, 48*, 323-335.

Stevens, S. S. (1936). A scale for the measurement of a psychological magnitude: Loudness. *Psychological Review, 43*, 405-416.

Stevens, S. S., Volkmann, J., & Newman, E. B. (2007). A scale for the measurement of the psychological magnitude pitch. *Journal of the Acoustical Society of America, 8*, 185-190.

Webb, A. L., Carding, P. N., Deary, I. J., MacKenzie, K., Steen, N., & Wilson, J. A. (2004). The reliability of three perceptual evaluation scales for dysphonia. *European Archives of Oto-Rhino-Laryngology, 261*, 429-434.

Wuyts, F. L., De Bodt, M. S., Molenberghs, G., Remacle, M., Heylen, L., Millet, B., . . . Van de Heyning, P. H. (2000). The dysphonia severity index: An objective measure of vocal quality based on a mutiparameter approach. *Journal of Speech, Language, and Hearing Research, 43*, 796-809.

CHAPTER 22

Evaluating Voice Quality

RAHUL SHRIVASTAV

PURPOSE

■ To assess an individual's voice quality during phonation and/ or speech.

THEORETICAL BACKGROUND

Voice disorders frequently result in changes to voice quality. Based on the American National Standards Institute (ANSI) definition of sound quality (ANSI, 1960) and the description by Titze (1994), voice quality may be described to include all attributes that serve to distinguish two voices with identical pitch, loudness, and phonetic category from each other. A change in voice quality is often the most noticeable symptom of a voice disorder and its remediation frequently is a major objective of voice treatment. For these reasons, clinical measurement of voice quality has been the focus of considerable research over the past few decades. Although significant progress has been made, an accurate, easy to implement, and universally accepted measurement scheme to quantify voice quality remains elusive. The following discussion summarizes some theoretical issues related to voice quality measurement, contemporary practices and their limitations, and some suggestions regarding measurement of voice quality in research and clinic.

More than 300 different terms have been identified to describe voice quality in speakers (Pannbacker, 1984). However, only a few of these, such as "breathiness," "roughness," and "strained" have received wide acceptance as being major subtypes of dysphonic voice quality. Some research into perceptual classification of dysphonic voice quality, such as using factor analyses (Isshiki & Takeuchi, 1970; Takahashi & Koike, 1976) further supports a three- to four-dimensional solution for dysphonic voice quality. A few other perceptual attributes, such as "pitch" or "regularity," often are critical parts of voice evaluation, but are not always considered voice *quality* per se. However, recent experimentation has shown that factors such as pitch may play a critical role in the perception of voice quality (Shrivastav & Camacho, 2010) and it is difficult to isolate the perception of vocal quality from other perceptual attributes of voice.

Evaluation of voice quality may take one of two broad approaches. First, voice quality may be measured "subjectively," where one or more listeners assign a score to the voice(s) being measured. Second, voice quality may be measured "objectively," in which a specific algorithm is applied to quantify certain aspects of a correlate of vocal production, such as the vocal acoustic signal, the inverse-filtered oral airflow signal (or its derivative), or the electroglottographic signal. Certain approaches, sometimes referred to as "multiparametric approaches" may use a combination of objective measures to generate a single parameter reflecting changes in voice quality. Some like the Dysphonia Severity Index (Wuyts et al., 2000) are based on regression functions computed from a variety of objective measures from a large number of patients, whereas others such as those described by Rihkanen, Leinonen, Hiltunen, and Kangas (1994) and Ritchings, McGillion, and Moore (2002) have applied more advanced signal processing and pattern recognition techniques for the same purpose.

Subjective approaches are probably the oldest method to quantify voice quality. As the name implies, this approach requires a judge (often the clinician) to listen to a client's voice and assign it a score that reflects his or her judgment of the voice. These judgments usually are assigned on a three- to seven-point rating scale to indicate gradations in voice quality. More recent recommendations, such as the Consensus Auditory Perceptual Evaluation of Voice (CAPE-V; Kempster, Gerratt, Verdolini Abbott, Barkmeier-Kraemer, & Hillman, 2009) favor the use of a "visual-analog" scale, where a continuous line may be used to obtain a finer gradation of voice quality changes. A number of authors have published formal tools for perceptual evaluation of voice (Andrews & Summers, 2002; Boone, McFarlane, & Von Berg, 2005; Hirano, 1981; Wilson, 1987), and some such as the GRBAS and CAPE-V have been used in a fairly large number of clinics worldwide. Another variation of rating scales is to use predetermined "anchors" that highlight a typical voice quality magnitude for one or more units on that scale (Eadie & Baylor, 2006; Gerratt, Kreiman, Antonanzas-Barroso, & Berke, 1993; Yiu, Murdoch, Hird, & Lau, 2002). Some other approaches, such as direct magnitude estimation or matching, sometimes have been used for research (Eadie & Doyle, 2002; Hillenbrand, Cleveland, & Erickson, 1994; Patel, Shrivastav, & Eddins, 2006) but have found limited utility in clinical practice. Subjective approaches are popular because they have relatively high construct validity, are easy and inexpensive to implement, and require minimal time and effort on the part of the clinician.

Nevertheless, subjective judgments have several limitations. A commonly recognized limitation is the poor reliability and agreement within and across multiple raters (Kreiman & Gerratt, 1998; Kreiman, Gerratt, Kempster, Erman, & Berke, 1993). The subjective score assigned to a given voice stimulus can vary significantly from one listener to another and even from one test to another. A number of factors that contribute to such variability have been identified. These include, among others, factors related to the test procedures themselves (Shrivastav, Sapienza, & Nandur, 2005), variability in instructions or definitions of voice quality, or listener training and experience (Bassich & Ludlow, 1986; Kreiman, Gerratt, & Precoda, 1990). Another limitation of commonly used subjective judgments, although not widely discussed in the literature, is the nature of the information obtained from such measurements. Even in the most tightly controlled experiments, most rating scale approaches provide only ordinal data and can only help judge whether the quality of one voice is better or worse than that of another (Shrivastav et al., 2005). Such data cannot be used to interpret *how much* the quality of one voice may be better or worse than another. Thus, it often is possible to say that a patient's voice quality has improved after therapy, but it is not possible to quantify the magnitude of improvement. Some of these limitations can be controlled or accounted for in an experimental setup (Shrivastav et al., 2005), but these errors are difficult to address in everyday clinical practice. This is because the procedures needed to derive the magnitude of change in a percept are often time consuming and not feasible during routine clinical care.

The second approach is to quantify voice quality by measuring some aspect(s) of a correlate of voice production (Baken & Orlikoff, 2000). The ubiquity of computers in modern clinics has made such objective measurement very popular, especially when these measures are obtained from the voice acoustic signal. A number of software products for analyses of voice are available at minimal costs and even specialized hardware, such as that for recording oral airflow, is now available at reasonable

costs. The common premise underlying all objective measurement of voice quality is that a change in vocal production, whether quantified via the acoustic, airflow, electroglottographic, or other signals, is directly related to a change in voice quality. Therefore, a number of researchers and clinicians have attempted to quantify voice quality by measuring a change in some parameters related to voice production. A large number of candidate measures have been proposed and tested, but few, if any, have been found to be universally successful in describing voice quality.

As voice quality by its very definition is a perceptual attribute, any objective measure for voice quality *has* to be validated against listener judgments. Much of the research on objective measures of voice quality attempts to do this by obtaining a linear correlation between proposed measures of voice quality and perceptual judgments from a panel of listeners. The findings are highly inconsistent across multiple experiments and typically show a low-to-moderate correlation between objective and perceptual data (Kreiman & Gerratt, 2000). Additionally, many objective measures lack specificity to a particular voice quality dimension and seem to be correlated best with overall judgments of the magnitude of dysphonia. This further limits their utility in research and clinical practice.

These limitations arise from a number of factors. One primary reason for the failure of most objective measures to correlate with voice quality judgments may be traced to their origin, which was to quantify changes in vocal production or merely to describe and quantify differences in the underlying signal characteristics itself (e.g., Deliyski, 1993). Over the years, many authors and clinicians have assumed that changes in voice production attributes also will result in corresponding (and linear) changes to voice quality. However, there is little evidence to support this assumption. Instead, there is considerable evidence showing that the auditory-perceptual process is not linear and often utilizes multiple acoustic cues in the formation of a percept (e.g., Klatt & Klatt, 1990; Repp, 1988; Shrivastav & Sapienza, 2003). Therefore, a simple linear correlation between one or more objective measure of voice and perceptual judgments of voice quality rarely shows good results. However, when some of the nonlinear and multidimensional aspects of the auditory-perceptual process are taken into account, objective measures specifically designed to predict voice quality show a much higher correspondence with listener judgments (Shrivastav & Camacho, 2010; Shrivastav & Sapienza, 2003).

Various multiparametric approaches to voice quality measurement also have specific limitations. One commonly used approach, the Dysphonia Severity Index (DSI; Wuyts et al., 2000) uses a combination of measures such as the highest fundamental frequency, the lowest intensity, the maximum phonation time, and short-term perturbation of fundamental frequency (jitter %) to predict the overall severity of dysphonia. Although the DSI has been shown to have significant clinical utility, the underlying measures do not necessarily measure voice *quality* itself and instead focus on measuring variables that covary with the severity of the dysphonia (note that most of the measures that constitute the DSI score may/are not directly related to *quality*). Thus, such multiparametric measurement schemes often lack the specificity to measure one or more subdimensions of dysphonic voice quality. Instead, these usually indicate the over-all change in the severity of dysphonia. A similar problem is encountered when using approaches that are based primarily on pattern-recognition algorithms using a variety of acoustic measures as input.

Summary

In summary, there is no standard or universally accepted protocol or tool for voice quality evaluation. By its very definition, voice quality is a perceptual phenomenon. Therefore, any attempts to quantify voice quality must either directly use listener judgments (which are often expensive, time-intensive, and prone to errors) or utilize an "objective" approach that is known to correlate with perceptual judgments (which, in the best cases, tend to be nonspecific and correlate only with a global change in dysphonia severity). Fortunately, despite these concerns, it is often possible to identify a suitable approach to measure voice quality in a way that allows a clinician or researcher to obtain the kind of information that he or she needs. However, it is necessary to understand the limitations of any measurement scheme so as to minimize the potential of making erroneous measurements or incorrect interpretation of resulting data. Obtaining meaningful measurements of voice quality requires clinicians and researchers to carefully identify the type of information they seek to obtain and to determine the degree of sensitivity and specificity that they need from their measurement. Once such requirements have been established, it is possible to select an approach that is suitable for the information needed. In the following sections, the terms "measurement" and "evaluation" often are used interchangeably and refer to the quantification of voice quality.

DESCRIPTION

Voice quality evaluation requires careful thought about a number of factors. Some critical issues are described below. Although voice quality evaluation can take many different forms, it is best to choose the protocol based on the specific needs or objectives of the measurement.

1. Stimuli

An important decision in the process of voice quality evaluation is the choice of stimuli. Stimuli selected for such measurement may include vowel(s) or speech (syllables/words/sentences). The duration of the stimuli may be relatively brief (as low as 400 to 500 ms) to relatively long (several seconds). There are some advantages of choosing speech (sentences, words, or even syllables) over vowels as stimuli. First, speech provides a better approximation to everyday conversational samples than vowels alone. Second, speech stimuli often allow evaluation of certain characteristics that can be easily missed when evaluating vowel stimuli. For example, the effect of phonetic context (coarticulation) on voice quality changes may not be evident from vowel samples. Furthermore, speech samples often show greater variability in voice quality than vowels and this variability may itself affect the perceived severity of the disorder. Thus, the severity of specific voice quality dimensions may be different for vowels and speech. For such reasons, speech is often the preferred stimulus for voice quality evaluation, especially when a clinician or researcher is interested in assessing a global or *holistic* change in voice quality. However, sometimes these very characteristics may be a disadvantage.

For instance, if a clinician or researcher is interested in evaluating the perception of a specific voice quality dimension, then the greater variability in speech stimuli (or even vowel stimuli of long duration) may prove to be a disadvantage. If the voice quality varies across the duration of the stimulus, it becomes difficult to determine whether the measurement value assigned to it reflects a specific part of the stimulus or some sort of an average (perhaps weighted in some manner).

Although there is no good rule of thumb for selecting the stimuli, speech stimuli are generally better for: (1) evaluating the overall or global magnitude of voice quality changes, or (2) when one seeks to obtain estimates of real-world issues related to voice quality. For these reasons, speech stimuli often are ideal for developing standard clinical evaluation protocols. In contrast, vowel stimuli often are preferred when: (1) one seeks to establish a relationship between perceived quality and vocal fold physiology, or (2) when voice quality is needed to validate other instrumental measures of voice (e.g., acoustic, EGG).

2. Instrumentation for Recording, Storage, and Playback

Another critical element for voice quality measurement is the equipment used for recording and playback. Easy access to computers and widespread use of digital formats for recording and playback has eliminated many of the limitations associated with analog systems. However, some problems remain and some additional limitations need to be recognized. Although not exhaustive, a few key issues are described below.

All recording and playback systems include a microphone, a medium for storage of data, and a transducer for playback of recorded data. Microphones vary greatly in their sensitivity and frequency response. Many commercially available microphones, especially those designed to be worn around the head, are designed to attenuate low frequency signals (the cutoff frequency may be as high as 250 Hz). Depending on the microphone and the measurement scheme used for voice quality evaluation, this may have an adverse affect on the results. For example, using a poor quality microphone may introduce additional noise to the voice signal, inappropriate microphone placement may affect its sensitivity, or variations in frequency response across microphones may affect specific measurements made from the recorded signals (see Švec & Granqvist, 2010, for details). Therefore, users should carefully evaluate the characteristics of the microphone used for recording and ensure that its fidelity is sufficiently good for their purpose. Users also should ensure that the microphone is suitably coupled to the recording device and that the impedance of the microphone matches the recording device. An impedance mismatch can alter the frequency response and sensitivity of the recording system.

Although the use of digital signals has eliminated many limitations of the older recording systems, one must be aware of the compression used for storing data. Digital sound files are essentially memory intensive and some sort of compression is almost always applied to reduce the size of the recordings when storing the data. Some compression techniques, such as the MP3 compression, are "lossy" and result in some loss of data. Others, such as the commonly used WAV format, are "lossless." Although MP3 and other lossy compression formats may be acceptable for certain goals, it is recommended that a lossless compression be used when storing digital recordings of voice. In recent years there has been a move toward recording data directly to a computer. This often is done using a "sound-card" on a personal computer. Although the overall quality of computer sound cards has improved greatly over the last few years, several limitations must be borne in mind when they are used to record voices. First, even though many sound-cards have very good specifications for sound *output*, they often lack the same rigor for sound input. Few sound cards offer a balanced XLR input for sound recordings. Second, many sound-cards, especially those used in laptops, suffer from significant noise interference such as that arising from the proximity of various computer components. Finally, the operating system and sound-card "driver" used in the computer sometimes can result in distortions in the recordings.

If voice quality evaluation needs a listening test, then playback of the sound file is essential. Voice stimuli may be played using headphone or speakers. Some researchers and clinicians prefer to use speakers for playback because of its "ecological validity" (i.e., its close approximation to everyday listening situations). However, others prefer headsets or earinserts because the frequency and temporal characteristics of headsets are more easily available and often more stringent than speaker systems. An additional limitation of using speakers is that effective sound pressure level at a listener's ear can vary significantly even with small head movements, thereby altering the level and the spectrum at the ear. Again, there is no simple rule to determine the best option for playback. Instead, users need to choose the right approach for the goals they wish to achieve when measuring voice quality.

3. Listeners

If voice quality is measured through listening tests, then the characteristics of listeners are an important variable that needs to be considered. Some clinicians and researchers prefer to obtain voice quality judgments through trained listeners and/or listeners who have considerable experience or exposure to dysphonic voice quality. It often is believed that such listeners may be more consistent and accurate in their judgments due to the uniformity of their experiences and closer agreement regarding the definition of various terms used to describe voice quality. However, this assumption has not prevailed in all empirical studies (e.g., Kreiman et al., 1990) and there is some debate about listener consistency for subjective judgments of voice quality. A different viewpoint is to test naïve listeners when evaluating voice quality (Chan & Yiu, 2006). One advantage of this approach is that voice quality measurement obtained from naïve listeners may provide better estimates of the average listener population. However, naïve listeners typically need clear explanation and definitions for various dimensions of voice quality and often benefit from some degree of training in the measurement task. It also is possible that naïve listeners are good at making global judgments of voice quality changes but are not as accurate as trained listeners when judging specific dimensions that require a more careful and precise evaluation.

Once again, there is no universal consensus or a simple rule of thumb to decide whether to test expert or naïve listeners for voice quality evaluation. Instead, one needs to choose listeners based on the overall goals for measurement. In our experience, we have observed that, when the listening test is conducted under carefully controlled experimental paradigms, the differences between trained/experienced listeners and naïve listeners are relatively small. Thus, the differences observed between trained and naïve listeners may reflect differences in the test-taking abilities across the two groups rather than differences in their ability to perceive voice quality changes itself.

4. Procedural Factors

Several other factors related to voice quality measurement are equally important, although often overlooked. These include, among others, factors such as listener training and instructions, listening or analyses environment, efforts to minimize fatigue and maximize attention, and measurement scheme. The following section describes some of these variables that can impact voice quality measurement significantly.

Assessing voice quality subjectively is not an easy task for many listeners, especially those who are not familiar with dysphonic voice quality or the test procedures used to obtain voice quality judgments. It is useful to provide clear definitions and even some practice with the task used for obtaining listener judgments. Additionally, when asked to rate or scale specific dimensions of voice quality (e.g., roughness, breathiness, strain), it is common for many listeners to default to making global judgments of dysphonia severity. This can be minimized by using clear instructions to specify the task at hand, practice exercises, and frequent reminders (possibly with examples) of the task at hand. Another approach is to use matching tasks (Gerratt & Kreiman, 2001; Patel, Shrivastav, & Eddins, 2010) that essentially force listeners to judge specific dimensions of voice quality instead of making more global judgments of dysphonia severity.

Controlling the listening environment can help minimize many errors in subjective judgments. For example, all listening tests should be done in a quiet environment that is free of distractions. If the listening test requires more than a few minutes, it is advisable to provide frequent rest periods to minimize fatigue and to ensure that listener's attention is at optimal levels. These also provide the experimenter ample opportunities to reinstruct the listener(s) about the listening task. If the experimenter tests multiple listeners and/or conducts the test over multiple test sessions, it also is critical to ensure that the test equipment remains consistent and properly calibrated.

The test or measurement procedures employed to obtain subjective judgments of voice quality are of critical importance because they have a significant impact on the kinds of information obtained from subjective data. Clinicians and researchers must give very careful attention to these details and choose a measurement procedure that is suitable for the information they seek to obtain. A typical protocol used for routine clinical evaluation rarely will give the precision of measurement that can be achieved even in a very simple experimental setup. However, the time- and resource- constraints in most clinics permit limited accuracy and precision. Although an exhaustive description of possible subjective measurement paradigms and their advantages is beyond the scope of this chapter, a few key aspects are described below.

1. There is a tradeoff between time required for testing and sensitivity and specificity of measurement. When a brief test time is critical (e.g., in a voice clinic), then one can only obtain an approximate measurement of voice quality. For example, the resolution of voice quality measurement using a typical clinical assessment protocol (such as the CAPE-V) is lower than that obtained using an experimental paradigm that uses an *n*-point rating scale or a paired-comparison task with multiple listeners and multiple presentations of each stimuli. However, the standard clinical protocol is considerably quicker to administer than other procedures.

2. There is a tradeoff between task difficulty and complexity of information obtained during measurement. A measurement paradigm that uses a relatively simple task, such as a simple *n*-point rating scale or a visual-analog scale typically will provide only ordinal data. Ordinal data allow one to rank order two or more voices in terms of their voice quality, but it does not indicate the magnitude of difference between these voices. In contrast, other measurement schemes such as direct magnitude estimation or matching can allow clinicians/researchers to obtain a ratio level measurement in which the magnitude of the difference between two or more voices can be interpreted. Needless to say, such tasks not only are more difficult for listeners, but also require greater test time.

3. Some variability (inter- and intralistener) is inherent to all perceptual tasks. The magnitude of variability that may be acceptable can vary depending on the goal of measurement. A number of factors affect the magnitude of variability. For example, more difficult tasks (e.g., direct magnitude estimation or matching) will result in greater variability of data compared to easier tasks (e.g., rating scale). Similarly, training, instructions, and practice can

alter the magnitude of variability. Variability also can be addressed through averaging multiple data points (e.g., Shrivastav et al., 2005).

4. The accuracy of subjective measurement is limited by the weakest element in the measurement process. As described in the preceding sections, subjective voice quality measurement is affected by a large number and variety of factors. The accuracy of such measurement is limited by the factors that impart the greatest variability or pose the strictest limitations. For example, one may design a very elegant measurement scheme for voice quality measurement that requires testing multiple listeners over multiple test sessions. However, the measurement is conducted in different locations using different computers and sound-cards and in environments that has frequent distractions. In this scenario, the benefits of the measurement scheme are severely limited by the variability associated with distractions and differences in the test equipment. Highly precise measurements can be achieved only when all such variables are carefully controlled.

CASE STUDIES

A few hypothetical examples are described to illustrate how one may go about choosing a suitable protocol for voice quality evaluation. These examples attempt to describe a variety of scenarios. Note that there may be multiple approaches to obtaining the same information and the protocols described here should not be viewed as the only suitable approach to voice quality evaluation.

1. I manage a very busy voice clinic and I have limited time or resources for voice quality evaluation. What is the best approach to measure voice quality during routine clinical evaluation?

Most voice clinics have limited time and resources for an exhaustive voice quality evaluation that offers high sensitivity and specificity. The general goal of such measurements typically is to establish a baseline that may be used for comparison against future assessment (e.g., following therapy or surgery). Sometimes, clinicians also use voice quality evaluation to validate other instrumental measures. Although high sensitivity and specificity is ideal, in this scenario, the clinician's time is the major limiting factor. Fortunately, ordinal data with relatively coarse sensitivity can still provide useful clinical information. Therefore, a clinician can use a simple rating scale or visual-analog procedure to quantify voice quality. To allow direct comparisons across patients or over time, it is recommended that a standard protocol be used across all patients and all assessment sessions. Either speech alone or both vowels and speech should be used as stimuli. Using a standard set of speech material will help minimize variability in judgments to some degree. A global judgment of dysphonia severity along with judgments on individual dimensions (such as breathiness, roughness, strain) will help get a complete picture of the dysphonic voice quality. A standard protocol such as the CAPE-V (Kempster et al., 2009) meets all such criteria and may serve as a good approach to measure voice quality in this scenario. However, the clinician must bear in mind that the information obtained through this protocol likely has relatively high variability and poor sensitivity and provides only ordinal data. Thus, when comparing this to another patient's data (or the same patient's data obtained at another time), the clinician may be unable to quantify small changes in voice quality or determine how *much* better (or worse) one voice was relative to another.

The clinician also may want to obtain some "objective" measures of voice quality. One good candidate is the cepstral peak prominence (Heman-Ackah et al., 2003; Hillenbrand & Houde, 1996), which appears to be reliable across a wide range of dysphonia. There are limited data on its sensitivity or specificity, but it appears to be highly correlated with breathiness (Hillenbrand & Houde, 1996; Shrivastav & Sapienza, 2003). Another possibility is to compute the Dysphonia Severity Index (DSI; Wuyts et al., 2000), which is correlated to the dysphonia severity. Note that this provides a general measure of the severity of dysphonia, without any information regarding changes in specific dimensions of dysphonic voice quality.

2. I wish to determine whether a new therapy protocol that I have designed improves voice quality for my patients. I have tried this protocol on 15 patients so far and want to ensure that its benefits on voice quality are as expected.

In this scenario, the need for expediency is replaced by a greater need for accuracy and sensitivity. Note that the primary goal here is only to determine whether voice quality has changed post-treatment.

Information regarding the *magnitude* of change following treatment does not appear to be critical. Therefore, a rating scale task (such as an *n*-point scale or a visual-analog scale) is a suitable approach. However, to minimize variability in listener judgments and improve sensitivity, it is recommended that the listening test be administered to multiple listeners who are presented multiple trials of each stimulus in random order. By averaging data across such repeated presentations, one can minimize errors arising from specific biases in the perceptual rating task (Shrivastav et al., 2005).

Depending on the nature of the therapy protocol, one may choose to obtain a global measure of dysphonia severity or a more specific measurement across one or more dimensions of dysphonic voice quality (or both). For example, a therapy protocol that is fairly generic in terms of its effects on vocal fold physiology may be best evaluated using a global measure of dysphonia severity. On the other hand, if the therapy protocol was designed specifically to improve glottal closure, then one may wish to evaluate breathiness instead of (or in addition to) a global measure of dysphonia severity. Likewise, the choice of stimuli for the listening tests, whether vowels or speech, may be dictated by the objectives of the therapy protocol and the questions that the clinician wishes to investigate.

3. I work in an interdisciplinary voice team. We have tried two different surgical approaches (A and B) to treat a particular problem. We wish to determine whether

the two approaches result in different voice quality outcomes. On informal listening, the differences seem to be small or none at all, but we feel that one approach is consistently better than another. What is the best method to measure voice quality?

As in the previous example, the need for expediency is replaced by the need for accuracy. The general goal of voice quality measurement is almost identical to that in the previous example as the researcher needs to determine whether voice quality following one treatment is better or worse than following another. Obtaining ordinal data appears sufficient as the researcher does not need to know the magnitude of change in voice quality. However, it appears that voice quality changes, if any, are likely to be fairly small. Thus, the measurement needs to have much greater sensitivity than may be obtained in a standard rating scale task described previously.

One approach to measurement is to use a paired-comparison task. In this task, listeners are presented pairs of stimuli and are asked to judge which of the two has better voice quality. The order of stimuli is randomized and each pair is presented multiple times in random order. To further correct for chance, a number of "catch trials" can be included. These contain two items from the same patient and the same surgical protocol. Accuracy and sensitivity can be measured using percent correct scores or through metrics such as the *d'*. Analysis of the resulting data can provide a highly sensitive measure of voice quality changes following the two surgical approaches.

As described previously, the decision to obtain judgments on overall dysphonia severity and/or specific dysphonia dimensions may be related to the objectives and expected outcomes of the surgical procedure. The researchers also may wish to compare voice quality outcome for each surgical procedure against the presurgical baseline (comparisons within-patients instead of across-groups). Depending on the magnitude of change, a rating scale task or a paired-comparison approach may be used for within-patient comparison.

4. I am interested in comparing voice quality outcomes from surgery (S) to that following surgery + voice therapy (S+VT). I know they both improve the voice quality, but I suspect that S+VT leads to at least 20% greater improvement in voice quality. What is the best approach to measure voice quality?

The primary question here requires determination of the magnitude of change in voice quality. Although rating scale approaches may show that voice quality outcome in the S+VT condition are better/worse than S, they cannot quantify the magnitude of change easily. A better approach to address this question is to use a direct magnitude estimation paradigm. In this procedure, a group of listeners is asked to use *any* number to identify the magnitude of dysphonia (or breathiness/roughness/strain). However, when making these judgments, they must maintain a ratio-level relationship across their judgments. Thus, for example, if one voice is given a score of 100, then another voice that has twice the breathiness must be given a score of 200. The stimuli need to be repeated multiple times and presented in random order to address variability associated with a variety of biases. The resulting scores are assumed to have ratio-level measurement properties, which can enable the researcher to compute the magnitude of change between the S and the S+VT conditions.

5. I am planning to complete a series of studies to evaluate how voice quality changes with age and specific neurologic conditions across different cultural groups. I wish to find out whether a specific drug changes the course of these changes, and to determine the magnitude of the change across various cultural groups. What is the best approach to measure voice quality?

This requires a fairly complex experimental design. Note that the researchers need to evaluate the magnitude of change in voice quality. Additionally, these measurements may be done at different times and possibly different locations. Furthermore, comparisons need to be made across multiple variables (age, neurologic condition, cultural groups).

A possible approach is to first obtain *all* voice samples (across all age groups, neurologic conditions, and cultural groups) and to conduct a direct magnitude estimation study that includes all of these samples. This would provide the magnitude of change across each variable of interest.

However, such a design often is unrealistic because the test time required to evaluate a large number of samples is very high.

One way around this problem is to divide the experiment into smaller experiments. For example, all voices from a single age and cultural group may be evaluated in a separate direct magnitude estimation task. This will enable the researcher to evaluate the magnitude of change in voice within an experimental group. However, the researcher cannot make a direct comparison of data across multiple experiments because the scores assigned in a direct magnitude estimation task are arbitrary and may vary from one experiment to another. For example, a voice assigned a score of 1000 in Experiment A may have a different magnitude of dysphonia than a voice with the same score in Experiment B.

To avoid this problem, the researcher may have to use a different approach. One possibility is to design the experiment in a way that some stimuli are repeated across multiple (or all) experiments. These stimuli may then be used to normalize the arbitrary scores in the direct magnitude estimation task, enabling a more direct comparison across experiments. Another approach is to use a matching task (Patel et al., 2010) where the voice quality of each stimulus is measured by comparing it against a standard reference that can be manipulated in a specific manner. As long as the reference signal and its manipulation remain consistent across experiments, a direct comparison of perceptual data can be made across experiments.

SUMMARY

Voice quality evaluation can be conducted in a variety of ways. There is no universal consensus on how voice quality should be evaluated. It is recommended that clinicians and researchers carefully assess the type of information sought from voice quality evaluation and select a protocol that is most suitable for their purposes.

REFERENCES

Andrews, M. L., & Summers, A. C. (2002). *Voice treatment for children and adolescents* (2nd ed.). San Diego, CA: Singular Thomson Learning.

ANSI. (1960). *USA Standard: Acoustical terminology (S1.1)*. New York, NY: Author.

Baken, R. J., & Orlikoff, R. F. (2000). *Clinical measurement of speech and voice* (2nd ed.). San Diego, CA: Singular.

Bassich, C. J., & Ludlow, C. L. (1986). The use of perceptual methods by new clinicians for assessing voice quality. *Journal of Speech and Hearing Disorders, 51*(2), 125–133.

Boone, D. R., McFarlane, S. C., & Von Berg, S. L. (2005). *The voice and voice therapy*. Boston, MA: Allyn & Bacon.

Chan, K. M.-K., & Yiu, E. M.-L. (2006). A comparison of two perceptual voice evaluation training programs for naïve listeners. *Journal of Voice, 20*, 229–241.

Deliyski, D. D. (1993). *Acoustic model and evaluation of pathological voice production*. Paper presented at the 3rd Conference on Speech Communication and Technology, EUROSPEECH'93, Berlin, Germany.

Eadie, T. L., & Baylor, C. R. (2006). The effect of perceptual training on inexperienced listeners' judgments of dysphonic voice. *Journal of Voice, 20*(4), 527–544.

Eadie, T. L., & Doyle, P. C. (2002). Direct magnitude estimation and interval scaling of pleasantness and severity in dysphonic and normal speakers. *Journal of the Acoustical Society of America, 112*(6), 3014–3021.

Gerratt, B. R., & Kreiman, J. (2001). Measuring voice quality with speech synthesis. *Journal of the Acoustical Society of America, 110*(5 Pt. 1), 2560–2566.

Gerratt, B. R., Kreiman, J., Antonanzas-Barroso, N., & Berke, G. S. (1993). Comparing internal and external standards in voice quality judgments. *Journal of Speech and Hearing Research, 36*(1), 14–20.

Heman-Ackah, Y. D., Heuer, R. J., Michael, D. D., Ostrowski, R., Horman, M., Baroody, M. M., . . . Sataloff, R. T. (2003). Cepstral peak prominence: a more reliable measure of dysphonia. *Annals of Otology, Rhinology and Laryngology, 112*(4), 324–333.

Hillenbrand, J., Cleveland, R. A., & Erickson, R. L. (1994). Acoustic correlates of breathy vocal quality. *Journal of Speech and Hearing Research, 37*(4), 769–778.

Hillenbrand, J., & Houde, R. A. (1996). Acoustic correlates of breathy vocal quality: Dysphonic voices and continuous speech. *Journal of Speech and Hearing Research, 39*(2), 311–321.

Hirano, M. (1981). *Clinical examination of voice*. Wien; New York: Springer-Verlag.

Isshiki, N., & Takeuchi, Y. (1970). Factor analysis of hoarseness. *Studia Phonologica, 5*, 37–44.

Kempster, G. B., Gerratt, B. R., Verdolini Abbott, K., Barkmeier-Kraemer, J., & Hillman, R. E. (2009). Consensus auditory-perceptual evaluation of voice: development of a standardized clinical protocol. *American Journal of Speech Language Pathology, 18*, 124–132.

Klatt, D. H., & Klatt, L. C. (1990). Analysis, synthesis, and perception of voice quality variations among female and male talkers. *Journal of the Acoustical Society of America, 87*(2), 820–857.

Kreiman, J., & Gerratt, B. R. (1998). Validity of rating scale measures of voice quality. *Journal of the Acoustical Society of America, 104*(3 Pt. 1), 1598–1608

Kreiman, J., & Gerratt, B. (2000). Measuring voice quality. In R. D. Kent & M. J. Ball (Eds.), *Voice quality measurement* (1st ed., pp. 73–102). San Diego, CA: Singular.

Kreiman, J., Gerratt, B. R., Kempster, G. B., Erman, A., & Berke, G. S. (1993). Perceptual evaluation of voice quality: Review, tutorial, and a framework for future research. *Journal of Speech and Hearing Research, 36*(1), 21–40.

Kreiman, J., Gerratt, B. R., & Precoda, K. (1990). Listener experience and perception of voice quality. *Journal of Speech and Hearing Research*, *33*(1), 103-115.

Pannbacker, M. (1984). Classification systems of voice disorders: A review of the literature. *Language, Speech and Hearing Services in Schools*, *15*, 169-174.

Patel, S., Shrivastav, R., & Eddins, D. A. (2006). Perceptual judgments of breathy voice quality using rating scale, magnitude estimation and matching tasks. *Journal of the Acoustical Society of America*, *119*, 3340.

Patel, S., Shrivastav, R., & Eddins, D. A. (2010). Perceptual distances of breathy voice quality: A comparison of psychophysical methods. *Journal of Voice*, *24*(2), 168-177.

Repp, B. H. (1988). Integration and segregation in speech perception. *Language and Speech*, *31*(3), 239-271.

Rihkanen, H., Leinonen, L., Hiltunen, T., & Kangas, J. (1994). Spectral pattern recognition of improved voice quality. *Journal of Voice*, *8*(4), 320-326.

Ritchings, R. T., McGillion, M., & Moore, C. J. (2002). Pathological voice quality assessment using artificial neural networks. *Medical Engineering and Physics*, *24*(7-8), 561-564.

Shrivastav, R., & Camacho, A. (2010). A computational model to predict changes in breathiness resulting from variations in aspiration noise level. *Journal of Voice*, *24*(4), 395-405.

Shrivastav, R., & Sapienza, C. M. (2003). Objective measures of breathy voice quality obtained using an auditory model. *Journal of the Acoustical Society of America*, *114*(4), 2217-2224.

Shrivastav, R., Sapienza, C. M., & Nandur, V. (2005). Application of psychometric theory to the measurement of voice quality using rating scales. *Journal of Speech, Language, and Hearing Research*, *48*(2), 323-335.

Svec, J. G, & Granqvist, S. (2010). Guidelines for selecting microphones for human voice production research. *American Journal of Speech-Language Pathology*, *19*, 356-368.

Takahashi, H., & Koike, Y. (1976). Some perceptual dimensions and acoustical correlates of pathologic voices. *Acta Oto-Laryngologica Supplement*, *338*, 3-24.

Titze, I. R. (1994). *Principles of voice production*. Englewood Cliffs, N.J.: Prentice-Hall.

Wilson, D. K. (1987). *Voice problems of children* (3rd ed.). Baltimore, MD: Williams & Wilkins.

Wuyts, F. L., De Bodt, M. S., Molenberghs, G., Remacle, M., Heylen, L., Millet, B., . . . Van de Heyning, P. H. (2000). The Dysphonia Severity Index: An objective measure of vocal quality based on a multiparameter approach. *Journal of Speech, Language, and Hearing Research*, *43*(3), 796-809.

Yiu, E. M.-L., Murdoch, B., Hird, K., & Lau, P. (2002). Perception of synthesized voice quality in connected speech by Cantonese speakers. *Journal of the Acoustical Society of America*, *112*(3 Pt. 1), 1091-1101.

CHAPTER 23

Auditory-Perceptual Voice Evaluation: A Practical Approach

KAREN M.-K. CHAN

PURPOSE

- To describe the type, nature, and severity of voice quality impairment.

THEORETICAL BACKGROUND

Auditory-perceptual voice evaluation refers to the procedure where a listener judges the perceptual voice quality of a voice sample based on the listener's subjective judgment. The listener usually judges the type and severity of the dysphonic qualities based on his or her training and experience. Auditory-perceptual voice evaluation is commonly used by voice scientists and clinicians (including speech pathologists and otolaryngologists) in voice-related research and voice clinics (e.g., Carding, Carlson, Epstein, Mathieson, & Shewell, 2000; Hammarberg, 2000; Ver-

dolini & Palmer, 1997). Experienced clinicians regard auditory-perceptual voice evaluation as an important diagnostic tool for treatment planning and outcome measurement (Behrman, 2005). Auditory-perceptual voice evaluation has been widely used in treatment efficacy studies (e.g., Holmberg, Hillman, Hammarberg, Södersten, & Doyle, 2001; Verdolini-Marston, Burke, Lessac, Glaze, & Caldwell, 1995; Ylitalo & Hammarberg, 2000) and studies on validation of instrumental measurement of voice (e.g., Piccirillo, Painter, Fuller, & Fredrickson, 1998; Rabinov, Kreiman, Gerratt, & Bielamowicz, 1995; Yu, Revis, Wuyts, Zanaret, & Giovanni, 2002). Despite the fact that perceptual voice evaluation is commonly used in research and in clinics, the reliability of perceptual voice evaluation frequently has been questioned (see review by Oates, 2009). Past studies have shown that voice scientists do not agree on which perceptual qualities (e.g., roughness, breathiness, harshness) are to be included in perceptual voice evaluation (Kreiman & Gerratt, 1996), which type of rating scale to be used (Kreiman & Gerratt, 1998), or whether training and experience in perceptual voice evaluation affects reliability (Eadie & Baylor, 2006; Kreiman, Gerratt, & Precoda, 1990).

DESCRIPTION OF AUDITORY-PERCEPTUAL VOICE EVALUATION

Auditory-perceptual voice evaluation approaches generally vary in four aspects:

- Terminologies used for describing the auditory-perceptual voice qualities;
- Type of rating scales used in the evaluation;
- Provision and types of anchors used for the evaluation; and
- Provision and type of training given prior to the evaluation.

These variations affect the reliability of the voice evaluation and make it difficult to compare data across clinicians and studies. Each of these areas is discussed below.

Terminologies Used for Describing Auditory-Perceptual Voice Quality

Voice quality is broadly defined as "everything in the acoustic signal that is not pitch or loudness" (Gerratt & Kreiman, 2000, p. 336). This definition indicates voice quality could include a vast range of perceptual correlates of an acoustic signal. A range of "labels" for describing different types of voice quality has been used in the literature. To name a few, these include breathy, harsh, hoarse, rough, strain, tremor, and vocal fry. Researchers have attempted to improve this situation by proposing a number of protocols for perceptual voice evaluation. The GRBAS scale (Hirano, 1981) and the Consensus Auditory-Perceptual Evaluation of Voice (CAPE-V) (Kempster, Gerratt, Verdolini-Abbott, Barkmeier-Kraemer, & Hillman, 2009) are two of the protocols more commonly used in clinical settings and voice research (Carding et al., 2000; Hammarberg, 2000). The GRBAS scale includes five perceptual parameters: overall severity (G), roughness (R), breathiness (B), asthenic (A), and strain (S). The G scale refers to the overall severity level of the dysphonic quality in the voice. The R scale refers to the perception of unclear voice with uneven quality and is thought to be a reflection of the irregular vibration of the vocal folds (Hirano, 1981; Laver, 1980). The B scale refers to the perception of audible expiratory air escape during phonation (Hirano, 1981) and is shown to be related to the incomplete closure of the vocal folds during phonation. The A scale refers to the perception of weakness in the voice. The S scale refers to the perception of tension and extraneous effort in the voice. Among the five perceptual parameters, the overall severity, breathiness, and roughness were rated with significantly higher reliability than the other two parameters (De Bodt, Wuyts, van de Heyning, & Croux, 1997; Dejonckere, Obbens, de Moor, & Wieneke, 1993).

The CAPE-V includes six perceptual parameters: the overall severity, roughness, breathiness, strain, pitch, and loudness. The definition of the overall severity, roughness, and breathiness are similar to those provided in the GRBAS scale. *Strain* in the CAPE-V refers to the perception of excessive vocal effort. For the pitch and loudness scales, the rater has to first describe whether it is too high/low or too loud/soft before indicating the severity. For each scale, the rater also needs to indicate whether the dysphonic quality is consistently or intermittently shown by the client. Karnell et al. (2007) found strong correlations between the grade, rough, breathy, and strain scales of the GRBAS scale and their counterparts in the CAPE-V. The CAPE-V further suggests that sustained vowels (/a/ and /i/), a set of standard sentences, and a running speech sample should be used to gather a representative sample of the client's voice for evaluation. For details of the speech sample, please refer to the CAPE-V instructions which are downloadable from the American Speech-Language-Hearing Association (http://www.asha.org/members/divs/div_3.htm).

Rating Scales

A second area in auditory-perceptual voice evaluation that varies greatly across studies and clinicians is the type of rating scales used for evaluation. Severity ratings in auditory-perceptual voice evaluation are often represented as points on an ordinal scale (De Bodt et al., 1997), equal-appearing scale (Yamaguchi, Shrivastav, Andrews, & Niimi, 2003), direct magnitude estimation (Eadie & Doyle, 2002), or a visual analogue scale (Yiu & Chan, 2003). Contradictory results have been found in the literature in support of each type of rating scale. The ordinal scale and the visual analogue scales are discussed below.

An ordinal scale refers to the scale that involves ordering or ranking of the different points on the scale. However, the scale neither specifies the distance between each point on the scale nor assumes that the intervals between the scale points are identical. An example of such scale is the use of the ordinal scale in the GRBAS as proposed by Hirano (1981). Each perceptual parameter was labeled as 0 to 3 to indicate the severity of the dysphonic quality, with "0" representing normal; "1" representing mild; "2" representing moderate; and "3" representing severe.

The visual analogue scale (VAS) assumes the intervals between scale points are equal. The VAS usually is represented as an undifferentiated line where both ends of the line are marked with descriptors. This scale assumes that the parameter being rated can be represented along a continuum. The CAPE-V is an example of a profile that uses the VAS. A 10-cm horizontal line is used to represent the severity of each of the dysphonic quality. The rater simply marks on each line to indicate the severity. A score is obtained by measuring the distance (in millimeters) between the start of the line on the left and the rater's mark.

Studies have attempted to compare the reliability in using different rating scales in perceptual voice evaluation. Wuyts, de Bodt, and van de Heyning (1999) concluded that the GRBAS scale should be used with an ordinal scale rather than with a VAS because listeners tend to score with the middle section of the VAS but not with the ordinal scale and that the ordinal scale offered higher reliability across listeners than the VAS. Yiu and Ng (2004) compared the ratings of roughness and breathiness between an equal appearing interval (EAI) scale and VAS. They found that naïve listeners rated roughness and breathiness with higher intrarater agreement when an EAI scale was used than when a VAS was used and the interrater reliability was similar with the two rating scales. The authors concluded that because the EAI scale showed higher intrarater agreement and is relatively simpler and more practical to use in clinics than the VAS, the EAI scale was suggested to be a more appropriate tool for rating roughness and breathiness. The EAI scale also has been used with matching anchors for each scale point (Yiu, Chan, & Mok, 2007), which may help to improve the reliability of auditory-perceptual evaluation of voice quality.

Use of Anchors

Anchors are a set of voice stimuli (natural or synthesized) that are considered to be representative of a certain voice quality at a particular severity level. They usually are available to the listeners throughout the process of auditory-perceptual voice evaluation. The use of anchors to improve the reliability in auditory-perceptual voice evaluation is based on a framework proposed by Kreiman and her colleagues (Kreiman, Gerratt, Kempster, Erman, & Berke, 1993). They proposed that listeners make use of the internal representations of voice quality in their memory when they carry out auditory-perceptual voice evaluation. Unfortunately, these internal representations are not stable and, therefore, would lead to poor reliability. The provision of anchors has been proposed to replace these unstable internal representations by allowing the listeners to compare the to-be-rated stimulus with the stable external anchors. Theoretically, this should lead to a higher reliability in the evaluation. Chan and Yiu (2002) found positive

anchor effect with inexperienced listeners when the listeners were rating roughness and breathiness. They found that listeners' intrarater agreement (± 1 cm on a 10-cm VAS) significantly improved from 56 to 70% when anchors were provided than when no anchor was provided. They also found that the interrater variance significantly reduced when anchors were provided. This finding supported the earlier hypothesis that the external anchors were able to compensate for the unstable internal representations during the evaluation. The external anchors also helped to "calibrate" the standards of evaluation across listeners, leading to lower inter-rater variability. Currently, there is a lack of well-defined and validated synthesized anchors to match with the two commonly used evaluation profiles mentioned above. Kempster et al. (2009) suggested that, to further improve the current version of CAPE-V, future studies could develop anchors to match with each rating scale. Samples of synthesized breathy and rough voice stimuli in a range of severity are available at <http://www.hku.hk/speech/voice-handbook>. The synthesis parameters used to develop these stimuli are validated in Yiu, Murdoch, Hird, and Lau (2002) and Chan and Yiu (2002) to represent breathiness and roughness.

Training

Training is another method commonly used to improve the reliability in auditory-perceptual voice evaluation. Some of the proposed training methods were based on the framework proposed by Kreiman et al. (1993) (e.g., Chan & Yiu, 2002; Martin & Wolfe, 1996). The aim of training programs is to consolidate the internal representations of the voice qualities (e.g., Chan & Yiu, 2002; Martin & Wolfe, 1996; Shewell, 1998). Positive training effects are found in numerous studies (Chan & Yiu, 2002, 2006; Eadie & Baylor, 2006; Martin & Wolfe, 1996; Shewell, 1998).

EQUIPMENT AND MATERIALS

Equipment

It is strongly recommended that clients' voice samples be recorded through high-quality audio-recording equipment in a sound treated room. This allows the clinician to listen to the voice samples again for reliability rating and for comparison with other voice samples from the same person or across a group of clients. In clinical situations, it often is useful to present the pre-training and post-training voice samples to the clients before they are discharged.

- Recording software: You can download Audacity, a free audiorecording and editing software, from http://audacity .sourceforge.net/ .
- Recording equipment:
  - A high-quality hand-held microphone with microphone stand or head-mounted microphone (e.g., Shure, Beta 54);
  - Professional grade external sound card that allows audio recording at a minimum sampling rate of 44 kHz (e.g., USB-powered Avid, Mbox 2)
- Playback equipment:
  - Professional grade headphone (e.g., Sennheiser, HD25, with a frequency response of 16 to 22,000 Hz (−3 dB))

Materials

We will use the CAPE-V (Kempster et al. , 2009) as the perceptual evaluation protocol. You will need the recording form of the CAPE-V. This can be downloaded from: http://www.asha.org/uploadedFiles /members/divs/D3CAPEVform.pdf

STEP-BY-STEP PROCEDURES

1. Make sure the microphone and sound card are plugged into the computer and turned on.

2. Launch *Audacity.*

3. Ask the client to position his or her mouth 10 cm away from the microphone and get ready for the recording.

   Instructions: *"We are about to start the recording. When you see my hand signal, please say "ah" with your usual voice. Try to extend it for about 5 seconds, I'll show you another signal to stop."*

4. When the client is ready, click on the **record** button (the red circle on the top menu) and signal the client to start.

5. When the client has sustained the vowel for approximately 5 seconds, show him or her the signal to stop.

6. Click on the **stop** button (the square button on the top menu) to stop the recording.

7. From the **FILE** menu, select **EXPORT AS WAV** and save the file in a designated folder.

8. To playback, click on the **play** button (the triangle button on the top menu).

9. Close the saved audio track before recording the next sound file. Close the track by clicking on the cross on the left-hand corner of the audio track.

10. Repeat steps 3 to 9 by replacing /a/ with /i/.

11. Next, instruct the client to read out the six sentences from the CAPE-V as naturally as possible. Save all of the sentences as one file or as separate files. If the client cannot read, ask him or her to repeat after the clinician.

    Instructions: *"Well done. Next we are going to record some sentences. Please read out the following sentences one by one using your regular voice."*

12. Repeat steps 4, 6, and 7 to record the sentences. Remember to close the saved audio track before recording a new one. Otherwise, both tracks will be exported as one combined sound file.

13. Collect a spontaneous speech sample from the client. To make this natural, you can start the recording before giving the following instruction.

    Instructions: *"OK, for the final recording, can you tell me about your voice problem or how your voice is functioning?"*

14. Once a 1-minute spontaneous speech is recorded, save the recording.

15. For each perceptual parameter, indicate the severity of that quality by marking a cross along the 10-cm line. Note whether that particular quality is consistently demonstrated in the client's voice or it only appears intermittently.

(**Precautions:** During the recordings, make sure that the background noise level is kept to a minimum and the recorded sound level is at an appropriate level. It should be noted that the CAPE-V is not restricted to the use of perceptual quality terms listed in the form. Additional terms may be used when appropriate.)

CASE STUDY

J.S. was a 26-year-old teacher. In her third year as a full-time teacher, J.S. noticed that her voice was getting hoarse and she was unable to sing high notes. She visited a laryngologist who examined her vocal folds. A vocal polyp was found on her left vocal fold and the laryngologist recommended that she consulted a speech pathologist for voice training. Throughout the assessment session, the speech pathologist noticed that J.S.'s voice was mildly rough and breathy. J.S. spoke with moderate degree of tension and her voice was low in pitch. She also talked a little too loudly at times and occasional pitch breaks were noticed. Figure 23–1 shows the auditory-perceptual voice evaluation profile that was obtained by the speech pathologist in the first assessment session. It was concluded that J.S.'s overall dysphonic severity was mild to moderate.

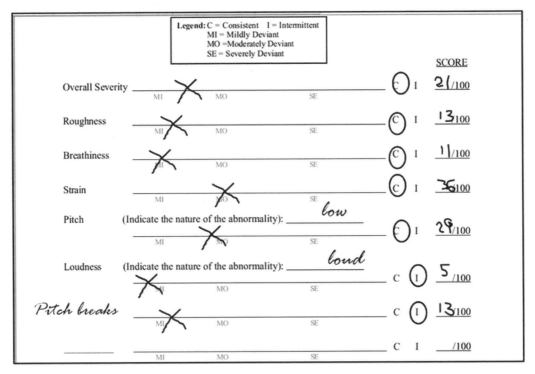

Figure 23–1. An example of a completed CAPE-V form.

REFERENCES

Behrman, A. (2005). Common practices of voice therapists in the evaluation of patients. *Journal of Voice, 19*, 454–469.

Carding, P., Carlson, E., Epstein, R., Mathieson, L., & Shewell, C. (2000). Formal perceptual evaluation of voice quality in the United Kingdom. *Logopedics, Phoniatrics and Vocology, 25*, 133–138.

Chan, K. M.-K., & Yiu, E. M.-L. (2002). The effect of anchors and training on the reliability of perceptual voice evaluation. *Journal of Speech, Language, and Hearing Research, 45*, 111–126.

Chan, K. M.-K., & Yiu, E. M.-L. (2006). A comparison of two perceptual voice evaluation training programs for naïve listeners. *Journal of Voice, 20*, 229–241.

De Bodt, M. S., Wuyts, F. L., Van de Heyning, P. H., & Croux, C. (1997). Test-retest study of the GRBAS scale: influence of experience and professional background on perceptual rating of voice quality. *Journal of Voice, 11*(1), 74–80.

Dejonckere, P. H., Obbens, C., de Moor, G. M., & Wieneke, G. H. (1993). Perceptual evaluation of dysphonia: reliability and relevance. *Folia Phoniatrica, 45*, 76–83.

Eadie, T. L., & Baylor, C. R. (2006). The effect of perceptual training on inexperienced listeners' judgments of dysphonic voice. *Journal of Voice, 20*(4), 527–544.

Eadie, T. L., & Doyle, P. C. (2002). Direct magnitude estimation and interval scaling of naturalness and severity in tracheoesophageal (TE) speakers. *Journal of Speech, Language and Hearing Research, 45*(6), 1088–1096.

Gerratt, B. R., & Kreiman, J. (2000). Theoretical and methodological development in the study of pathological voice quality. *Journal of Phonetics, 28*, 335–342.

Hammarberg, B. (2000). Voice research and clinical needs. *Folia Phoniatrica et Logopaedica, 52*(1–3), 93–102.

Hirano, M. (1981). *Clinical examination of voice* (Vol. 5). Vienna, Austria: Springer-Verlag.

Holmberg, E. B., Hillman, R. E., Hammarberg, B., Södersten, M., & Doyle, P. (2001). Efficacy of a behaviorally based voice therapy protocol for vocal nodules. *Journal of Voice, 15*(3), 395–412.

Karnell, M. P., Melton, S. D., Childes, J. M., Coleman, T. C., Dailey, S. A., & Hoffman, H. T. (2007). Reliability of clinician-based (GRBAS and CAPE-V) and patient-based (V-RQOL and IPVI) documentation of voice disorders. *Journal of Voice, 21*, 576–590.

Kempster, G. B., Gerratt, B. R., Verdolini-Abbott, K., Barkmeier-Kraemer, J., & Hillman, R. E. (2009). Consensus auditory-perceptual evaluation of voice: Development of a standardized clinical protocol. *American Journal of Speech-Language Pathology, 18*, 124–132.

Kreiman, J., & Gerratt, B. R. (1996). The perceptual structure of pathologic voice quality. *Journal of the Acoustical Society of America, 100*(3), 1787–1795.

Kreiman, J., & Gerratt, B. R. (1998). Validity of rating scale measures of voice quality. *Journal of the Acoustical Society of America, 104*(3), 1598–1608.

Kreiman, J., Gerratt, B. R., Kempster, G. B., Erman, A., & Berke, G. S. (1993). Perceptual evaluation of voice quality: Review, tutorial, and a framework for future research. *Journal of Speech and Hearing Research, 36*, 21–40.

Kreiman, J., Gerratt, B. R., & Precoda, K. (1990). Listener experience and perception of voice quality. *Journal of Speech and Hearing Research, 33*, 103–115.

Laver, J. (1980). *The phonetic description of voice quality*. Cambridge, UK: Cambridge University Press.

Martin, D. P., & Wolfe, V. I. (1996). Effects of perceptual training based upon synthesized voice signals. *Perceptual and Motor Skills, 83*, 1291–1298.

Oates, J. (2009). Auditory-perceptual evaluation of disordered voice quality: Pros, cons and future directions. *Folia Phoniatrica et Logopaedica, 61*, 49–56.

Piccirillo, J. F., Painter, C., Fuller, D., & Fredrickson, J. M. (1998). Multivariate analysis of objective vocal function. *Annals of Otology, Rhinology, and Laryngology, 107*(2), 107–112.

Rabinov, C. R., Kreiman, J., Gerratt, B. R., & Bielamowicz, S. (1995). Comparing reliablity of perceptual ratings of roughness and acoustic measures of jitter. *Journal of Speech and Hearing Research, 38*, 26–32.

Shewell, C. (1998). The effect of perceptual training on ability to use the vocal profile analysis scheme. *International Journal of Language and Communication Disorders, 33*, S322–S326.

Verdolini-Marston, K., Burke, M. K., Lessac, A., Glaze, L., & Caldwell, E. (1995). Preliminary study of two methods of treatment for laryngeal nodules. *Journal of Voice, 9*, 74–85.

Verdolini, K., & Palmer, P. M. (1997). Assessment of a "profiles" approach to voice screening. *Journal of Medical Speech-Langauge Pathology, 5*, 217–232.

Wuyts, F. L., de Bodt, M. S., & Van de Heyning, P. H. (1999). Is the reliability of a visual analog scale higher than an ordinal scale? An experiment with the GRBAS scale for the perceptual evalution of dysphonia. *Journal of Voice, 13*(4), 508–517.

Yamaguchi, H., Shrivastav, R., Andrews, M. L., & Niimi, S. (2003). A comparison of voice quality ratings made by Japanese and American listeners using the GRBAS Scale. *Folia Phoniatrica et Logopaedica, 55*(3), 147–157.

Yiu, E. M.-L., Chan, K. M.-K., & Mok, R. S.-M. (2007). Reliability and confidence in using a paired comparison paradigm in perceptual voice quality evaluation. *Clinical Linguistics and Phonetics, 21*(2), 129–145.

Yiu, E. M.-L., & Chan, R. M. M. (2003). Effect of hydration and vocal rest on the vocal fatigue in amateur Karaoke singers. *Journal of Voice, 17*(2), 216–227.

Yiu, E. M.-L., Murdoch, B., Hird, K., & Lau, P. (2002). Perception of synthesised voice quality in connected speech by Cantonese speakers. *Journal of the Acoustical Society of America, 112*(3), 1091–1101.

Yiu, E. M.-L., & Ng, C.-Y. (2004). Equal appearing interval and visual analogue scaling of perceptual roughness and breathiness. *Clinical Linguistics and Phonetics, 18*(3), 211–229.

Ylitalo, R., & Hammarberg, B. (2000). Voice characteristics, effects of voice therapy, and long-term follow-up of contact granuloma patients. *Journal of Voice, 14*(4), 557–566.

Yu, P., Revis, J., Wuyts, F. L., Zanaret, M., & Giovanni, A. (2002). Correlation of instrumental voice evaluation with perceptual voice analysis using a modified visual analog scale. *Folia Phoniatrica et Logopaedica, 54*(6), 271–281.

SECTION VII

Quality of Life Evaluation

CHAPTER 24

Patient-Reported Outcomes in Voice Disorders

BARBARA H. JACOBSON AND RICHARD I. ZRAICK

PURPOSE

- To assess the experience of patients with voice disorders in various aspects of their lives.

THEORETICAL BACKGROUND

Traditionally, clinical diagnosis in voice disorders follows the process of collecting data from the client, creating a hypothesis of how the disorder developed, testing that hypothesis by developing a plan to manage the voice disorder, and then reassessing the disorder after treatment by collecting more data. The initial data collection consists of taking a history, making perceptual judgments, performing an instrumental assessment, and assigning a rating based on the American Speech-Language-Hearing Association National Outcomes Measurement System (ASHA NOMS; ASHA, 2003). A hypothesis is created by determining the conditions, behaviors, and events that precipitated the voice disorder. The potential for effective behavioral voice therapy is compared to

medical and surgical management options. Using this hypothesis and calculating a prognosis, strategies are developed to achieve changes in voice use and voice production with the aim of ameliorating or managing the disorder. Finally, the initial measures are repeated to document the degree of change (in perceptual, instrumental, and functional parameters) after completing voice therapy.

As we have moved into the era of emphasis on evidence-based practice, we have expanded our perspective on what components are essential to "best practice" in the diagnosis and treatment of voice disorders. Certainly, we continue to use our clinical expertise, but Sackett and colleagues (2000) argue that we must also include the patient's values as well as current best evidence to provide excellent services to patients. The fund of knowledge on best practice continues to evolve slowly in our field. Assessing and assuming the patient's perspective on his or her voice disorder also continues to evolve. Patient-reported outcomes are the best way to incorporate the concept of patient values and experience into our assessment process. These values are represented by the preferences, environment, culture, and attitudes toward health and well-being that we develop as adults.

The most well-known framework of health was developed by the World Health Organization (WHO). The *International Classification of Impairments, Disabilities, and Handicaps (ICIDH)* was published in 1980 as an attempt to categorize potential outcomes from diseases and disorders. In the original conceptualization of the ICIDH, a disease or disorder causes a loss or abnormality of an anatomic, physiologic, or psychologic structure or function or *impairment*. In the field of voice disorders, a unilateral vocal fold paralysis can be considered to be an impairment (i.e., unilateral damage to the recurrent laryngeal nerve). The impairment then impacts the daily functioning of the individual. Certain tasks or skills are impacted by the impairment resulting in a *disability*. For the person with vocal fold paralysis, she might not be able to produce adequate loudness. Finally, the WHO framework defines the impact of impairment and disability on individuals' social roles in their environment. This relates particularly to the attitudes and responses of others to the impairment and disability. For our patient with a vocal fold paralysis, she might have difficulty in her elementary teaching job as she cannot produce adequate loudness to be heard in the classroom, playground, and lunchroom. She might be frustrated when she tries to place an order at a drive-through window. Her mother with a hearing impairment could have difficulties

understanding her on the telephone. When examining these examples, it is clear that an external observer would be aware of the impairment and disability, but might not be able to appreciate the handicap, as that is reflected in a more "global" experience of the individual.

The initial WHO framework as designed was intended to provide a guide for developing treatments that would impact the three components in the continuum as needed. This ensured that whatever intervention was planned, these three aspects of disorder and disease would be addressed. For our patient with vocal fold paralysis, this means that not only would some sort of medialization be attempted, but that modifications might be made to her environment (e.g., amplification for classroom use) that would help her to maximize the benefit of surgery. She also might require voice therapy to "unload" the vocal mechanism if she were using excessive extrinsic laryngeal muscle effort to produce voice. Outcome measures would include not only acoustic and aerodynamic measures of voice, but also some assessment of the patient's satisfaction with her voice and the process of rehabilitation as well as her feelings about how the results affected her emotional state.

Professionals who used the ICIDH to inform their clinical or research endeavors complained about several aspects of the classification system. It is primarily a medical model, with the focus on disease and disorder. This "medcentric" approach primarily relies on the perspective of the clinician. It is a simplistic framework that may not account for all the conditions or experiences of health. In 2001, the WHO published a revised framework called the *International Classification of Functioning, Disability, and Health (ICF)*. The emphasis is on disability, health, and the influence of environmental and personal factors that provide a context for the individual (Figure 24–1).

This new formulation of how various health states impact populations and individuals determines what questions we ask and how we describe what happens when someone has a voice disorder. When developed thoughtfully and with perspective, patient-reported outcomes measures for persons with voice disorders reflect the scope of their communication experiences.

TOOLS FOR MEASURING PATIENT-REPORTED OUTCOMES (PRO)

An outcome is the amount of change in the physical, mental, and social states that compromise health as the result of treatment or nontreatment (WHO, 1997). In the past, physical aspects of an illness or condition have received the most attention. In recent years, the mental and social aspects have been recognized as important indicators of a patient's quality of life. Patient-reported outcomes assess various parameters of a patient's experience of health. A patient-reported outcome is the measurement of any aspect of a patient's health status that comes directly from the patient. These include (in no particular hierarchical order) general well-being, function, symptoms, satisfaction, and global quality of life. The term "patient-reported outcomes" (PRO) has superseded the term "quality of life" in much of the literature. This term emphasizes the patient-focused construct as well as the practical shift to using PRO to evaluate disease and disorder states and to evaluate and compare treatments.

There is considerable support for use of PRO in evidence-based medicine. For

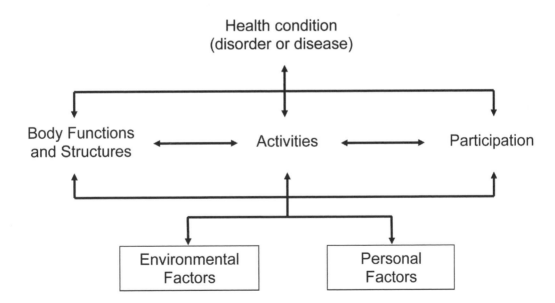

Figure 24–1. World Health Organization (WHO) International Classification of Functioning, Disability, and Health (ICF) (2001).

example, patient-reported outcomes have predictive value for survival in cancer patients. The amount of social support and levels of symptom distress are prognostic factors for survival (Degner & Sloan, 1995; Silliman, Dukes, Sullivan & Kaplan, 1998). Patients with cancer who report that they are doing well in general and have a good appetite live longer (Hobday et. al., 2002). Finally, patients with advanced cancer who report a higher quality of life live longer than those who report less favorable status (Sloan et al., 1998). The potential to discover associations such as these can help us to plan treatments that directly impact on well-being and subsequently positively affect the resolution of the patient's disease or disorder.

Measuring PRO in General Health

In 1987 the Medical Outcomes Survey (Tarlov, Ware, Greenfield, Nelson, Perrin, & Zubkoff, 1989) was administered to a variety of individuals across the United States. From this initial effort, a "short form" was developed that consisted of 36 items that covered a variety of domains. These domains included physical functioning, role limitations (physical), social functioning, bodily pain, general health, role limitations (emotional), vitality, mental health, and change in health status. These items ultimately were combined into two summary scales: physical health and mental health. The SF-36 has been used to assess attitudes about well-being for patients with a wide variety of medical diagnoses. Although the SF-36 contains generic health measures, it has been validated for use with many populations. There are standardized general population norms for the standard (4 week

recall) and acute (1 week recall) forms. Reliability ranges from 0.6 to 0.9 for the subscales of the SF-36.

There are now two shorter versions of the SF-36, the SF-12 (Quality Metric Corp., Lincoln, NE) and the SF-8 (Quality Metric Corp., Lincoln, NE). Both have been shown to provide valid and reliable data for assessing health status. However, score precision can be sacrificed when a scale is shortened to allow for less "burden" on the respondent. The SF-36 best represents the domains of health that were developed empirically in the original Medical Outcomes Survey (Tarlov et al., 1989). It is psychometrically sound. However, it generates an unwieldy amount of data for large scale studies and may be too difficult for fragile patients to complete. The SF-12 has been shown to be the best scale for large studies. On the other hand, analysis of SF-12 data may miss some potentially significant information and it may be less sensitive to change. Finally, the SF-8 is brief and comprehensive but is not designed to detect small group-level differences.

Several investigators have examined the impact of voice disorders on general health status as measured by the SF-36 (Cohen, Dupont, & Courey, 2006). Patients with dysphonia typically score lower (i.e., worse) than normal speakers. Patients with neurogenic voice disorders demonstrate more handicap than patients without dysphonia and are slightly more affected than other voice-disordered patients. In general, patients with voice disorders have scores that are similar to patients with chronic diseases such as heart failure, angina, sciatica, or chronic obstructive pulmonary disease.

The National Institutes of Health (NIH) has developed the Patient-Reported Outcomes Measurement Inventory System (PROMIS). This initiative is part of the

NIH Roadmap, which is designed to move scientific and medical discoveries from the bench to the clinic. The primary aim of PROMIS is to create ways to measure patient-reported symptoms. A consortium of six sites has commenced work since 2004 to create item banks, develop questionnaires, and establish a computerized testing system. The Web site for PROMIS (www.nihpromis.org) contains the core elements of the system and describes the various stages of development of items and population administration. Some of the instruments available assess health status in the areas of emotional distress, fatigue, pain, physical function, social satisfaction, sleep, and global health. The project has moved into its second phase (Wave II) and serves as an excellent resource for all phases of PRO development and assessment.

Measuring PRO in Voice Disorders

Interest in reporting outcomes in voice disorders began in the 1940s. Published articles noted that various voice therapy techniques were effective for certain types of disorders. However, there was no formal analysis to demonstrate efficacy or effectiveness. Most of this literature was of the "how I do it" variety with limited reporting of specific measures and no standardized reporting of auditory-perceptual analysis. Instrumental analysis was evident in the 1970s, although formal experimental studies were not developed until the 1990s. Some functional and patient satisfaction outcomes were presented in research published in the 1980s, but quality of life measures were not used in reporting outcomes until the 1990s (Zraick & Risner, 2008). As researchers and clinicians began to be interested in the patient

perspective, they developed ways of eliciting information that reflected how patients looked at their voice disorders.

Initially, clinicians elicited information about patients' attitudes toward their voice disorders when collecting history during the assessment process. They might ask patients how their voice disorder affected them in their daily activities. They might get reflections on how frustrated patients were with their voices. They would get reports from the patients about their physical symptoms. These anecdotal reports were helpful in providing some idea of the impact of a voice disorder on a particular patient, but they did not allow for comparison from pretreatment status to post-treatment status. Clinicians could not compare one patient to another with the same type of voice disorder. Treatment efficacy or effectiveness comparisons were not possible.

Izdebski et al. (1984) reported an epidemiologic study of 200 individuals with spasmodic dysphonia compared to 200 controls. They collected information on medical history, voice history, job functioning, and satisfaction with care. In 1984, Llewellyn-Thomas and colleagues developed a linear analogue self-assessment of voice quality in laryngeal cancer. This measure was designed to assess symptoms and functional status for patients undergoing radiation treatment for laryngeal cancer and compare their pretreatment responses to those collected after radiation treatment. There was a group of 16 scales anchored at each end by statements such as, "able to speak without any effort" and "able to speak only with great effort." Other scales measured perceived symptoms such as dryness. Other functions that were assessed included the ability to sing, talk on the telephone, and whistle. Psychometric analysis demonstrated that this instrument met standards of feasibility, reliability and sensitivity to change. A follow-up study (Sutherland et al., 1984) found that patients and physicians did not agree on status related to functional ability. This highlighted the importance of collecting data directly from patients.

Smith et al. (1996) developed the Voice Clinic Questionnaire, which collected demographic information, medical and social history, and information about quality of life related to voice disorders. Some of the questions were, "How much do voice problems limit your job?," "How much do voice problems make you feel sad or depressed?" Respondents marked their answers as "not at all," "very little," "moderately," "very much," and "extremely." This essentially was a symptoms inventory survey. However, it attempted to collect information systematically for group comparisons.

In the field of audiology, standardized and validated patient-focused instruments have a long history (Jacobson & Newman, 1990; Newman, Jacobson, & Spitzer, 1996; Newman, Weinstein, Jacobson, & Hug, 1990; Ventry & Weinstein, 1982). In the field of voice disorders, clinicians were looking for patient-focused measures that would be easy to use in their practices. These measures had to be reliable, relatively easy to administer, easy to score, and stand up to psychometric scrutiny. These measures would help to answer the following questions: Did my particular treatment technique work? Did it change a particular aspect of the patient's daily functioning? Did the patient's perception of his/her problem differ from mine? Did this particular quality of life measure correspond to other tests or measures that one might take in the assessment of pre- or post-treatment status?

A number of voice-disordered quality of life (VDQOL) instruments are available to clinicians and researchers working with voice-disordered patients (Table 24–1). The choice of which instrument to administer often is driven by the clinician's personal preference and dynamics of clinical practice. Regardless of which instrument is used, the clinician should be aware that variables such as life events and experiences, personality factors, and the effects of adaptation may influence reported subjective well-being (O'Connor, 2004). Review of Table 24–1 indicates that the available scales can be grouped and categorized using criteria such as patient age (e.g., adult versus child), rater (e.g., patient versus parent or other proxy), and patient population (e.g., singer versus nonsinger). The following sections review the instruments that are appropriate for use with adults and pediatric patients.

Voice Handicap Index (VHI)

The Voice Handicap Index was created in response to a realization that there was no standardized measure of how patients felt about their voice disorders. It was developed by Jacobson and colleagues (1997) at Henry Ford Medical Center in Detroit, Michigan. Other quality of life measures (e.g., SF-36) have been surveyed, but many of these were quite general. Jacobson et al. aimed to have an instrument that was specific to a certain population of patients. They surveyed the histories of past patients to collect statements that patients had made regarding their complaints and effects of the voice disorders on their lives. A list of 85 items related to the experiences of voice-disordered patients was generated. Several of the items were redundant in that they had essentially the same meaning, but were worded differently.

Three domains were created a priori that reflected the underlying focus of

Table 24–1. Major Voice-Disordered Quality of Life (VDQOL) Instruments

Instrument Name and Acronym	Developers
Voice Handicap Index (VHI)	Jacobson et al. (1997)
Voice Handicap Index–10 (VHI-10)	Rosen et al. (2004)
Voice Handicap Index–Partner (VHI-P)	Zraick et al. (2007)
Pediatric Voice Handicap Index (pVHI)	Zur et al. (2007)
Singing Voice Handicap Index (SVHI)	Cohen et al. (2007)
Vocal Performance Questionnaire (VPQ)	Carding et al. (1999)
Voice Disability Coping Questionnaire (VDCQ)	Epstein et al. (2009)
Voice Symptom Scale (VoiSS)	Deary et al. (2003)
Voice Activity and Participation Profile (VAPP)	Ma & Yiu (2001)
Voice-Related Quality of Life (V-RQOL)	Hogikyan & Sethuraman (1999)
Pediatric Voice-Related Quality of Life (PVRQOL)	Boseley et al. (2006)
Voice Outcome Survey (VOS)	Gliklich et al. (1999)
Pediatric Voice Outcome Survey (PVOS)	Hartnick (2002)

each statement. These domains were "functional," "emotional," and "physical." Functional items were related to the impact of the voice disorder. A sample functional item was, "My voice problem causes me to miss work." Emotional items reflected affective responses to the voice disorders. A sample item in the emotional domain was, "I feel annoyed when people ask me to repeat." Finally, in the physical domain, statements addressed laryngeal discomfort and voice quality characteristics. A sample item in this domain was, "I feel as though I have to strain to produce voice." An ordinal scale was used for gathering responses. They were "never" (0 points), "almost never" (1 point), "sometimes" (2 points), "almost always" (3 points), and "always" (4 points).

The 85-item alpha version was reduced in size in four ways. Items with poor internal consistency were elimi-nated. Statements that demonstrated a gender bias were removed. Items that were redundant were eliminated if they had a poorer internal consistency than their counterparts. Finally, items that were answered "never" by more than 50% of respondents were eliminated. Four items were retained for the beta version because of their high face validity. They represented information that we wanted to collect. They were, "The sound of my voice varies throughout the day," "My voice sounds creaky and dry," "My voice problem causes me to lose income," and "I run out of air when I talk."

The resulting beta version contained 30 items with 10 items in each subscale. Test-retest reliability for the entire instrument was 0.92. From test-retest data, critical difference scores were calculated. That is, what was the difference from the first to second administration that might indicate that some clinically significant change had occurred? Some variability in responses was expected even in the absence of treatment due to normal fluctuations in perceptions of their voices by the subjects. Analysis indicated that a critical difference of 18 points on the total scale was necessary to demonstrate a real change in self-perception of voice handicap. A change of 8 points was needed for each individual subscale. The change could be in either positive or negative direction.

Finally, patients' scores on the VHI were compared to their self-perceived severity of voice problems. This served to measure an aspect of construct validity as there was no other available instrument for comparison. The correlation between the two measures was 0.60. Relative severity of voice handicap was also calculated using these two measures. A mild severity was indicated by responses between 0 and 40. A moderate self-perceived handicap was indicated by scores between 41 and 60. A severe level of handicap was indicated by a score of 61 to 120. In collecting these data, subjects often noted that they did not know how "bad" their voice disorder was until they completed the VHI.

There are several limitations to the VHI. In the original study, the VHI was not administered to a cohort of individuals without voice disorders. Without this, there may be an artificial "floor" effect. In the development of the VHI-10 (Rosen, Lee, Osborne, Zullo, & Murry, 2004), a group of control subjects had a mean VHI score of 8.75. Based on this report, a score of 9 or below might be considered to reflect a "normal" level of self-perceived voice handicap. No factor analysis was performed in the process of developing the VHI. Rosen et al. (2004) noted that a single factor accounted for the majority of

the variance in VHI scores. This might be considered to be "voice handicap."

Several meta-analyses have examined various aspects of psychometric adequacy of the VHI. Eadie et al. (2006) reviewed six instruments for their ability to measure communication participation, one of the constructs of the ICF. Four voice disorder-specific measures were included in that group. For the VHI, 23% of the items assessed communication participation. In 2002, the Agency for Healthcare Research and Quality (AHRQ) published a review of instruments that might be suitable for use in determining disability in communication disorders. In the area of voice disorders, the VHI and the KayPENTAX Multidimensional Voice Program (KayPENTAX Corp., Lincoln Park, NJ) met criteria for reliability, validity, and presence of normative data. It is important to note that AHRQ reports are considered to be "current" for 5 years. Franic et al. (2005) evaluated the VHI along with other voice-related self-report measures. Results are detailed later in this chapter.

To date, the VHI has been translated into at least 15 languages. Verdonck-de Leeuw and colleagues (2008) found that VHI scores were equivalent across "European" languages when examining various translations. It is important to remember that, when translations are attempted for any validated instrument, the translated instrument should meet similar measures of validity and reliability of the original version. Forward and backward translations are also important to retain the integrity of the measure.

The Voice Handicap Index-10 (VHI-10)

The VHI-10 is a shorter representation of the VHI. It was developed by Rosen and colleagues (Rosen et al., 2004). In their study, expert consensus review and subsequent item analysis of the VHI was performed using the VHI responses of 100 dysphonic patients and 159 control subjects. The VHI-10 was formed from the 10 most robust VHI items, chosen in part by a panel of expert clinicians to be "clinically relevant" for both the assessment of voice-related handicap and responsiveness to treatment. Statistical analysis comparing the validity of the VHI-10 to that of the VHI was performed with 819 patients representing a wide spectrum of voice disorders. Rosen et al. reported that there was no statistically significant difference between the VHI and the VHI-10 scores and that, irrespective of diagnosis, the two versions were highly correlated. Rosen et al. (2004) concluded that, "the VHI-10 is a powerful representation of the VHI that takes less time for the patient to complete without loss of validity" (p. 1549). The VHI-10 has good internal consistency (Deary, Webb, MacKenzie, Wilson, & Carding, 2004) and recently was used in a multiparametric study of patient-related outcomes after therapy for functional dysphonia (Morsomme et al., 2010). Like the VHI, the VHI-10 also has been translated for use with non-English speakers with voice disorders (Amir et al., 2006; Lam et al., 2006).

The Voice-Related Quality of Life (V-RQOL) Measure

Developed by Hogikyan and Sethuraman (1999), the V-RQOL instrument asks the patient to assess their quality of life in the context of their voice disorder. The V-RQOL contains 10 items and provides a standard score. The V-RQOL was validated on 109 patients and 21 speakers with normal voice. It has been reported to have

acceptable reliability, validity, and sensitivity to change (Franic et al., 2005). It has been used with a variety of adult patient populations (Golub, Chen, Otto, Hapner, & Johns, 2006). The V-RQOL has been translated for non-English users (Behlau, Hogikyan, & Gasparini, 2007; Gasparini & Behlau, 2009). The V-RQOL and the VHI are reported to be highly correlated in certain patient populations (Kazi et al., 2007; Portone, Hapner, McGregor, Otto, & Johns, 2007)

The Voice Outcome Survey (VOS)

Gliklich and colleagues (1999) developed the VOS as a brief (5-item), valid, reliable, and highly sensitive outcome measure in patients with unilateral vocal fold paralysis. An expert panel consisting of physicians and voice therapists, in addition to patients with vocal fold paralyses, provided input. Raw scores on the VOS are transformed to a scale of 0 (worst) to 100 (best) for ease of interpretation. Low scores describe a relatively poor VDQOL; high scores describe a better VDQOL. In their study of 56 patients, Gliklich et al. reported that the VOS was found to correlate highly with subscales of the Short-Form 36 (Tarlov et al., 1989; Ware & Sherbourne, 1992) and with selected acoustic voice parameters. However, Franic et al. (2005) question the reliability of the VOS and its limited applicability. The VOS has been translated recently for non-English users (Fang, Li, Gliklich, Chen, & Wang, 2007).

The Vocal Performance Questionnaire (VPQ)

The VPQ was developed by Carding and colleagues and has been used as an outcome measure in a number of treatment studies (Carding, Horsley, & Docherty,

1999; Dejonckere, Obbens, de Moor, & Wieneke, 1993; Dejonckere et al., 2001; Meek, Carding, Howard, & Lennard, 2008). The VPQ is designed such that it enables patients to consider aspects of their own vocal performance and rate the severity of that aspect with regard to their normal voice usage (Lee, Drinnan, & Carding, 2005). The VPQ contains 12 items. With a numerical value of 1 to 5 assigned for every item, a total severity score is calculated for each patient. The range of possible total scores is 12 (normal voice functioning as perceived by the patient) to 60 (severely limited voice functioning). In a study by Deary and colleagues (2004), the psychometric properties of the VPQ were examined and compared to those of the VHI-10. It was reported that the VPQ has good internal consistency and reliability, and appears to assess the same constructs as the VHI-10. Deary et al. concluded that the VPQ may be useful in clinical settings where time constraints limit the ability to administer longer instruments such as the VHI (p. 233).

The Voice Activity and Participation Profile (VAPP)

The VAPP is a 28-item self-report instrument developed by Ma and Yiu (2001) from interviews with dysphonic patients and speech-language pathologists. As described by Ma and Yiu (p. 511), the VAPP evaluates the perception of voice problem, activity limitation, and participation restriction using the WHO International Classification of Impairments, Disabilities and Handicaps-2 framework (WHO, 1997). The VAPP attempts to quantify the following domains: self-perceived severity of voice problem, effects on job, effects on daily communication, effects on social communication, and effects on emotion. The VAPP requires patients to use visual analog scaling to respond. In Ma and Yiu's initial study, the VAPP was administered to 40 patients with dysphonia and 40 control subjects with normal voices. Results showed that the dysphonic group reported significantly more severe voice problems, limitation in daily voice activities, and restricted participation in activities than the control group. They also showed that the perception of a voice problem by the dysphonic subjects correlated positively with the perception of limitation in voice activities and restricted participation. However, the self-perceived voice problem had little correlation with the degree of voice-quality impairment measured acoustically and perceptually. The data also showed that the aggregate scores of activity limitation and participation restriction were positively correlated, and the extent of activity limitation and participation restriction was similar.

In a more recent study, Ma and Yiu (2007) compared their original visual analog scaling response method for the VAPP to that of equal-appearing interval scaling (Guyatt, Townsend, Berman, & Keller, 1987; Zraick & Liss, 2000). Thirty-two individuals with dysphonia rated their self-perceived activity limitation and participation restriction using both response methods. Test-retest reliabilities were similar for both methods. The overall extents of activity limitation and participation restriction were similar for both rating methods. Ma and Yiu concluded that either response method is valid, noting that patients may favor equal-appearing interval scaling because of its relative ease of use (p. 74). The VAPP has been translated for use with non-English speakers with voice disorders (e.g., Sukanen et al., 2007).

The Voice Symptom Scale (VoiSS)

The VoiSS was developed by Deary and colleagues in a series of studies (Deary, Wilson, Carding, & MacKenzie, 2003; Scott, Robinson, Wilson & Mackenzie, 1997) involving nearly 500 patients. The VoiSS is a 30-item questionnaire that addresses three areas: impairment, emotion, and related physical symptoms. Wilson and colleagues (2004) compared the structure and content of the VoiSS to the VHI by having 319 patients complete both instruments. It was reported by Wilson et al. that the VoiSS has a more valid underlying content structure than the VHI, and presents no item redundancy. Wilson et al. suggested that further examination of the content structure of the VHI is necessary, concluding that, " . . . the VoiSS is psychometrically the most robust and extensively validated self-report voice measure available" (p. 169). The VoiSS recently was used in a study of perceived vocal morbidity in a problem asthma clinic (Stanton, Sellars, Mackenzie, McConnachie, & Bucknall, 2009), where it was reported that patients with functional or structural laryngeal abnormality had significantly worse VoiSS scores than patients with normal larynges.

The Voice Disability Coping Questionnaire (VDCQ)

The impact of voice disability is more wide ranging than simply restriction in voice. Voice disorders may have pervasive effects on the individual's life beyond the vocal impairment itself. In an attempt to understand the coping process in persons with voice disorders, Epstein and colleagues (2009) developed the Voice Disability Coping Questionnaire (VDCQ), a disease-specific coping measure that elicits how patients cope with voice problems. This instrument was validated on 80 patients presenting with muscle tension dysphonia (MTD) and adductor spasmodic dysphonia (ADDSD). Each patient completed the 28-item VDCQ as part of an initial assessment protocol before intervention, within a longitudinal study. Four coping subscales were identified: social support, passive coping, avoidance, and information seeking. It was reported by Epstein et al. that avoidance and passive coping were found to be used by the ADDSD group significantly more than the MTD group (p. 209). The authors concluded that the VDCQ was a valid and reliable instrument that differentiated between clinical groups and that facilitated a patient-centered approach, both of which enhanced the understanding of voice disorders.

The Pediatric Voice Outcome Survey (PVOS)

Hartnick (2002) altered the VOS such that individual item structure was modified to reflect parent proxy administration rather than self-administration. He administered the PVOS to 108 caregivers of children from 2 to 18 years old who had undergone tracheotomy or had achieved surgical decannulation, and reported that children with tracheotomies had poorer VOS scores than children who had been decannulated. A follow-up study by Hartnick and colleagues (2003) reported normative data obtained from 385 parents of children and adolescents aged 2 to 18 years from a broad pediatric otolaryngology population. In a more recent study (Mirasola, Braun, Blumin, Kerschner, & Merati, 2008), the PVOS was administered to 20 patients with paradoxic vocal fold dysfunction (PVFD) and age-matched healthy controls. It was reported that PVOS scores were not significantly different between the two groups and that the overall PVOS did not show a significant decline in the self-reported VDQOL in persons with PVFD.

Pediatric Voice-Related Quality-of-Life (PVRQOL) Survey

Boseley and colleagues (2006) developed the 10-item PVRQOL from the adult V-RQOL. Individual item structure was altered to reflect parent proxy administration rather than self-administration. The PVRQOL was jointly administered with the Pediatric Voice Outcomes Survey (PVOS) (Hartnick, 2002) to 104 caregivers of children with a variety of dysphonia etiologies. The physical-functional scores on the PVRQOL agreed most closely with the PVOS whereas the social-emotional scores correlated to a lesser degree but were still significant. Blumin and colleagues (2008) examined the impact of gender and age on voice related quality of life in children without voice complaints using the PVRQOL and reported no significant difference between age groups or gender, although a diminished PVRQOL score was reported for boys as compared to girls (p. 229). In a follow-up study conducted by Merati and colleagues (2008), the PVRQOL scores of healthy children from Blumin et al. (2008) were compared to those of children with vocal nodules, vocal fold paralysis, and paradoxical vocal fold disorder. Merati et al. (2008) reported that children with the aforementioned common disorders demonstrated statistically significant impairment than age-matched children for total PVRQOL, as well as for the social-emotional and physical-functional domains (p. 259).

Pediatric Voice Handicap Index (pVHI)

In an attempt to understand parental proxy ratings of voice handicap, Zur and colleagues (2007) developed the pVHI, a 23-item modification and extension of the VHI. This instrument was validated on 45 normal children and 33 voice-disordered children before and after laryngotracheal reconstruction. These speakers also completed another questionnaire consisting of 10 open-ended questions regarding the impact of the child's voice quality on overall communication, development, education, social life, and family circumstances. The two groups were reported by Zur et al. to differ greatly on the pVHI subscale and total scores, with the correlations between pVHI subscale and total scores being similar to those reported in the original VHI validation study (Jacobson et al., 1997). It was further reported by Zur et al. that the pVHI had good internal consistency and high test-retest reliability (p. 78). The results of Zur et al. are consistent with previous studies from the general medical literature which report that parental proxy ratings can provide clinically useful information (Sneeuw, Sprangers, & Aaronson, 2002; Spieth & Harris, 1996).

The Voice Handicap Index-Partner (VHI-P)

The VHI-P was introduced by Zraick and colleagues (2007) in a study which examined partner proxy ratings of voice handicap. In this study, the items on the full-length VHI were rewritten from the point of view of the patient's primary communication partner. The VHI was then administered to 20 patients with moderate dysphonia and the VHI-P was administered to their communication partners. Zraick et al. reported that patients and their communication partners were in close agreement about the degree of voice handicap. It was further reported that patients and their partners were in close agreement on each of the three VHI subscales (physical, functional, and emotional), and that in all cases the physical domain was perceived by both patients and their partners to be most handicapped. The results of Zraick et al. are consistent with previous studies from the general medical literature which report that partner proxy ratings can be a useful alternative or collaborative source of patient's self-perception (Sneeuw et al., 2002).

Singing Voice Handicap Index (SVHI)

The SVHI was developed by Cohen and colleagues (2007) to assess the physical, emotional, social and economic impact of voice problems on singers, a population with more self-reported voice problems and more vocal disability than nonsingers (Cohen, Noordzij, Garrett, & Ossoff, 2008; Murry, Zschommler, & Prokop, 2009; Rosen & Murry, 2000). The SVHI is a 36-item survey that was validated on 112 dysphonic and 129 normal singers, both professional and nonprofessional. Cohen et al. reported that dysphonic singers had worse SVHI scores than normal singers and that the SVHI had high test-retest reliability and internal consistency. It was further reported by Cohen et al. that the correlation between the SVHI and self-rated singing voice impairment was moderate. The responsiveness of the SVHI to treatment-related changes in patients' singing voices was not evaluated in this initial study (p. 406). However, in a follow-up study by Cohen and colleagues (2008),

the responsiveness of the SVHI was examined in 30 singers from a tertiary voice clinic. These patients completed the SVHI at initial presentation, at pretreatment and at post-treatment. Cohen et al. reported that patients had lower SVHI scores post-therapy compared with the initial SVHI scores and that the change in SVHI scores from initial to post-treatment evaluation was greater than the change from initial to pretreatment evaluation (p. 1705). It also was reported that the SVHI treatment responsiveness correlated well with that of the VHI which was administered concurrently.

PSYCHOMETRIC CONSIDERATIONS

Voice-disordered quality of life (VDQOL) can be used as a gauge by which success of voice therapy is measured (Benninger, Gardner, Jacobson, & Grywalski, 1997; Speyer, Wieneke, & Dejonckere, 2004). In a recent survey of diagnostic practices of experienced voice clinicians (Behrman, 2005), 94% responded that VDQOL instruments are important for assessment of treatment outcomes, and 81% considered the data from such instruments important in defining overall therapy goals (p. 460). As Ma and Yiu (2001) stated, "The impact of a voice disorder on an individual is more than a mere visible abnormality of the larynx or audible deviant voice quality. The daily activities and social function of an individual are often affected as well" (p. 511).

Many of the instruments described in this chapter are reported to be psychometrically sound, that is, they are reliable (produce consistent and reproducible data) and valid (measure what is intended to be measured). Franic and colleagues (2005) conducted a comprehensive review of the psychometric properties of four VDQOL instruments: the VHI, the VAPP, the V-RQOL, and the VOS. These instruments were evaluated based on 11 measurement standards related to item information, versatility, practicality, breadth and depth of health measure, reliability, validity, and responsiveness. Franic et al. reported that none of the instruments met all psychometric criteria, although the VHI and the V-RQOL fared best. VHI showed preferable measurement characteristics on item information, practicality, and reliability, whereas V-RQOL showed preferable responsiveness properties. Franic et al. suggested the use of V-RQOL total or dimension scores for group-level decision making and the use of total VHI score for individual-level decision making.

Branski and colleagues (2010), intrigued by the findings of Franic et al. (2005), sought to examine why none of the existing VDQOL instruments met all psychometric criteria. It was hypothesized by Branski et al. that the psychometric deficiencies were associated with deficits in the development process for each instrument. As one might imagine, each instrument was developed by using varying methods and standards. For example, only the adult scales reflect input from expert clinicians. Only the VHI, VHI-10, V-RQOL, and the VoiSS were refined over multiple administrations to new patient cohorts, with the VHI and the VoiSS considered by Branski et al. to be the most rigorous in this regard. The three pediatric scales were derived from existing adult scales. As Branski et al. stated, " . . . It is unclear whether the domains used to assess QOL in dysphonic adults assess QOL in children; measures developed for

adults may fail to assess specific aspects of QOL that are important to children" (p. 5). Branksi et al. also identified a trend of translating existing QOL instruments for use with non-English speakers, cautioning that cross-linguistic validation must be ensured. Branski et al. concluded that none of the QOL instruments currently used meet all of the current standards for instrument development (Scientific Advisory Committee of the Medical Outcomes Trust, 2002), and they offered suggestions for more rigorous development of new scales and refinement/extension of existing scales.

FUTURE DIRECTIONS

The emphasis on demonstrating treatment effectiveness and efficacy in the field of voice disorders is the impetus for developing measures that are psychometrically rigorous, clinically valid, and efficiently incorporated into any practice settings. There is no doubt that reimbursement will be driven by quality indicators in clinical practice that include patient-reported outcomes. Although several instruments currently address some of these benchmarks, clearly there are ways that new approaches can fulfill all these criteria. Further refinement of existing measures, development of other types of scales, and integration of innovative administration and analysis methodology offer us the opportunity to evaluate service delivery to our patients and provide best practice.

The instruments described in this chapter all have some degree of psychometric power. They illustrate the need to provide comprehensive validity for any measure that purports to assess outcomes from the patient perspective. Crucial elements include reliability (test-retest, internal consistency, across interviewers), validity (content-related, construct, predictive), ability to detect change specific to a time interval, and interpretability (difference in a score that is evidence of a treatment benefit) (FDA, 2006). Ultimately, patient reported outcomes in voice must measure communication participation as one of their key constructs.

Most of the inventories that have been created are directed at the general populations of adult voice disordered patients. With the exception of the SVHI, scales have been standardized on patients with a variety of voice disorders and it is important to know the subject pool that was used for standardization. Some may have included patients with laryngectomy (e.g., VHI) or resonance disorders. Some clinics have a patient mix with a large number of individuals with spasmodic dysphonia or paradoxical vocal fold motion. It is of clinical *and* research interest to have scales that address the specific experiences of these patients. In addition to disorder-specific measures, age-specific inventories can be useful in the evaluation and treatment of older adults. As the population worldwide ages and continues to remain active in the community, there is a need to understand what older adults regard as communication well-being. Although there are some pediatric-focused scales, younger children have different communication needs from adolescents. If a certain client population represents a cross-section of age, then current pediatric scales are appropriate. However, inventories with a more narrow focus (e.g., adolescents) would produce more meaningful data. Other categories of patients whose particular attitudes are not explicitly addressed in the development of instruments are those with diverse cultural backgrounds. No research

has explored cultural perspectives on communication well-being. Consequently, there are no PRO measures in voice disorders that address cultural differences and similarities in communication requirements and attitudes.

Although the concept of a single total scale score is appealing in reporting the outcomes of intervention, it also may serve a purpose to produce a qualitative analysis of multiple responses. This is dependent on the needs of a particular clinical or research endeavor. Such an analysis could help in developing profiles for particular voice disorders. This could be applicable to differentiate muscle tension dysphonia from spasmodic dysphonia, for example. These analyses involve making associations between responses for well-validated scales with other behavioral factors. It is possible that attitudes about health status as it relates to voice disorders may have a bearing on important considerations for positive treatment outcomes including motivation, compliance, and locus of control.

Technology offers several options for the administration of PRO. Traditionally, pencil/paper techniques have been used to collect data. However, several institutions offer online administration through the Internet or computer administration via a clinic kiosk. Essentially, the only limitation is that the responses have to be sent over a secured connection. For scales with linear analogue scales, a sliding cursor can be used to register responses. It is conceivable that a smartphone application will be available in the future for patients to send in data in real time, as they encounter communication experiences that challenge their voice production.

In contrast to a detailed analysis, it has been demonstrated that a single question can be adequate to assess patient-reported outcomes (Buchanan, O'Mara, Kelaghan, & Minasian, 2005; Sloan et al., 2001). The appropriately designed item will have enough power to measure the effect of intervention and can be used as a predictive measure associated with other outcomes. If the objective is to assess the overall construct of effective communication or communication participation, then a single question is adequate. Regardless of the type of scale, patient-reported outcomes are a critical element of assessment that bring us closer to achieving results that are meaningful to patients.

CASE STUDY

J.B. is a 23-year-old female graduate student who presented with a 2-year history of poor voice quality and vocal fatigue. Indirect laryngoscopy revealed mild edema and erythema of the vocal folds and irregular vocal fold edges, suggestive of vocal hyperfunction. She expressed concerns about how her dysphonia might affect future employment opportunities and interpersonal relationships. She repeatedly had tried, but unsuccessfully, to self-

treat her dysphonia with a loosely defined and applied approach of vocal hygiene.

J.B. was seen for direct voice therapy once a week for 60 minutes for a total of 8 weeks. The focus of therapy was reduction of voice use as described by van der Merwe (2004). A number of clinical outcome measures were obtained before, during, and at the end of therapy, including indirect laryngoscopy, acoustic analyses, aerodynamic analyses, auditory-perceptual ratings, and VHI and VHI-P scores. J.B. completed the VHI and her primary communication partner completed the VHI-Partner. Thus, both primary and supplemental information was obtained about voice handicap.

Table 24–2 shows the raw score, subscale scores, and range as reported by the patient and her partner on the VHI and VHI-P. Review of Table 24–2 reveals that the VHI/VHI-P raw scores, as well as the VHI/VHI-P subscale scores, were significantly lower at the end of therapy than at the beginning. These findings corresponded with a positive change in all other outcome measures, including a post-therapy questionnaire addressing satisfaction with therapy. After graduation J.B. got a job as a teacher and became a newlywed.

Table 24–2. Pre- and Post-Treatment Voice Handicap Index (VHI) and VHI-Partner (VHI-P) Scores

Dimension	Baseline VHI	Baseline VHI-P	Week 8 VHI	Week 8 VHI-P	Maintenance VHI	Maintenance VHI-P
Total Score	20	20	3	2	3	2
Subscale—Functional	1	0	0	0	0	0
Subscale—Physical	16	14	3	2	3	2
Subscale—Emotional	3	6	0	0	0	0
Range	0–20	0–20	0–3	0–2	0–3	0–2

REFERENCES

Agency for Healthcare Research and Quality. (2002). Criteria for determining disability in speech-language disorders. *Evidence Report/Technology Assessment, 52.*

American Speech-Language-Hearing Association. (2003). *National Outcomes Measurement System (NOMS): Adult speech-language pathology user's guide.* Rockville, MD: Author.

Amir, O., Tavor, Y., Leibovitzh, T., Ashkenazi, O., Michael, O., Primov-Fever, A., & Wolf, M. (2006). Evaluating the validity of the Voice Handicap Index-10 (VHI-10) among Hebrew speakers. *Otolaryngology-Head and Neck Surgery, 135*(4), 603–607.

Behlau, M., Hogikyan, N., & Gasparini, G. (2007). Quality of life and voice: Study of a Brazilian population using the Voice-Related Quality of Life measure. *Folia Phoniatrica et Logopaedica, 59*(6), 286–296.

Behrman, A. (2005). Common practices of voice therapists in the evaluation of patients. *Journal of Voice, 19*(3), 454–469.

Benninger, M. S., Gardner, G. M., Jacobson, B. H., & Grywalski, C. (1997). New dimensions in measuring voice treatment outcomes. In R. T. Sataloff (Ed.), *Professional voice: The science and art of clinical care* (2nd ed., pp. 789–794). San Diego, CA: Singular Publishing Group.

Blumin, J. H., Keppel K. L., Braun N. M., Kerschner, J. E., & Merati, A. L. (2008). The impact of gender and age on voice related quality of life in children: Normative data. *International Journal of Pediatric Otorhinolaryngology, 72*(2), 229–234.

Boseley, M. E., Cunningham, M. J., Volk, M. S., & Hartnick, C. J. (2006). Validation of the Pediatric Voice-Related Quality-of-Life Survey. *Archives of Otolaryngology-Head and Neck Surgery, 132*(7), 717–720.

Branski, R. C., Cukier-Blaj, S., Pusic, A., Cano, S. J., Klassen, A., Mener, D., . . . Kraus, D. H. (2010). Measuring quality of life in dysphonic patients: A systematic review of content development in patient-reported outcomes measures. *Journal of Voice, 24*(2), 193–198.

Buchanan, D. R., O'Mara, A. M., Kelaghan, J. W., & Minasian, L. M. (2005). Quality-of-life assessment in the symptom management trials of the National Cancer Institute-Supported Community Clinical Oncology Program. *Journal of Clinical Oncology, 23*(3), 591–598.

Carding, P. N., Horsley, I. A., & Docherty, G. J. (1999). A study of the effectiveness of voice therapy in the treatment of 45 patients with nonorganic dysphonia. *Journal of Voice, 13*(1), 72–104.

Cohen, S. M., Dupont, W. D., & Courey, M. S. (2006). Quality-of-life impact of non-neoplastic voice disorders: A meta-analysis. *Annals of Otology, Rhinology, and Laryngology, 115*, 128–134.

Cohen, S. M., Jacobson, B. H., Garrett, C. G., Noordzij, J. P., Stewart, M. G., Attia, A., . . . Cleveland, T. F. (2007). Creation and validation of the Singing Voice Handicap Index. *Annals of Otology, Rhinology and Laryngology, 116*(6), 402–406.

Cohen, S. M., Noordzij, J. P., Garrett, C. G., & Ossoff, R. H. (2008). Factors associated with perception of singing voice handicap. *Otolaryngology-Head and Neck Surgery, 138*(4), 430–434.

Cohen, S. M., Witsell, D. L., Scearce, L., Vess, G., & Banka, C. (2008). Treatment responsiveness of the Singing Voice Handicap Index. *Laryngoscope, 118*(9), 1705–1708.

Deary, I. J., Webb, A., MacKenzie, K., Wilson, J. A., & Carding, P. N. (2004). Short, self-report voice symptom scales: Psychometric characteristics of the Voice Handicap Index-10 and the Vocal Performance Questionnaire. *Otolaryngology-Head and Neck Surgery, 131*(3), 232–235.

Deary, I. J., Wilson, J. A., Carding, P. N., & MacKenzie, K. (2003). VoiSS: A patient-derived voice symptom scale. *Journal of Psychosomatic Research, 54*(5), 483–489.

Degner, L. F., & Sloan, J. A. (1995). Symptom distress in newly diagnosed ambulatory cancer patients and as a predictor of survival in lung cancer. *Journal of Pain and Symptom Management, 10*(6), 423–431.

Dejonckere P. H., Bradley, P., Clemente, P., Cornut, G., Crevier-Buchman, L., Friedrich, G., . . . Woisard, V. (2001). A basic protocol for functional assessment of voice pathology, especially for investigating the efficacy of phonosurgical treatments and evaluating new assessment techniques. *European Archives of Otorhinolaryngology, 258*(2), 77–82.

Dejonckere, P. H., Obbens, C., de Moor, G. M., & Wieneke, G. H. (1993). Perceptual evaluation of dysphonia: Reliability and relevance. *Folia Phoniatrica et Logopaedica, 45*(2), 76–83.

Eadie, T. L., Yorkston, K. M., Klasner, E. R., Dudgeon, B. J., Deitz, J. C., Baylor, C. R., . . . Amtmann, D. (2006). Measuring communicative participation: A review of self-report instruments in speech-language pathology. *American Journal of Speech-Language Pathology, 15,* 307–320.

Epstein, R., Hirani, S. P., Stygall, J., & Newman, S. P. (2009). How do individuals cope with voice disorders? Introducing the Voice Disability Coping Questionnaire. *Journal of Voice, 23*(2), 209–217.

Fang, T. J., Li, H. Y., Gliklich, R. E., Chen, Y. H., & Wang, P. C. (2007). Assessment of Chinese-version voice outcome survey in patients with unilateral vocal cord paralysis. *Otolaryngology-Head and Neck Surgery, 136*(5), 752–756.

Food and Drug Administration. (2006). Draft guidance for industry on patient-reported outcome measures: Use in medicinal product development to support labeling claims. *Federal Register, 71,* 5862–5863.

Franic, D. M., Bramlett, R. E., & Bothe, A. C. (2005). Psychometric evaluation of disease specific quality of life instruments in voice disorders. *Journal of Voice, 19*(2), 300–315.

Gasparini, G., & Behlau, M. (2009). Quality of life: Validation of the Brazilian version of the Voice-Related Quality of Life (V-RQOL). *Journal of Voice, 23,* 76–81.

Gliklich, R. E., Glovsky, R. M., & Montgomery, W. W. (1999). Validation of a voice outcome survey for unilateral vocal cord paralysis. *Otolaryngology-Head and Neck Surgery, 120,* 153–158.

Golub, J. S., Chen, P. H., Otto, K. J., Hapner, E., & Johns III, M. M. (2006). Prevalence of perceived dysphonia in a geriatric population. *Journal of the American Geriatrics Society, 54*(11), 1736–1739.

Guyatt, G. H., Townsend, M., Berman, L. B., & Keller, J. L. (1987). A comparison of Likert and visual analog scales for measuring change in function. *Journal of Chronic Disease, 40*(12), 1129–1133.

Hartnick, C. J. (2002). Validation of a pediatric voice quality-of-life instrument: The Pediatric Voice Outcome Survey. *Archives of Otolaryngology-Head and Neck Surgery, 128,* 919–922.

Hartnick, C. J., Volk, M. S., & Cunningham, M. J. (2003). Establishing normative voice-related quality of life scores within the pediatric otolaryngology population. *Archives of Otolaryngology-Head and Neck Surgery, 129,* 1090–1093.

Hobday, T. J., Kugler, J. W., Mahoney, M. R., Sargent, D. J., Sloan, J. A., Fitch, T. R., . . . Goldberg, R. M. (2002). Efficacy and quality-of-life data are related in a phase II trial of oral chemotherapy in previously untreated patients with metastatic colorectal carcinoma. *Journal of Clinical Oncology, 20,* 4574–4580.

Hogikyan, N. D., & Sethuraman, G. (1999). Validation of an instrument to measure Voice Related Quality of Life (V-RQOL). *Journal of Voice, 13*(4), 557–569.

Izdebski, K., Dedo, H. H., & Boles, L. (1984). Spastic dysphonia: A patient profile of 200 cases. *American Journal of Otolaryngology, 5,* 7–14.

Jacobson, B., & Bush, C. (1996, November). *Voice Handicap Index (VHI) and clinicians' perceptual judgments.* Poster presented at the ASHA Convention. Seattle, WA.

Jacobson, B. H., Johnson, A., Grywalski, C., Silbergleit, A., Jacobson, G., Benninger, M. S., & Newman, C. W. (1997). The Voice Handicap Index (VHI): Development and validation. *American Journal of Speech Language Pathology, 6,* 66–70.

Jacobson, G. P., & Newman, C. W. (1990). The development of the Dizziness Handicap Inventory. *Archives of Otolaryngology-Head and Neck Surgery, 116*(4), 424–427.

Kazi, R., De Cordova, J., Singh, A., Venkitaraman, R., Nutting, C. M., Clarke, P., . . . Harrington, K. J. (2007). Voice-related quality of life in laryngectomees: assessment using the VHI and V-RQOL symptom scales. *Journal of Voice, 21*(6), 728–734.

Lam, P. K., Chan, K. M., Ho, W. K., Kwong, E., Yiu, E. M., & Wei, W. I. (2006). Cross-cultural adaptation and validation of the Chinese Voice Handicap Index-10. *Laryngoscope, 116*(7), 1192–1198.

Lee, M., Drinnan, M., & Carding, P. (2005). The reliability and validity of patient self-rating of their own voice quality. *Clinical Otolaryngology, 30*(4), 357–361.

Ma, E. P.-M., & Yiu, E. M.-L. (2001). Voice activity and participation profile: Assessing the impact of voice disorders on daily activities. *Journal of Speech, Language, and Hearing Research, 44,* 511–524.

Ma, E. P.-M., & Yiu, E. M.-L. (2007). Scaling voice activity limitation and participation restriction in dysphonic individuals. *Folia Phoniatrica et Logopaedica, 59,* 74–82.

Meek, P., Carding, P. N., Howard, D. H., & Lennard, T. W. J. (2008). Voice change following thyroid and parathyroid surgery. *Journal of Voice, 22*(6), 765–772.

Merati, A. L., Keppel, K., Braun, N. M., Blumin, J. H., & Kerschner, J. E. (2008). Pediatric Voice-Related Quality of Life: Findings in healthy children and in common laryngeal disorders. *Annals of Otology, Rhinology, and Laryngology, 117*(4), 259–262.

Mirasola, K. L., Braun, N., Blumin, J. H., Kerschner, J. E., & Merati, A. L. (2008). Self-reported voice-related quality of life in adolescents with paradoxical vocal fold dysfunction. *Journal of Voice, 22*(3), 373–378.

Morsomme, D., de la Bardonnie, M. F., Verduyckt, I., Jamart, J., & Remacle, M. (2010). Subjective evaluation of the long-term efficacy of speech therapy on dysfunctional dysphonia. *Journal of Voice, 24*(2), 178–182.

Murry, T., Zschommler, A., & Prokop, J. (2009). Voice handicap in singers. *Journal of Voice, 23*(3), 376–379.

Newman, C. W., Jacobson, G. P., & Spitzer, J. B. (1996). Development of the Tinnitus Handicap Inventory. *Archives of Otolaryngology-Head and Neck Surgery, 122*(2), 143–148

Newman, C. W., Weinstein, B. E., Jacobson, G. P., & Hug, G. A. (1990). The Hearing Handicap Inventory for Adults: Psychometric adequacy and audiometric correlates. *Ear and Hearing, 11*(6), 430–433.

O'Connor, R. (2004). *Measuring quality of life in health.* New York. NY: Elsevier Science.

Portone, C. R., Hapner, E. R., McGregor, L., Otto, K., & Johns III, M. M. (2007). Correlation of the Voice Handicap Index (VHI) and the Voice-Related Quality of Life Measure (V-RQOL). *Journal of Voice, 21*(6), 723–727.

Rosen, C. A., Lee, A. S., Osborne, J., Zullo, T., & Murry, T. (2004). Development and validation of the Voice Handicap Index-10. *Laryngoscope, 114*(9), 1549–1556.

Rosen, C. A., & Murry, T. (2000). Voice Handicap Index in singers. *Journal of Voice, 14*(3), 370–377.

Sackett, D. L., Straus, S. E., Richardson, W. S., Rosenberg, W., & Haynes, R. B. (2000). *Evidence-based medicine: How to practice and teach EBM* (2nd ed.). New York, NY: Churchill Livingstone.

Scientific Advisory Committee of the Medical Outcomes Trust. (2002). Assessing health status and quality-of-life instruments: Attributes and review criteria. *Quality of Life Research, 11*(3), 193–205.

Scott, S., Robinson, K., Wilson, J. A., & Mackenzie, K. (1997). Patient reported problems associated with dysphonia. *Clinical Otolaryngology, 22*(1), 37–40.

Silliman, R. A., Dukes, K. A., Sullivan, L. M., & Kaplan, S. H. (1998). Breast cancer care in older women: Sources of information, social support, and emotional health outcomes. *Cancer, 83*(4), 706–711.

Sloan, J. A., Loprinzi, C. L., Kuross, S. A., Miser, A. W., O'Fallon, J. R., Mahoney, M. R., . . . Vaught, N. L. (1998). Randomized comparison of four tools measuring overall quality of life in patients with advanced cancer. *Journal of Clinical Oncology, 16,* 3662–3673.

Sloan, J. A., Loprinzi, C. L., Novotny, P. J., Barton, D. L., Lavasseur, B. I., & Windschitl, H. (2001). Methodologic lessons learned from hot flash studies. *Journal of Clinical Oncology, 19*(23), 4280–4290.

Smith, E., Verdolini, K., Gray, S., Nichols, S., Lemke, J., Barkmeier, J., . . . Hoffman, H. (1996). Effect of voice disorders on quality of life. *Journal of Medical Speech-Language Pathology, 4,* 223–244.

Sneeuw, K. C. A., Sprangers, M. A. G., & Aaronson, N. K. (2002). The role of healthcare providers and significant others in evaluating the quality of life of patients with chronic disease. *Journal of Clinical Epidemiology, 55*(11), 1130–1143.

Speyer, R., Wieneke, G. H., & Dejonckere, P. H. (2004). Self-assessment of voice therapy for chronic dysphonia. *Clinical Otolaryngology, 29*(1), 66–74.

Spieth, L. E., & Harris, C. V. (1996). Assessment of health-related quality of life in children and adolescents: An integrative review. *Journal of Pediatric Psychology, 21*(2), 175–193.

Stanton, A. E., Sellars, C., Mackenzie, K., McConnachie, A., & Bucknall, C. E. (2009). Perceived vocal morbidity in a problem asthma clinic. *Journal of Laryngology and Otology, 123*(1), 96–102.

Sukanen, O., Sihvo, M., Rorarius, E., Lehtihalmes, M., Autio, V., & Kleemola, L. (2007). Voice Activity and Participation Profile (VAPP) in assessing the effects of voice disorders on patients' quality of life: validity and reliability of the Finnish version of VAPP. *Logopedics, Phoniatrics and Vocology, 32*(1), 3–8.

Sutherland, H. J., Llewellyn-Thomas, H., Hogg, S. A., Keane, T. J., Harwood, A. R., Till, J. E., & Boyd, N. F. (1984). Do patients and physicians agree on the assessment of voice quality in laryngeal cancer? *Journal of Otolaryngology, 13,* 325–330.

Tarlov, A. R., Ware, J. E., Greenfield, S., Nelson, E. C., Perrin, E., & Zubkoff, M. (1989). The medical outcomes study: An application of methods for monitoring the results of medical care. *Journal of the American Medical Association, 262,* 925–930.

U.S. Department of Health and Human Services FDA Center for Drug Evaluation and Research, U.S. Department of Health and Human Services FDA Center for Biologics Evaluation and Research, U.S. Department of Health and Human Services FDA Center for Cervices and Radiological Health. (2006). Guidance for industry: Patient-reported outcome measures: use in medical product development to support labeling claims: draft guidance. *Health Quality of Life Outcomes, 4,* 79.

van der Merwe, A. (2004). The voice use reduction program. *American Journal of Speech-Language Pathology, 13*(3), 208–218.

Ventry, I. M., & Weinstein, B. E. (1982). The Hearing Handicap Inventory for the Elderly: a new tool. *Ear and Hearing, 3*(3), 128–134.

Verdonck-de Leeuw, I. M., Kuik, D. J., De Bodt, M., Guimaraes, I., Holmberg, E. B., Nawka, T., . . . Woisard, V. (2008). Validation of the Voice Handicap Index (VHI) by assessing equivalence of European translations. *Folia Phoniatrica et Logopaedica, 60,* 173–178.

Ware, J. E., & Sherbourne, C. D. (1992). The MOS 36-Item Short-Form Health survey (SF-36): I. Conceptual framework and item selection. *Medical Care, 30*(6), 473–483.

Wilson, J. A., Webb, A. L., Carding, P. N., Steen, I. N., Mackenzie, K., & Deary, I. J. (2004). The Voice Symptom Scale (VoiSS) and the Voice Handicap Index (VHI): A comparison of structure and content. *Clinical Otolaryngology, and Applied Sciences, 29,* 169–174.

World Health Organization. (1997). *International classification of impairment, disability and handicap–Beta-1: A manual*

*of dimensions of disablement and partic-
ipation*. Geneva, Switzerland: Author.

World Health Organization. (2001). *International Classification of Functioning, Disability, and Health*. Geneva, Switzerland:
Author.

Zraick, R. I., & Liss, J. M. (2000). A comparison
of equal-appearing interval scaling and
direct magnitude estimation of nasal voice
quality. *Journal of Speech, Language, and
Hearing Research, 43*, 979–988.

Zraick, R. I., & Risner, B. Y. (2008). Assessment
of quality of life in persons with voice disorders. *Current Opinion in Otolaryngology
and Head and Neck Surgery, 16*, 188–193.

Zraick, R. I., Risner, B. Y., Smith-Olinde, L.,
Gregg, B. A., Johnson, F. L., & McWeeny, E.
K. (2007). Patient versus partner perception of voice handicap. *Journal of Voice,
21*, 485–494.

Zur, K. B., Cotton, S., Kelchner, L., Baker, S.,
Weinrich, B., & Lee, L. (2007). Pediatric
Voice Handicap Index (pVHI): A new tool
for evaluating pediatric dysphonia. *International Journal of Pediatric Otorhinolaryngology, 71*(1), 77–82.

Index